Principles of
ALS Care

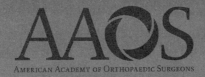

AMERICAN ACADEMY OF ORTHOPAEDIC SURGEONS

Author:

Nicholle Brock
Fire Fighter/Paramedic
MedicsPrep
Atlanta, Georgia

Contributing Author:

Brian J. Williams, BS, NREMT-P, CCEMT-P
EMS Chief
Pembina Ambulance
Pembina, North Dakota

Medical Editor:

Benjamin Gulli, MD
Northwest Orthopedic Surgeons
Minneapolis, Minnesota

JONES AND BARTLETT PUBLISHERS
Sudbury, Massachusetts
BOSTON   TORONTO   LONDON   SINGAPORE

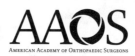

World Headquarters
Jones and Bartlett Publishers
40 Tall Pine Drive
Sudbury, MA 01776
978-443-5000
info@jbpub.com
www.jbpub.com

Jones and Bartlett Publishers Canada
6339 Ormindale Way
Mississauga, Ontario L5V 1J2
Canada

Jones and Bartlett Publishers International
Barb House, Barb Mews
London W6 7PA
United Kingdom

Jones and Bartlett's books and products are available through most bookstores and online booksellers. To contact Jones and Bartlett Publishers directly, call 800-832-0034, fax 978-443-8000, or visit our website, www.jbpub.com.

Substantial discounts on bulk quantities of Jones and Bartlett's publications are available to corporations, professional associations, and other qualified organizations. For details and specific discount information, contact the special sales department at Jones and Bartlett via the above contact information or send an email to specialsales@jbpub.com.

Editorial Credits
Chief Education Officer: Mark W. Wieting
Director, Department of Publications: Marilyn L. Fox, PhD
Managing Editor: Barbara A. Scotese
Associate Senior Editor: Gayle Murray

AAOS Board of Directors, 2009-2010
Joseph D. Zuckerman, MD
President

John J. Callaghan, MD
First Vice President

Daniel J. Berry, MD
Second Vice President

Frederick M. Azar, MD
Treasurer

Thomas C. Barber, MD
Richard J. Barry, MD
Leesa M. Galatz, MD
M. Bradford Henley, MD, MBA
Michael L. Parks, MD
E. Anthony Rankin, MD
William J. Robb, III, MD
Michael F. Schafer, MD
David D. Teuscher, MD
Paul Tornetta III, MD
G. Zachary Wilhoit, MS, MBA
Karen L. Hackett, FACHE, CAE (*Ex-Officio*)

Production Credits
Chief Executive Officer: Clayton Jones
Chief Operating Officer: Don W. Jones, Jr.
President, Higher Education and Professional
    Publishing: Robert W. Holland, Jr.
V.P., Design and Production: Anne Spencer
V.P., Manufacturing and Inventory Control: Therese Connell
Publisher: Kimberly Brophy
Acquisitions Editor—EMS: Christine Emerton
Managing Editor: Carol B. Guerrero
Associate Editor: Karen Greene
Production Manager: Jenny L. Corriveau

Associate Production Editor: Sarah Bayle
Director of Marketing: Alisha Weisman
Director, Public Safety Group: Matthew Maniscalco
Cover Design: Kristin E. Parker
Interior Design: Anne Spencer
Senior Photo Researcher and
    Photographer: Christine Myaskovsky
Composition: diacritech
Printing and Binding: Courier Companies
Cover Printing: Courier Companies

Library of Congress Cataloging-in-Publication Data
Brock, Nicholle.
   Principles of ALS care / Nicholle Brock ; contributing author, Brian J. Williams.
      p. ; cm.
   Includes bibliographical references and index.
   ISBN-13: 978-0-7637-6581-1 (pbk.)
   ISBN-10: 0-7637-6581-3 (pbk.)
   1. Emergency medicine. I. Williams, Brian J. (Brian Jeremy), 1976- II. American Academy of Orthopaedic Surgeons. III. Title.
   [DNLM: 1. Emergencies. 2. Emergency Treatment—methods. 3. Wounds and Injuries—physiopathology. 4. Wounds and Injuries—therapy. WB 105 V773p 2010]
   RC86.7.V56 2010
   616.02'5—dc22
                                    2009014469

6048
Printed in the United States of America
13 12 11 10 09   10 9 8 7 6 5 4 3 2 1

Contents

Acknowledgments

Jones and Bartlett Publishers would like to thank the following individuals for their review of the manuscript:

Rick Barton, BS, CCEMT-P, NREMT-P
Gundersen Lutheran Medical Center
La Crosse, Wisconsin

Brandon R. Beck, AS, NREMT-P
Gadsden State Community College
Gadsden, Alabama

J. R. Behan, MICT, CCEMT-P
Supervisor
Finney County Emergency Medical Service
Garden City, Kansas

Mark Bird, RN, BSN, CCRN, EMT-P
Manatee Technical Institute
St. Petersburg, Florida

Bradley Dean, BBA, NREMT-P
Davidson County Emergency Services
Lexington, North Carolina
Wake Forest University Baptist Medical
    Center—Trauma Department
Winston-Salem, North Carolina
Randolph Community College
Asheboro, North Carolina
Alamance Community College
Graham, North Carolina

Robert M. Hawkes, MS, PA-C, NREMT-P
Southern Maine Community College
South Portland, Maine

Jeremy H. Huffman, AAS, EMT-P
Southwestern Community College
Asheville, North Carolina

David Brian Jones, MSN, ACNP, BC, EMT-P
Macungie, Pennsylvania

**Daniel Kane, MEd, BSN, RN, CEN, CCRN,
    CFRN, EMT-P**
Massachusetts General Hospital—Institute
    of Health Professions
Billerica, Massachusetts

Judy Larsen, RN, EMT-P
City of Brookfield Paramedic Training
    Center
Brookfield, Wisconsin

Thomas T. Levins, BSN, RN, CCRN, CFRN
University of Pennsylvania Health System
PennSTAR Flight
Blue Bell, Pennsylvania

Jim Mobley, RN, BSN, CEN, CFRN, NREMT-P, FP-C
Program Director, Regional One Air
    Medical Service
Spartanburg, South Carolina

Tina Nuckols, BSN, RN, CEN, CCEMT-P
Aiken, South Carolina

Jeffrey Rockett, AA, AS, EMT-P
Nature Coast EMS
Inverness, Florida

Joshua Tanner, FF/NREMT-P
EMS Coordinator
ALERT Academy
Big Sandy, Texas

Timothy Whitaker, NREMT-P, FP-C, CMTE
Allen Medical Center
Stark State College
Oberlin, Ohio

Brian J. Williams, BS, NREMT-P, CCEMT-P
EMS Chief
Pembina Ambulance
Pembina, North Dakota

The author would like to thank the following individuals for sharing their wisdom and experience and helping to make this book a success:

James Augustine, MD
Washington, District of Columbia

James Potts, MD
Meharry Medical College
Nashville, Tennessee

Regina V. Clark, EdD
Kennesaw State University
Atlanta, Georgia

Brandy Slade, RN
Savannah, Georgia

Gwinnett Ladsen, MD
Meharry Medical College
Nashville, Tennessee

Preparatory

CHAPTER 1

The Cellular Environment

It is important to remember when treating your patients that at the cellular level you are trying to aid the body in maintaining homeostasis (stability, equilibrium) or return it to a homeostatic state. An understanding of basic cellular structure and function—as well as of the cellular environment and how alterations in that environment can lead to disease—is critical in restoring homeostasis.

The Cell

Cells are the basic structural and functional units of the human body. There are many different types of cells, such as muscle cells, nerve cells, and blood cells. This basic unit of life consists of **protoplasm**, a fluid made up of many compounds, such as water, proteins, lipids, ions, and amino acids. The protoplasm of a cell is composed of three vital parts:

- A nucleus
- Cytoplasm
- The cell surface membrane

The parts of the cell are illustrated in **Figure 1-1** and discussed in the next sections.

Components of the Cell

Nucleus

The **nucleus** controls all normal cell activities, such as growth and metabolism. It contains the following:

- **Chromatin:** Genetic material and chromosomes, which make up proteins
- **Nucleoli:** Spherical structures that play a part in the building of ribonucleic acid (RNA)

Cytoplasm

The protoplasm that surrounds the nucleus is called the **cytoplasm**. It plays a part in cell division and forms the larger part of the human cell. It fills the cell, giving it shape, and contains **organelles**. Organelles are specialized structures that perform specific functions. In addition to the nucleus, the cell's organelles include:

- Centrioles
  - Paired cylindrical structures located near the nucleus
  - Job description: Play an important role in cell division
- Endoplasmic reticulum (ER)
  - Two forms: Rough ER and smooth ER. The surface of rough ER is coated with ribosomes; the surface of smooth ER is not.
  - Job description: Rough ER—building of proteins; smooth ER—building of lipids.
- Golgi complex
  - Membrane-bound, stacked structures located near the nucleus
  - Job description: Packages and processes proteins and lipids (fats) synthesized by the cell, synthesis (of substances such as phospholipids), packages materials for transport (in vesicles), produces lysosomes

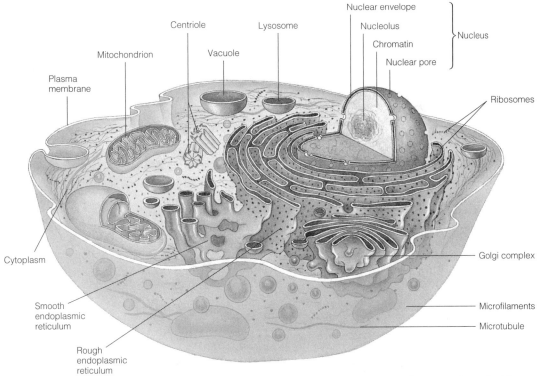

Plasma membrane · Mitochondrion · Centriole · Vacuole · Lysosome · Nuclear envelope · Nucleolus · Chromatin · Nuclear pore · Nucleus · Ribosomes · Golgi complex · Cytoplasm · Smooth endoplasmic reticulum · Rough endoplasmic reticulum · Microfilaments · Microtubule

Figure 1-1 The structure of a cell. The cell is divided into nuclear and cytoplasmic compartments. The cytoplasm is packed with organelles, the specific structures in the cell that carry out a variety of functions.

- Lysosomes
  - Vesicles containing digestive enzymes
  - Job description: Destruction of damaged cells and degradation of bacteria
- Mitochondria
  - Small, rodlike structures
  - Job description: Contain enzymes that form adenosine triphosphate (ATP), the energy source of the body
- Ribosomes
  - Composed of ribosomal RNA and protein
  - Often linked together in chains called polyribosomes or polysomes
  - May be dispersed randomly throughout the cytoplasm or attached to the surface of rough ER
  - Job description: Create proteins
- Vacuoles: Contain water and food substances

Cell Surface Membrane

The cell surface membrane, also called the plasma membrane, is a semipermeable membrane that surrounds the cell and protects the components within the cytoplasm. It controls which substances enter and leave the cell.

Structures of the cell membrane include the following:

- Flagella and cilia
  - Hairlike projections from some human cells
  - Cilia are relatively short and numerous
  - The flagellum is relatively long and there is typically only one
  - Job description: Varies depending on the type of cell. For example, cells of the trachea contain cilia to move dust particles, and a sperm cell contains a flagellum that helps propel it in its search for the egg.

- Villi
  - Outward projections of cell membrane
  - Job description: Increase surface area of a cell; aid in the absorption of nutrients, as in the small intestine

Substance Movement Across the Cell Membrane

Passive and active transport are the two processes by which water and dissolved particles move across the cell membrane. **Passive transport** requires no expenditure of energy by the cells. This process consists of two movements, osmosis and diffusion.

- **Osmosis** is the movement of a solvent (water) across a semipermeable membrane from an area of low solute concentration to an area of higher solute concentration (**Figure 1-2**).
- **Diffusion** is the movement of a solute (substance) from an area of high solute concentration to an area of lower solute concentration; this process continues until the concentration of substances is uniform throughout the cell (**Figure 1-3**). The rate of diffusion is influenced by several factors:
  - Concentration gradient
  - Cross-sectional area through which diffusion occurs
  - Temperature
  - Molecular weight of a substance
  - Distance through which diffusion occurs

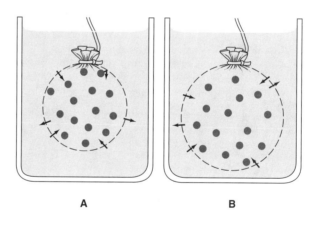

● Sucrose molecules

Figure 1-2 Osmosis is movement of solvent (water) from an area of low solute concentration to an area of higher solute concentration. **A.** For example, immerse a bag of sugar water into a solution of pure water. **B.** Water diffuses into the bag, where there is higher solute (sugar) concentration, causing it to swell.

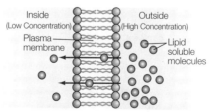

Figure 1-3 Diffusion is the movement of solute from an area of high solute concentration to an area of lower solute concentration.

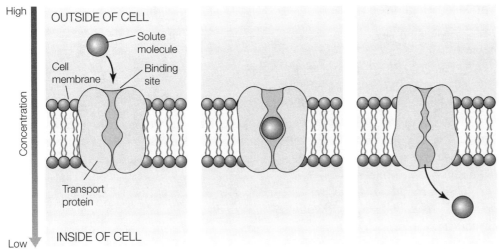

Figure 1-4 Facilitated diffusion. The movement of a substance through a cell membrane with the assistance of carrier proteins.

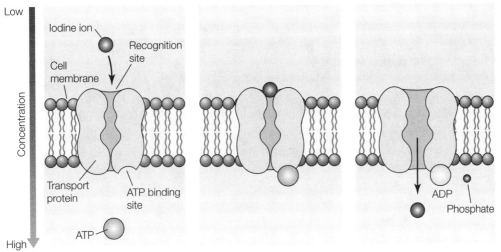

Figure 1-5 Active transport. The movement of a substance through a cell membrane against the osmotic gradient, with the assistance of carrier proteins and ATP (a form of energy).

Facilitated diffusion is the movement of a specific molecule across a cell membrane from an area of high concentration to an area of low concentration using a specific carrier protein (**Figure 1-4**).

Active transport is the movement of a substance (particles) across a cell membrane from an area of low concentration to an area of higher concentration, using a helper protein. The energy for active transport comes from ATP created in the mitochondria. (**Figure 1-5**). Helper proteins are proteins that combine with solutes on one side of the membrane, change their shape to pass through the membrane, and release the solute molecule.

Composition of Body Fluids

The average adult is made up of 50% to 70% fluid. Infants are made up of about 60% fluid, and older adults about 55%. Fluid inside the body cells is called **intracellular fluid**; it makes up about 40% of total body weight. Fluid outside the body cells, called **extracellular fluid**, composes about 20% of body weight. One type of extracellular fluid is **interstitial fluid**, which is found between cells and outside the vascular bed.

Alterations in Fluid Balance

__Edema__ is the accumulation of excess fluid in the interstitial spaces. It can be caused by several factors:

- A defect in fluid distribution (not necessarily an excess of fluid)
- A decrease in plasma osmotic pressure
- An increase in hydrostatic pressure
- An increase in capillary permeability. Increased capillary permeability can be caused by inflammation, the immune response as a result of a trauma, or allergic reaction
- An obstruction in the lymph system (the system of vessels that carries excess interstitial fluid into the circulation)
- Retention of sodium and water. The increase in sodium and water retention can increase the circulating fluid volume, ultimately causing a fluid volume overload. Two conditions associated with sodium and water retention are renal failure and congestive heart failure (CHF).

Dehydration

Dehydration occurs when the body's fluid volume is depleted. There are three types of dehydration:

- __Isotonic dehydration__ is the excessive loss of equal amounts of sodium and water. It results from severe or excessive vomiting or diarrhea.
- __Hypernatremic dehydration__ occurs when the body loses more water than sodium. Causes include excess use of diuretics, increased intake of sodium and decreased intake of water, and diarrhea.
- __Hyponatremic dehydration__ occurs when the body loses more sodium than water. Causes include increased water intake, diuretics, and sodium loss from renal disorder.

Dehydration is discussed in depth in Chapter 11.

Fluid Replacement

To reverse the effects of dehydration, fluid replenishment needs to be initiated. There are three types of fluid replacement solutions:

- __Isotonic:__ A solution that has the same solute concentration as the body's blood, plasma, and other fluids. Excellent for patients with severe blood loss or fluid loss from excessive vomiting. It replaces extracellular fluid. It may be prescribed for patients with chloride loss equal to or greater than sodium loss. Examples of isotonic solutions are lactated Ringer's solution and normal saline.
- __Hypertonic:__ A solution that has a higher solute concentration and lower water concentration than that inside the cell. This solution causes a cell to shrink. It is effective in drawing tissue fluid into the vascular space and therefore useful for reducing infusion volumes and postresuscitation pulmonary issues. An example of a hypertonic solution is D_5 0.45% normal saline.
- __Hypotonic:__ A solution that has a lower solute concentration and higher water concentration than that inside the cell. This solution causes a cell to expand or swell. It provides salt, water, and calorie replacement, especially in situations of dehydration. Examples of hypotonic solutions are 0.45% normal saline, 2.5% dextrose in water, and D_5 (although it is technically an isotonic solution, it contains properties consistent with hypotonic solutions).

Cellular Metabolism

Metabolism is the combination of all chemical processes that take place in the body, resulting in growth, generation of energy, body heat, elimination of wastes, and other bodily functions; catabolism is the breakdown phase, in which larger molecules are converted to smaller ones.

Because cells require energy for processes such as active transport, synthesis, impulse conduction (nerve cells), and contraction (muscle cells), they must be able to process, store, and release that energy as needed. The body's sources of "fuel" or energy are carbohydrates (mostly **glucose** [$C_6H_{12}O_6$]), fats, and proteins. Ultimately, glucose serves as the main cell "food," whether taken in orally, parenterally, or made from conversion of stored fats and proteins.

Once glucose, amino acids, and fats are absorbed from the gastrointestinal tract, the body metabolizes them to produce energy. Some glucose is stored in the liver as **glycogen**, which is catabolized when necessary to raise the blood glucose level.

Glucose, fat, and proteins are used to generate energy via the process of cellular respiration. This pathway is totally different from respiration in the lungs. Cellular respiration is a biochemical process that occurs in the mitochondria and results in the production of energy in the form of **adenosine triphosphate (ATP)** molecules. ATP molecules form the "energy food" for all of the body's functions.

Understanding Acid-Base Balance

The measurement of hydrogen ion concentration of a solution is called **pH**. Normal body functions depend on an acid–base balance that remains within the normal physiologic pH range of 7.35 to 7.45. The mathematical formula for calculating pH is $pH = -\log [H]$, where "log" refers to the base-10 logarithm and [H] refers to the hydrogen ion concentration. Changes in the pH are exponential, not linear. For example, a change in the pH from 7.40 to 7.20 results in a 10^2 (ie, 100-fold) change in the acid concentration.

To maintain the delicate acid–base balance, the body relies on its buffer systems. **Buffers** are molecules that modulate changes in pH. In the absence of buffers, the addition of acid to a solution will cause a sharp change in pH. In the presence of a buffer, the pH change will be moderated or may even be unnoticeable in the same situation. Because acid production is the major challenge to pH homeostasis, most physiologic buffers combine with hydrogen.

Buffer systems include proteins, phosphate ions, and bicarbonate (HCO_3^-). The large amounts of bicarbonate produced from the carbon dioxide (CO_2) made during metabolism create the body's most important extracellular buffer system. Hydrogen and bicarbonate ions combine to form carbonic acid, which readily dissociates into water and carbon dioxide:

$$H + HCO_3 \leftrightarrow H_2CO_3 \leftrightarrow H_2O + CO_2$$

In the bicarbonate buffer system, excess acid (H) combines with bicarbonate (HCO_3), forming H_2CO_3. This compound rapidly dissociates into water and CO_2, which is then exhaled. Because the acid is eliminated as water and CO_2, the total pH does not change significantly. A similar process occurs with the production of metabolic base (bicarbonate).

Acidosis Versus Alkalosis

When the buffering capacity of the body is exceeded, acid–base imbalances occur. A blood pH greater than 7.45 is called **alkalosis**; a blood pH less than 7.35 is called **acidosis**.

If the pH is too low (acidosis), neurons become less excitable and CNS depression results. Patients become confused and disoriented. If CNS depression progresses, the respiratory centers cease to function, leading to the person's death.

If pH is too high (alkalosis), neurons become hyperexcitable, firing action potentials at the slightest signal. This condition first manifests as sensory changes, such as numbness or tingling, then as muscle twitches. If alkalosis is severe, muscle twitches turn into sustained contractions (tetanus) that paralyze respiratory muscles.

Disturbances of acid–base balance are associated with disturbances in potassium balance, in part because of the kidney transport system that moves H and K in opposite directions. In acidosis, the kidneys excrete H and resorb K. Conversely, when the body goes into a state of alkalosis, the kidneys resorb H and excrete K. A potassium imbalance usually shows up as disturbances in excitable tissues, especially the heart.

Metabolic Versus Respiratory Acid–Base Imbalances

Acid–base disturbances are classified into two general categories: metabolic and respiratory. Each is then broken down into acidosis and alkalosis.

Metabolic acidosis is an accumulation of abnormal acids in the blood for any of several reasons (eg, sepsis, diabetic ketoacidosis, salicylate poisoning). Initially, the Pa_{CO_2} (partial pressure of carbon dioxide) is not affected, but the pH is decreased. Later, the body compensates for the metabolic abnormality by hyperventilating, leading to excretion of CO_2 and compensatory respiratory alkalosis. For example, patients with diabetic ketoacidosis often experience *Kussmaul respirations* (deep, rapid, sighing ventilations), in which they hyperventilate to "blow off" CO_2 and decrease the acidosis.

Metabolic alkalosis is rarely seen in an acute condition, but is very common in chronically ill patients, especially those undergoing nasogastric suction. It involves either a buildup of excess metabolic base (eg, chronic antacid ingestion) or a loss of normal acid (eg, through vomiting or nasogastric suctioning). The pH is high and the Pa_{CO_2} unchanged initially. On a chronic basis, the body compensates by slowing ventilation and increasing the Pa_{CO_2}, thereby creating a compensatory respiratory acidosis.

Respiratory acidosis occurs when CO_2 retention leads to increased Pa_{CO_2} levels. It also occurs in situations of hypoventilation (eg, heroin overdose) or intrinsic lung diseases (eg, asthma or COPD) (**Figure 1-6**).

Excessive "blowing off" of CO_2 with a resulting decrease in the Pa_{CO_2} causes respiratory alkalosis. Although often called hyperventilation, many potentially serious diseases (eg, pulmonary embolism, acute myocardial infarction, severe infection, diabetic ketoacidosis) may be responsible for increased ventilatory levels.

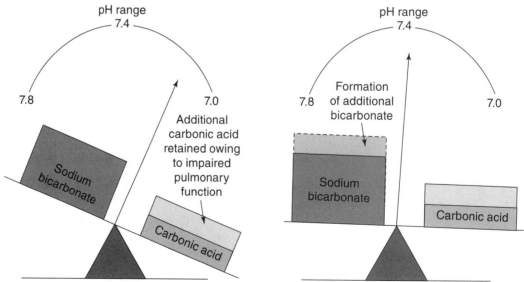

Figure 1-6 A. Derangement of acid-base balance in respiratory acidosis. **B.** Compensation by formation of additional bicarbonate.

Arterial blood gas values (ABGs) can help determine whether a particular disorder is respiratory or metabolic in nature (**Table 1-1**).

Table 1-1 Arterial Blood Gas Values

	Normal Values
pH	7.35-7.45
$Paco_2$	35-45 (amount of CO_2 gas dissolved in the arterial blood)
Pao_2	> 80 (amount of oxygen dissolved in the arterial blood)
Hco_3^-	22-26 (carbonic acid)
Sao_2	94-99%

One easy technique to remember this is the ROME mnemonic: **r**espiratory **o**pposite, **m**etabolic **e**qual. If the pH value is opposite the $Paco_2$ value (either high or low), it is a respiratory problem. If the pH value is equal to the Hco_3^- value, it is a metabolic problem.

Vital Vocabulary

acidosis A blood pH of less than 7.35—a pathologic condition resulting from the accumulation of acids in the body.

active transport The movement of molecules across a cell membrane from an area of low concentration to an area of higher concentration, using a helper protein and ATP to move the substance against a concentration gradient.

adenosine triphosphate (ATP) An organic compound that is the energy source in cells.

alkalosis A blood pH of greater than 7.45—a pathologic condition resulting from the accumulation of bases in the body.

buffers Molecules that modulate changes in pH to keep it in the physiologic range.

cytoplasm The protoplasm surrounding the nucleus, which plays a part in cell division and forms the larger part of the human cell.

diffusion A process in which molecules move from an area of high concentration to an area of lower concentration.

edema A condition in which excess fluid accumulates in tissues, manifested by swelling.

extracellular fluid The water outside the cells; accounts for approximately 20% of body weight.

facilitated diffusion The movement of a specific molecule across a cell membrane from an area of high concentration to an area of low concentration using a helper protein.

glucose The main "food" used by cells for energy.

glycogen The storage form of glucose occurring mainly in the liver and muscles.

hypernatremic dehydration Occurs when the body loses more water than sodium; causes include excess use of diuretics, increased intake of sodium and decreased intake of water, excessive sodium loss, and diarrhea.

hypertonic A solution that has a greater concentration of sodium than does the cell; the increased osmotic pressure can draw water out of the cell and cause it to collapse.

hyponatremic dehydration Occurs when the body loses more sodium than water; causes include increased water intake, diuretics, and sodium loss from renal disorder.

hypotonic A solution that has a lower concentration of sodium than does the cell; the increased osmotic pressure lets water flow into the cell, causing it to swell and possibly burst.

interstitial fluid The water bathing the cells; accounts for about 10% of body weight; includes special fluid collections, such as cerebrospinal fluid and intraocular fluid.

intracellular fluid The water contained inside the cells; normally accounts for 40% of body weight.

isotonic A solution that has the same concentration of sodium as does the cell. In this case, water does not shift, and no change in cell shape occurs.

isotonic dehydration The excessive loss of equal amounts of sodium and water. It results from severe or excessive vomiting or diarrhea.

nucleus A cellular organelle that contains the genetic information. The nucleus controls the function and structure of the cell.

organelles Internal cellular structures that carry out specific functions for the cell.

osmosis The movement of water across a semipermeable membrane (for example, the cell wall) from an area of lower to higher concentration of solute molecules.

passive transport The process by which water and dissolved particles move across the cell membrane, requiring no expenditure of energy by the cells; consists of two movements, osmosis and diffusion.

pH The measurement of hydrogen ion concentration of a solution.

protoplasm A fluid made up of many compounds, such as water, proteins, lipids, ions, and amino acids, that composes the basic units of life.

CHAPTER 2

Assessment and Documentation

Patient Assessment and Management Procedures

As an emergency care provider, you treat patients who are seriously ill or injured, and you are often the highest trained professional on the scene. You must size up the scene; take appropriate steps to ensure the safety of yourself, your crew, and the patient; assess the condition of the patient; and take the appropriate corrective measures quickly and efficiently (**Figure 2-1**). An accurate patient assessment is one of the most important skills you will perform. With precious few minutes to waste, an accurate and thorough assessment can save your patient's life. Remember that patient assessment begins when you receive the call from dispatch. You should begin to analyze the dispatch information as you are en route to the scene.

Scene Size-up

Scene size-up consists of the following components:

- Assess scene safety.
- Ensure body substance isolation (BSI) by use of personal protective equipment (PPE).
- Consider the mechanism of injury (MOI) or nature of illness.
- Determine the number of patients.
- Consider additional resources.
- Consider cervical spine (c-spine) immobilization.

Initial/Primary Assessment

Initial/primary assessment includes the following steps:

Approach and Form a General Impression

You should begin forming a general impression as soon as you see your patient. How does the patient look? How is he or she acting? What does the environment tell you? For infants and children, bend down to their eye level before conducting a hands-on assessment. Do not hover over the patient.

Assess Mental Status

Assess level of consciousness using <u>AVPU</u>:

A: **A**lert to person, place, time, and event

V: Responsive to **v**erbal stimuli

P: Responsive to **p**ain

U: **U**nresponsive

Assess mental status and neurologic function using the <u>**Glasgow Coma Scale**</u> (**Table 2-1**).

Check the Patient's Airway

Ensure that the airway is patent and clear. Correct any airway or breathing problems that you encounter. If necessary, open the airway:

- Position the patient, considering possible c-spine injury.
  - Head tilt–chin lift maneuver (nontrauma patients)
  - Jaw-thrust maneuver (trauma patients)

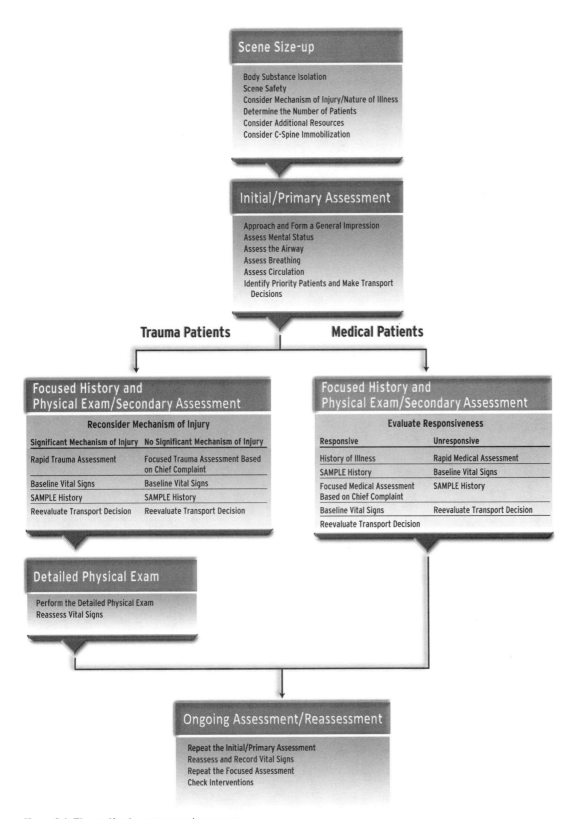

Figure 2-1 The patient assessment process.

- Suction.
- Use an airway adjunct if unable to maintain the airway with manual maneuvers.
- Expose your patient to determine any life-threatening injuries such as gross bleeding or paradoxical motion (asymmetric chest wall movement that lessens respiratory efficiency).

Table 2-1 Glasgow Coma Scale

Eye Opening		Best Verbal Response		Best Motor Response	
Spontaneous	4	Oriented and converses	5	Follows commands	6
To verbal command	3	Disoriented and confused	4	Localizes pain	5
To pain	2	Inappropriate words	3	Withdraws to pain	4
No response	1	Moans or makes unintelligible sounds	2	Decorticate flexion	3
		No response	1	Decerebrate extension	2
				No response	1

Scores:
14-15: Mild dysfunction
11-13: Moderate to severe dysfunction
10 or less: Severe dysfunction (The lowest possible score is 3.)

Assess the Patient's Breathing

"Look (inspect), listen (auscultate), and feel (palpate)." If the patient is breathing at a rate of less than 8 breaths/min or greater than 30 breaths/min, consider assisting ventilations.

Assess the Patient's Circulation

- Assess the pulse rate, quality, and rhythm: Palpate the radial artery in responsive patients and the carotid or femoral arteries in unresponsive children and adults. The following outlines a rough estimate of palpable systolic blood pressures:
  - Carotid = 60 mm Hg
  - Femoral = 70 mm Hg
  - Radial = 80 mm Hg
- Assess skin temperature, condition (**Tables 2-2** and **2-3**), and capillary refill. Control major bleeding *now*.
  - Apply direct pressure over the wound.
  - Elevate injury above the level of the heart.
  - Apply tourniquet if other interventions are not effective.

Techniques for Assessing Breathing

"Look, listen, and feel."

- Look for chest rise and fall; note depth and symmetry of respirations.
- Listen for breath sounds with a stethoscope. Correct any breathing problems immediately. If possible, establish a baseline pulse oximetry reading, and *then* administer oxygen. However, do not withhold oxygen from a patient in distress.
- Feel for air movement–place your cheek or the palm of your hand near the patient's mouth.

Identify Priority Patients and Make Transport Decisions

Patients with the following conditions are priority patients who require rapid transport:

- Signs of shock
- Unresponsive
- Increased work of breathing
- Unable to follow commands

Table 2-2 Inspection of the Skin

Skin Color	Possible Cause
Red	• Fever • Allergic reaction • Carbon monoxide poisoning
White (pallor)	• Excessive blood loss/shock • Fright
Blue (cyanosis)	• Hypoxemia
Mottled	• Constricted blood vessels from drop in cardiac output

Table 2-3 Palpation of the Skin

Skin Condition	Possible Cause
Hot, dry	• Excessive body heat (heatstroke)
Hot, wet	• Reaction to increased internal or external temperature
Cool, dry	• Exposure to cold
Cool, wet	• Shock

- Hypotension with chest pain
- Severe pain
- Multisystem trauma

Focused History and Physical Exam/Secondary Assessment

Trauma Patients

Evaluate injuries. The following are mechanisms that can produce life-threatening injuries:

- Ejection from any vehicle
- Death of another patient in same compartment
- Fall from more than three times the patient's height
- Vehicle rollover
- High-speed motor vehicle crash
- Vehicle-pedestrian collision
- Motorcycle crash
- Penetrating wounds to the head, chest, or abdomen

If the patient has multisystem trauma, identify all injuries and prioritize by their severity and the need to address. Any trauma patient who is unresponsive or has an altered mental status needs immediate transport to a trauma center.

Do not be distracted by highly visible injuries that are not necessarily the greatest threat.

Ensure that the patient's c-spine is manually immobilized in the neutral in-line position. Perform a rapid trauma assessment on all trauma patients with a significant MOI, quickly inspecting each part of the body and using the patient's chief complaint and symptoms to guide your assessment.

For responsive trauma patients who do not have a significant MOI, obtain vital signs and a SAMPLE history and reconsider your transport decision.

DCAP-BTLS

Look for DCAP-BTLS during the physical exam:
- **D**eformities
- **C**ontusions
- **A**brasions
- **P**unctures/**P**enetrations
- **B**urns
- **T**enderness
- **L**acerations
- **S**welling

Medical Patients

Evaluate responsiveness.

For responsive patients:

- Determine chief complaint (**OPQRST**) and history of present illness (**SAMPLE history**).
- Perform focused medical assessment based on chief complaint.
- Assess vital signs.
- Reconsider transport decision.

For unresponsive patients:

- Perform a rapid medical assessment.
- Assess vitals signs.
- Determine history of present illness (SAMPLE) using family members or bystanders.
- Reconsider transport decision.

Detailed Physical Exam

Perform a detailed physical exam when time allows, usually en route if there is an extended transport time.

- Assess the patient's mental status.
- Assess the patient's level of consciousness.
- Inspect and palpate each part of the body.
- Reevaluate the patient's vital signs and assess trends in any changes.

SAMPLE History

The SAMPLE history is obtained as part of the assessment of every patient. The following questions should be asked:

- **S**igns and symptoms: Signs and symptoms at onset? Evaluate for pathophysiologic changes.
- **A**llergies: Are you allergic to any medications, food, or environmental factors?
- **M**edications: Are you taking any medications? Prescription or herbal? Dosage?
- **P**ertinent past history: History of medical problems? Recent surgeries or hospitalizations?
- **L**ast oral intake: When did you last eat or drink? What was consumed?
- **E**vents leading up to the illness or injury: What made you call 9-1-1?

OPQRST

OPQRST is another mnemonic device that can help you remember questions to ask when you are obtaining a patient's history:

- **O**nset: When did the pain or illness start?
- **P**rovocation/**P**alliation: What makes the pain or illness worse? What makes the pain or illness better?
- **Q**uality: Can you describe the pain to me? Sharp, dull, or burning?
- **R**egion/**R**adiation: Can you point to where you feel the pain? Does it spread or go anywhere else?
- **S**everity: How bad is the pain on a scale of 0 to 10, with 10 being the worst?
- **T**iming: Has the pain been intermittent or chronic?

Ongoing Assessment/Reassessment

Reassess unstable patients every 5 minutes. Reassess stable patients every 15 minutes.

- Repeat the initial/primary assessment.
- Reassess and record vital signs.
- Repeat the focused physical exam/secondary assessment.
- Recheck interventions.

Legal and Ethical Issues for the EMS Provider

As an EMS provider, you must stay within your scope of practice. The scope of practice outlines the care you are able to provide for the patient; this scope varies from state to state.

Standards of care are different than scope of practice. The manner in which you must act or behave is called a standard of care.

Unlike a friend, family member, or bystander at the scene of an emergency, as an ALS provider, you may have a duty to act. Your duty to act includes:

- Providing care and transport according to the national, state, and local protocols
- Responding and rendering care to any patients in need of treatment
- Obeying federal, state, and local laws and regulations

If you fail to act as a reasonable, prudent person with similar training and experience would act under similar circumstances, with similar equipment, and in the same place, you may be guilty of negligence.

Four Components of Negligence

The four components of **negligence** are as follows:

- **Duty to act:** You have a duty to act reasonably within the standards of training when you are dispatched to a call.
- **Breach of duty:** You do not act within an expected and reasonable standard of care.
- **Damages:** Physical or psychological harm to your patient in some noticeable way.
- **Cause:** The actions or lack of action directly caused the injury or damage.

Important Medicolegal Concepts

The following are important medicolegal concepts:

- **Abandonment** is the termination of care without the patient's consent and without making any provisions for continuing care at the same or higher level. You cannot discontinue care without sufficient reason or turn a patient's care over to a person with less training without creating the potential for liability for abandonment.
- **Advance directive** refers to a written document that specifies medical care should the person become unable to make medical decisions. Types of advance directives include:
  - Living wills
  - Do not resuscitate orders (DNRs)
- **Assault** is threatening or attempting to inflict offensive physical contact.
- **Battery** is unlawfully touching a person. If a patient who is legally able to refuse care is treated without consent, the patient has grounds for criminal charges or civil suit against the EMT for battery.
- **Emancipated minors** are under the legal age in a given state but because of other circumstances can be legally treated as adults.
- **Expressed consent** is a type of informed consent that occurs when the patient does something, either by telling you or by taking some sort of action, that demonstrates he or she is giving you permission to provide care.
- **Implied consent** assumes that a person unable to give consent would consent to care and transport to a medical facility.
- **Informed consent** is a patient's voluntary agreement to be treated after being told about the nature of the disease, the risks and benefits of the proposed treatment, alternative treatments, and given the choice of refusing treatment.
- **Kidnapping** is moving a patient from one place to another without the patient's consent. If you restrain a person without proper justification, you could also be charged with false imprisonment. Both of these may result in civil or criminal liability.
- **Minors** cannot consent to or refuse medical care; consent must be obtained from a parent or legal guardian of the patient; in the case of life-threatening emergencies, consent may be implied.

Communication

When communicating with dispatch, medical direction, hospitals, police, or any other services, know that the Federal Communication Commission assigns, licenses, and regulates radio frequencies. Be sure to follow the following guidelines:

- **Do's**
  - Speak clearly and slowly.
  - Hold the microphone 2" to 3" away from your mouth.
  - Wait 1 second before speaking.
  - Acknowledge your unit.
  - Be brief and courteous.
  - Use confirmation words such as "affirmative" and "negative."
  - Get confirmation that the transmission was received.
- **Don'ts**
  - Use codes.
  - Mention the patient's name or any identifiable information regarding your patient.
  - Use profanity.

When giving a report to the hospital, include the following information:

- Your unit and service
- Patient's age, race, and sex
- Patient's chief complaint
- Patient's medical history
- Patient's mental status, along with baseline vital signs and other pertinent information
- Care rendered and status of treatment

Be sure to update any changes once you arrive at the hospital.

Documentation

Remember that documentation is just as important as patient care. If you don't write it down, it didn't happen. Use the SOAP method (subjective, objective, assessment, and plan [for treatment]), a simple, logical method for documenting patient care. Many other methods for narrative documentation also exist, such as reporting in chronological order, use of the CHARTE method, and the body system approach.

Patient Care Report

- Write neatly.
- Spell correctly.
- Do make conclusions.
- Be sure to document the events in a clear manner so that if you read it 10 years from now you could remember the incident.
- Write down the pertinent negatives.
- *Do not make false statements.*
- In case you make an error, strike it through one time, initial it, and correct it.

Patient Refusal Forms

Who can refuse treatment?

- Any mentally competent adult who is alert and oriented to person, place, time, and event

Who can't refuse treatment or transport?

- Minors
- Patients with an altered mental status

When a patient refuses care, make certain to follow all guidelines, have a witness, and document the situation. Do your best to convince patients to seek medical attention and always advise that if they need care after your departure, they may recall EMS later.

Vital Vocabulary

abandonment Unilateral termination of care by a prehospital provider without the patient's consent and without making provisions for transferring care to another medical professional with skills at the same level or higher.

advance directive A written document that expresses the wants, needs, and desires of a patient in reference to future medical care; examples include living wills, do not resuscitate (DNR) orders, and organ donation cards.

assault To create in another person a fear of immediate bodily harm or invasion of bodily security.

AVPU A method of assessing mental status by determining whether a patient is **a**wake and alert, responsive to **v**erbal stimuli, responsive to **p**ain, or **u**nresponsive.

battery Unlawfully touching a person; this includes providing emergency care without consent.

emancipated minors Persons who are under the legal age of consent in a given state but, because of other circumstances, have been legally declared adults by the courts.

expressed consent A type of informed consent that occurs when the patient does something, either through words or action, that demonstrates permission to provide care.

Glasgow Coma Scale An evaluation tool used to determine a patient's neurologic status, which evaluates three categories: eye opening, verbal response, and motor response; effective in helping to determine the extent of neurologic injury.

implied consent Assumption, on behalf of a person unable to give consent, that he or she would want life-saving treatment initiated.

informed consent A patient's voluntary agreement to be treated after being told about the nature of the disease, the risks and benefits of the proposed treatment, alternative treatments, and the choice of no treatment at all.

kidnapping Moving a patient from one place to another without the patient's consent, or restraining a person without proper justification; both may result in civil or criminal liability.

minors Persons who are not yet legally considered adults. Patients who are minors cannot consent to or refuse medical care; consent must be obtained from a parent or legal guardian of the patient; in the case of life-threatening emergencies, consent may be implied.

negligence Professional action or inaction on the part of the prehospital care provider that does not meet the standard of ordinary care expected of similarly trained and prudent prehospital care providers or that results in injury to the patient.

OPQRST A mode of patient questioning used to evaluate the specific details of the medical emergency and determine the chief complaint.

SAMPLE history A mode of patient questioning used to determine the history of the present illness; links the current medical emergency with the patient's preexisting medical conditions.

CHAPTER

3

Pharmacology

The goal of emergency pharmacology in the prehospital setting is to reverse, prevent, or control various diseases and conditions in order to stabilize the patient's condition. It is vital that you have a strong understanding of pharmacology and pharmacokinetics. The drugs and doses given in this chapter comply with nationally accepted guidelines. However, you must always follow the local protocols approved by your medical director. Remember that all medications are toxic if given to the wrong patient or in the wrong quantities. Never administer medication without the authorization of medical direction through approved standing orders or by direct verbal communication with online medical control.

Federal Drug-Related Legislation

- **Pure Food and Drug Act (1906):** The first federal legislation enacted to protect the public from mislabeled, poisonous, or otherwise harmful foods, medications, and alcoholic beverages.
- **Harrison Narcotic Act (1914):** Limited the use of addictive drugs by regulating the importation, manufacture, sale, and use of opium, cocaine, and cocaine derivatives.
- **Federal Food, Drug, and Cosmetic Act (1938):** Required drug makers to label their products, indicating any potentially habit-forming ingredients or possible side effects; authorized the establishment of the Food and Drug Administration (FDA) to enforce and set premarket safety standards for drugs.
- **1951 Durham-Humphrey amendments to the 1938 act, also referred to as the prescription drug amendments:** Required written or verbal prescription from a physician, dentist, or veterinarian to dispense dangerous drugs and created a category of medications known as over the counter (OTC).
- **The Narcotic Control Act (1956):** Increased the penalties for violation of the Harrison Narcotic Act; made the possession of heroin illegal, and outlawed marijuana.
- **Controlled Substances Act (1970):** Because of their high abuse potential, controlled substances became strictly regulated by the federal government. However, because not all controlled substances carry the same potential for abuse, five schedules were created, with each schedule requiring a different level of security and record keeping. The Controlled Substances Act replaced the Harrison Narcotic Act.

Schedule Created by the Controlled Substances Act of 1970

- **Schedule I:** Highest abuse potential; user may develop severe dependence; no accepted medical indications. Examples: Heroin, lysergic acid diethylamide, mescaline.
- **Schedule II:** Very high abuse potential, but with accepted medical indications. Examples: Opium, cocaine, morphine, oxycodone, codeine, methadone, secobarbital, amphetamines.
- **Schedule III:** Less abuse potential than Schedule I and II drugs, but may lead to moderate or low physical dependence; accepted medical indications. Examples: Limited opioids or combined with noncontrolled substances, such as hydrocodone–acetaminophen combination (Vicodin) or acetaminophen (Tylenol) with codeine.

- **Schedule IV:** Low abuse potential; limited psychological or physical dependence, or both; medically accepted. Examples: Phenobarbital, diazepam, lorazepam.
- **Schedule V:** Lowest abuse potential; may lead to limited physical or psychological dependence. Examples: Cough or cold remedies, medications used to treat diarrhea.

Medication Names

A drug (a chemical compound) becomes a medication when it is approved for use by the FDA for purposes of preventing, diagnosing, or treating illness or disease. Thousands of over-the-counter or prescription-only medications are available, and hundreds of new ones are marketed each year in the United States alone. To minimize the potential for confusion, all medications are assigned four names, as follows:

- **Chemical name:** Describes the drug's chemical composition.
- **Generic name (or nonproprietary name):** A general name for a drug, suggested by the original manufacturer. Usually derived from the chemical name but shorter and simpler.
- **Official name:** Once the generic name has been approved by the US Adopted Names Council and the drug has been approved by the FDA, the name is listed in the *United States Pharmacopeia* (USP) and becomes the drug's official name.
- **Brand name (or trade name):** Unique name under which the manufacturer registers the drug with the FDA. Use of the registration mark (®) in the upper-right corner of the trade name indicates that it has been registered as a trademark. Brand names may also be signified by capitalizing the first letter.

Sources of Drugs

- **Plant extracts:** Oldest source; for example, digitalis, used for heart failure, is made from the dried leaves of purple foxglove
- **Animal extracts:** For example, insulin is made from animal pancreas, primarily pig
- **Minerals:** Inorganic sources such as magnesium sulfate, sodium chloride (NaCl), and calcium chloride (CaCl)
- **Synthetic:** Laboratory made, alternative source; for example, synthetic forms of vitamins, steroids, narcotics

Drug Profile

Federal law requires that manufacturers package every medication with a drug profile that contains all pertinent information about that drug. Components of the drug profile are as follows:

- **Drug names:** The generic and trade names; sometimes the chemical name and a drawing of the drug molecule are included as well.
- **Drug classification:** All medications are categorized according to a specific classification based on the medication's effect on the patient and its mechanism of action. Know the qualities of each class of drugs as well as the medications that fall under that type.
- **Mechanisms of action:** A description of how the medication achieves its desired effect (eg, by binding to a receptor site, changing cell properties, combining with other chemicals, or altering a normal metabolic pathway).
- **Indications:** Appropriate condition or conditions for which the drug should be used based on what has been approved by the FDA.
- **Pharmacokinetics:** A description of how the medication is absorbed, distributed, and eliminated from the body (useful for determining best route of administration); also expected time of onset and duration of action.

> **Tip**
>
> What's in a name? When it comes to knowing your medications, plenty. Here are the four names for the antiarrhythmic amiodarone:
>
> - Chemical name: 2-butyl-3-benzofuranyl-4-[2-(diethylamino)-ethoxy]-3.5-diiodophenyl ketone hydrochloride
> - Generic name: amiodarone
> - Trade names: Cordarone, Pacerone
> - Official name: amiodarone USP

- **Side effects/adverse reactions:** The undesired, but often predictable, effects of the medication. All drugs have side effects, which must be discussed with the patient and weighed against the benefits of administering the drug.
- **Routes of administration:** How the drug is given to the patient (ie, enteral versus parenteral).
- **Doses:** Amount of drug to be given for a particular condition; factors to take into consideration (eg, patient's age and weight).
- **Contraindications:** Conditions for which the drug should *not* be given. If a medication is given when a contraindication is present, it is likely to cause predictable harm to the patient.
- **Special considerations:** How the drug may affect pediatric, geriatric, or pregnant patients.

Tip

Medication errors are the leading cause of patient safety errors in health care! Remember the six "rights" of medication administration:

1. The right patient
2. The right dose
3. The right route
4. The right time
5. The right medication
6. The right documentation

Guidelines for Safe and Effective Drug Administration to Patients

- Know the precautions and contraindications for all medications you administer, including those that relate to the particular patient being treated. Precautions also include drug interactions.
- Practice proper administration procedures.
- Know the side effects and interactions of the drug and how to observe and document those side effects.
- Maintain knowledge of current medications and uses.
- Know the pharmacokinetics and pharmacodynamics of the medications.
- Have current reference materials available. Don't trust your memory in an emergency!
- Take a careful drug history, including any over-the-counter medications, recreational drugs, or herbal or folk remedies.
- Consult with medical control when required or for clarification regarding medication administration.
- Know the six "rights" of medication administration.

FDA Rating Scale for Assessing Risk to Fetus and Mother

- Remember special considerations for pregnant patients. Certain drugs may harm the fetus (teratogenic).
  - Pregnant patients: Teratogenic drugs may harm the fetus.
    - Pass through the placenta to the fetus
    - Accumulate to toxic levels due to the fetus's inability to metabolize
    - Pass through to infant by breast milk
- **Category A:** Adequate, well-controlled studies in pregnant women have not shown an increased risk of fetal abnormalities.
- **Category B:** Animal studies have revealed no evidence of harm to the fetus; however, there are no adequate and well-controlled studies in pregnant women.
  or
  Animal studies have shown an adverse effect, but adequate and well-controlled studies in pregnant women have failed to demonstrate a risk to the fetus.
- **Category C:** Animal studies have shown an adverse effect, and there are no adequate and well-controlled studies in pregnant women.
  or
  No animal studies have been conducted, and there are no adequate and well-controlled studies in pregnant women.

- **Category D:** Adequate well-controlled or observational studies in pregnant women have demonstrated a risk to the fetus. However, the benefits of therapy may outweigh the potential risk.
- **Category X:** Adequate well-controlled or observational studies in animals or pregnant women have demonstrated positive evidence of fetal abnormalities. The use of the product is contraindicated in women who are or may become pregnant.

Special Populations

Pediatric Patients

- The skin of pediatric patients is thinner, resulting in less fat to absorb medication and causing drugs to be more potent, with the potential for systemic toxicity.
- Absorption of oral medications may be slower as a result of less gastric acid, low enzyme levels, and longer gastric emptying time.
- Diminished plasma protein concentrations result in less binding of drugs, which causes a free, active drug compared to the same dose in an adult.

Geriatric Patients

- Absorption of oral medications may be slower due to decreased gastrointestinal motility.
- Geriatric patients may be taking multiple medications, which may interact and modify each other's effects.
- Decreased plasma protein alters the way the medication is distributed in the system.

Pharmacokinetics

Pharmacokinetics is the study of the metabolism and action of medications within the body, with emphasis on absorption time, duration of action, distribution throughout the body, and method of excretion. Drugs diffuse across the cell membrane.

There are two types of transport across the cell membrane:

- **Active transport:** Requires energy
  - This energy is achieved by breaking down adenosine triphosphate (ATP) and adenosine diphosphate (ADP) (ie, the sodium-potassium pump).
  - Larger molecules, such as glucose, use facilitated diffusion.
- **Passive transport:** The way most drugs travel through the body
  - Diffusion: Movement of solute; higher to lower concentration
  - Osmosis: Movement of solution; lower to higher concentration
  - Filtration: Molecules across membrane; higher to lower concentration

Absorption

Absorption is the transfer of a medication from its site of administration to target tissues and organs. Most absorption takes place in the small intestine because of its large surface area and permeable membrane. The ultimate goal is to achieve a therapeutic concentration of the medication in the blood, which depends on the rate and extent of absorption. The rate and extent of absorption in turn depend on the ability of the medication to cross the cell membrane. Factors that affect the rate and extent of absorption include the following:

- **Blood flow:** Administration into areas of the body with rich blood supply and a good vascular system enhances absorption. Decreased blood flow may lower the concentration gradient across the intestinal mucosa and reduce absorption by passive diffusion.

- **Route given:** Intravenous (IV) administration has a faster absorption rate than intramuscular (IM), which has a faster absorption rate than subcutaneously (SubQ/SC/SQ). Medications administered orally (PO) must pass through the digestive tract. The thick mucous layer of the stomach limits absorption.
- **Medication concentration:** The higher the concentration, the faster the absorption.
- **Effects of pH:** The pH of a medication affects its ability to ionize (or become electronically charged). Most medications reach a state of equilibrium between their ionized and nonionized forms, facilitating their absorption.
- **Gastric emptying:** This limits the rate of absorption. Food, mainly fatty foods, slows gastric emptying.
- **Bioavailability:** The amount of the drug that is still active after it reaches the target tissue.
- **Timed release:** Medications with enteric coatings are formulated to not dissolve until they reach the duodenum. This enteric coating allows the medication to pass through the acidic stomach and reach the alkaline intestines before onset of action.
- **Nature of nontarget cells:** The medication must pass through nontarget cells on its way to the target cells; the size of the surface area of nontarget cells affects absorption (the larger the surface area, the greater the absorption).
- **Lipid soluble:** Medications that are lipid (fat) soluble move easily and directly across the cell membrane because the membrane is made of phospholipids.
- **Aqueous soluble:** Aqueous (water) soluble drugs move across cell membranes through aqueous channel proteins.
- **Ionization of drug:** Affected by the drug's pH.

Distribution

- The process by which medication moves throughout the body.
- Blood is the primary vehicle.
- Medication in the bloodstream may become bound to plasma proteins; this drug-protein complex cannot be used by the body, so its formation lowers the therapeutic concentration of the drug.
    - Amount of free drug is always proportional to the amount of bound drug; as the free drug is used and eliminated, drug-protein complexes break down and release more free drug.
    - Molecules of medication may become bound to the plasma protein albumin, which is too large to diffuse out of the bloodstream and essentially "kidnaps" drug molecules.
    - A single layer of capillary endothelial cells, the blood–brain barrier allows only lipid-soluble medications to enter the brain and cerebrospinal fluid.
    - The placental barrier does not permit *most* non–lipid-soluble medications to pass to the fetus; however, you must understand which medications can be given to a pregnant patient and in which situations.

Biotransformation

- Biotransformation is the manner in which the body metabolizes medications (ie, breaks drugs into different chemicals, or **metabolites**).
- First-pass metabolism: Although every tissue has some ability to metabolize drugs, the liver is the principal organ of drug metabolism. Other tissues that display considerable activity include the gastrointestinal tract, the lungs, the skin, and the kidneys.

- Following oral administration, many drugs (eg, isoproterenol, meperidine, pentazocine, morphine) are absorbed intact from the small intestine and transported first via the portal system to the liver, where they undergo extensive metabolism. Some orally administered drugs (eg, clonazepam, chlorpromazine) are more extensively metabolized in the intestine than in the liver. Thus, intestinal metabolism may contribute to the overall first-pass effect.

Elimination

- The remnants of the drug in the body, which may be toxic or inactive metabolites, are eliminated.
- Most drugs are excreted in the urine.
- Renal excretion occurs via two major processes.
  - **Glomerular filtration:** Allows drugs to pass into urine
  - **Tubular excretion:** Active carrier process for cations and anions

Drug Routes

- **Enteral:** Absorption somewhere along the gastrointestinal tract, including PO, orogastric/nasogastric tube, sublingual, buccal, and rectal
- **Parenteral:** Any route that is not the gastrointestinal tract; usually administered via needle or syringe; includes IV, intraosseous, endotracheal, umbilical, IM, SubQ, inhalation/nebulized, topical, transdermal, intranasal, instillation, and intradermal

Drug Forms

- Solid drug forms
  - Pills
  - Tablets
  - Capsules
  - Suppositories
  - Powders
  - Ointments
  - Extracts
  - Patches
- Liquid drug forms
  - Suspensions
  - Solutions
  - Elixirs
  - Emulsions
  - Syrups
  - Tinctures
  - Spirits
- Gaseous drug form
  - Inhaled

Pharmacodynamics

Also known as the mechanism of action, pharmacodynamics is the way in which a medication produces the intended response.

Theories of Drug Action

Medications operate in the body in one of four ways:

- Binding to a receptor site (most prevalent in the prehospital setting)
  - **Agonists** stimulate the receptor site to cause a normal response.
  - **Antagonists** inhibit normal response by blocking chemical mediators.
- Changing the physical properties of the cell, typically by changing the osmotic balance
- Combining with other chemicals, such as to neutralize the effect of a harmful chemical
- Altering a normal metabolic pathway, such as by interrupting the cell's normal growth process

Pharmacologic Classifications

Table 3-1 and **Table 3-2** list pharmacologic classifications.

Table 3-1 Pharmacologic Classifications by Receptor Type

Tissue	Receptor Subtype	Agonists	Antagonists
Heart	beta-1	Norepinephrine, epinephrine, dobutamine	Atenolol, metoprolol
Vascular smooth muscle	beta-2	Epinephrine, salbutamol, terbutaline, salmeterol	Butoxamine
Airway smooth muscle	beta-2	Terbutaline, salbutamol, salmeterol, zinterol	Butoxamine
Smooth muscle contraction	alpha-1	Norepinephrine, epinephrine, phenylephrine, oxymetazoline	Prazosin, doxazosin
Inhibition of transmitter release; hypotension; anesthesia; vasoconstriction	alpha-2	Clenbuterol, alpha-methylnoradrenaline, dexmedetomidine, mivazerol, clonidine	Yohimbine, idazoxan, atipamezole, efaroxan, rauwolscine

Table 3-2 Pharmacologic Classifications by Drug

Drug	Action	Used for	Examples
ACE inhibitors	Slow (inhibit) the activity of the enzyme angiotensin, which decreases the production of angiotensin II	Congestive heart failure; treatment of left ventricular function; hypertension	Lisinopril, captopril, enalapril, ramipril, benazepril, quinapril
Adrenergics	Adrenergic receptor sites: *Alpha-receptor site* Vasoconstriction Iris dilation Intestinal relaxation Intestinal sphincter contraction Bladder sphincter contraction *Beta-receptor site* Vasodilation (beta-2)	Positive chronotrope; positive inotrope; positive dromotrope; increase renal function (shock patients)	Epinephrine, norepinephrine, dobutamine, dopamine, isoproterenol, albuterol, racemic epinephrine, metaproterenol

Table 3-2 Pharmacologic Classifications by Drug (Continued)

Drug	Action	Used for	Examples
	Cardioacceleration (beta-1) Intestinal relaxation (beta-2) Uterine relaxation (beta-2) Bronchodilation (beta-2)		
Adrenocorticoids	Natural hormone secreted by the adrenal cortex whose main function is to assist in metabolism of carbohydrates, lipids, and proteins	Arthritis; allergic reactions	Cortisone
Alpha-1 adrenergic blockers; antiadrenergics; sympatholytics	Block the postsynaptic alpha-1 adrenergic receptors of the vascular smooth muscle; dilate the arterioles and veins to decrease blood pressure and improve blood flow	Hypertension	Doxazosin, prazosin, trimazosin
Amphetamines	Increase release of excitatory neurotransmitters; decrease levels of norepinephrine, dopamine, and serotonin	Drowsiness; fatigue; appetite suppressant	Methylphenidate
Analgesics	Block pain signals within the central nervous system (CNS)	Pain relief	Ketorolac, aspirin, morphine, oxymorphone, nalbuphine, fentanyl
Adjunctive medications that enhance the effects of other analgesics	Limited or no analgesic properties	Enhance the effects of other analgesics	Benzodiazepines, diazepam, lorazepam, midazolam, antihistamines, promethazine, caffeine
Anesthetics, general	Create a state of unconsciousness or dissociation so patient is unaware of painful stimuli	Surgical procedures	Diprivan, brevital
Anesthetics, local	Block peripheral nerve impulses	Surgical procedures	Lidocaine, novocaine
Antianginal drugs	Relax smooth vascular muscles	Angina pectoris	Nitrates
Antianxiolytics/ Antiepileptics	Hyperpolarize the membrane of the CNS neurons, which decreases their response to stimuli—GABA is the chief inhibitory neuro-transmitter	Status epilepticus; sedation; anticonvulsant	Hydroxyzine, droperidol, diazepam, midazolam, lorazepam, alprazolam

Continues

Table 3-2 Pharmacologic Classifications by Drug (Continued)

Drug	Action	Used for	Examples
Antiarrhythmics: Overall	Restore normal rhythm and conduction by; • Decreasing or increasing conduction velocity • Altering the excitability of cardiac cells by changing the duration of the effective refractory period • Suppressing abnormal automaticity	Arrhythmias	Bretylium, digoxin, quinidine, digitoxin
Antiarrhythmics: Class 1A (sodium channel blockers)	Decrease rate of sodium entry into the cell during depolarization; prolong duration of the action potential; depress phase 0 of the action potential, slowing conduction	Ventricular arrhythmias; Wolff-Parkinson-White syndrome; paroxysmal atrial fibrillation	Procainamide, quinidine, disopyramide
Antiarrhythmics: Class 1B (sodium channel blockers)	Decrease rate of sodium entry into the cell during depolarization; shorten the action potential; depress phase 0 of the action potential, slowing conduction	Ventricular tachycardia; atrial fibrillation	Lidocaine, phenytoin, mexiletine
Antiarrhythmics: Class 2 (beta-adrenergic blockers)	Depress polarization of phase 4	Reduce occurrence of tachyarrhythmias	Atenolol, esmolol, labetalol, propranolol
Antiarrhythmics: Class 3 (potassium channel blockers)	Prolong repolarization	Ventricular tachycardias; atrial fibrillation	Amiodarone
Antiarrhythmics: Class 4 (calcium channel blockers; cardiac glycosides)	Slow conduction velocity to increase atrioventricular node refractory period	Prevent recurrence of paroxysmal supraventricular tachycardia; reduce ventricular rate in patients with atrial fibrillation	Verapamil, diltiazem
Antiarrhythmics: Class 5	Direct nodal inhibition	Supraventricular arrhythmias	Digoxin, adenosine
Antiasthmatics	Bronchodilation	Prevent asthma attacks	Cromolyn
Anticholinergics	Block cholinergic receptors; oppose the parasympathetic nervous system	Asystole; asthma; pulseless electrical activity; symptomatic bradycardia; organophosphate poisoning	Atropine sulfate, ipratropium bromide, promethazine, diphenhydramine, hydroxyzine
Anticoagulants	Slow or prevent blood coagulation	Ischemic strokes; atrial fibrillation	Heparin, warfarin

Table 3-2 Pharmacologic Classifications by Drug (Continued)

Drug	Action	Used for	Examples
Antidepressants: Selective serotonin reuptake inhibitors, monoamine oxidase inhibitors, tricyclic antidepressants	Inhibit the transport of norepinephrine and serotonin; prevent the reuptake of serotonin; do not affect dopamine or norepinephrine; have anticholinergic properties	Depression; mood disorders	Sertraline, paroxetine, phenelzine, imipramine, amitriptyline, desipramine, nortriptyline
Antihistamines	Block H_1 receptors; block the effects of histamine I allergic reactions (H_2 blockers block gastric acid production and secretion)	Allergies; anaphylaxis	Diphenhydramine, loratadine, meclizine, cimetidine, famotidine, ranitidine
Antihyperglycemics	Decrease blood glucose levels; aid in conversion of glucose to glycogen; stimulate release of insulin from beta cells of the pancreas; increase release of glucagon and liver glucose	Hyperglycemia	Insulin, pioglitazone, lasartan, metformin, sitagliptin
Antihypertensives	Decrease blood pressure by blocking beta-adrenergic receptors	Hypertension	Clonidine, propranolol, nitroprusside, nitroglycerin, labetalol
Antihypoglycemics	Increase the level of circulating blood glucose by releasing glycogen from the liver; increase positive inotropic and chronotropic effects; smooth muscle relaxation (glucagon only)	Antihypoglycemia	Glucagon, dextrose
Anti-inflammatories	Decrease inflammation and cerebral edema	Inflammation	Dexamethasone, methylprednisone, ketorolac
Antitussives	Suppress dry cough	Cough suppressant	Dextromethorphan
Benzodiazepine antagonist	Competitively binds with benzodiazepine receptors and reverses benzodiazepine's effects	Benzodiazepine overdose	Flumazenil
Beta-1 adrenergic blockers	Bind to the beta-adrenergic receptors to block the sympathetic nervous system response; negative inotropic effect;	Atrial fibrillation and flutter; ventricular tachycardias	Labetalol, metoprolol, nadolol, propranolol

Continues

Table 3-2 Pharmacologic Classifications by Drug (Continued)

Drug	Action	Used for	Examples
	negative chronotropic effect; prolong action potential duration and refractory period		
Beta-2 adrenergic agonists	Bronchodilation	Anaphylaxis; chronic obstructive pulmonary disease; asthma	Terbutaline, racemic epinephrine, metaproterenol, aminophylline, albuterol, epinephrine
Butyrophenones	Produce a state of tranquility; depress the central nervous system (CNS)	Antipsychotic	Haloperidol, droperidol
Calcium channel blockers	Slow or inhibit the influx of calcium molecules passing through the cell membrane; reduce automaticity and conduction in the cardiac and smooth muscles *Potent vasodilator of coronary vessels:* Increase coronary blood flow; reduce coronary vasospasm *Vasodilator of peripheral vessels:* Decrease peripheral vascular resistance *Negative inotropic effect:* Decrease myocardium oxygen consumption *Negative chronotropic effect:* Slow conduction of the SA node reducing myocardium oxygen consumption	Angina	Verapamil, nifedipine, diltiazem
Cardiac glycosides	Positive inotropic effect by increasing the refractory period of the AV node and increasing total peripheral resistance	Congestive heart failure; atrial flutter; atrial fibrillation; paroxysmal supraventricular tachycardia	Digoxin
Central nervous system stimulants	Increase release or effectiveness of excitatory neurotransmitters; decrease release or effectiveness of inhibitory neurotransmitters	Used to treat conditions lacking adrenergic stimulation	Benzphetamine, diethylpropion
Depolarizing	Prevent stimulation of muscle fibers by acetylcholine	Short-term paralysis	Succinylcholine
Diuretics	Increase the rate of urine excretion;	Heart failure; hypertension; kidney disease	Furosemide, bumetanide

Table 3-2 Pharmacologic Classifications by Drug (Continued)

Drug	Action	Used for	Examples
	decrease the extra-cellular fluid volume to produce a negative extracellular fluid balance		
Dopaminergics	Restore balance of dopamine and acetylcholine; increase stimulation of dopamine receptors and decrease stimulation of acetylcholine receptors	Parkinson disease	Levodopa, amantadine, bromocriptine, MAOIs
Electrolyte modifiers	Electrolytes	Electrolyte imbalance	Calcium gluconate, calcium chloride, magnesium sulfate
Ganglionic blocking agents	Produced by competitive antagonism with acetylcholine only at nicotinic receptors in the autonomic ganglia	Hypertension	Trimethaphan, mecamylamine
Gases	Cellular perfusion; pain relief; bronchodilation	Cellular perfusion	O_2
Glucocorticoids	Suppress tissue inflammation, inhibit swelling to the spinal cord in a traumatic injury	Allergic reaction, inflammation, autoimmune disorders	Methylprednisolone, dexamethasone
H_2 histamine antagonists	Block the histamine receptors in the stomach, decreasing acid production by the cells	Used in the treatment of acid-related GI conditions	Cimetidine
Inotropics	Increase cardiac contractility	Cardiac	Adrenaline, dopamine, dobutamine, norepinephrine
Methylphenidate	Stimulates the ability to concentrate	Attention deficit disorder	Methylphenidate
Methylxanthines	Bronchial smooth muscle relaxer that helps dilate constricted airways, stimulates diuresis to relieve congestion, and acts as a mild cardiac and CNS stimulant	Asthma; treating certain tachycardias	Caffeine, theophylline, adenosine
Muscarinic cholinergic antagonists	Block muscarinic receptors so they cannot bind with acetycholine Atropine dose levels Decrease dose = decrease secretions from salivary glands, bronchial glands, and sweat glands;	Useful in reversing overdoses of muscarinic agonists; sedation; antiemetic; asthma	Atropine, scopolamine, ipratropium bromide

Continues

Table 3-2 Pharmacologic Classifications by Drug (Continued)

Drug	Action	Used for	Examples
	decrease gastric motility and stomach acid secretions Moderate = increase heart rate, mydriasis, blurry vision		
Narcotic antagonists	Block opioid receptors and reverse opioids' effects	Narcotic overdose	Nalmefene, naloxone
Neuromuscular blocking agents	Block the release of acetylcholine on the presynapse and postsynapse	Paralysis	Pancuronium, rocuronium, succinylcholine, vecuronium
Nondepolarizing	Block the binding of acetylcholine to its receptors	Long-term paralysis	Vecuronium
Nonopioid analgesics	Antipyretic, anti-inflammatory properties; also inhibit synthesis of prostaglandin	Pain	Ketorolac, acetaminophen, ibuprofen, salicylates
Opioid agonist-antagonists	Agonists because they reduce pain response; antagonists because they have fewer respiratory depressants and addictive side effects	Analgesia	Pentazocine, nalbuphine, butorphanol
Opioid analgesic agonists	Bind to opiate receptors and cause analgesia, euphoria, sedation, miosis, and a decrease in cardiac preload and afterload	Severe pain	Sublimaze, morphine, meperidine
Opioid antagonists	Reverse the effects of opioid analgesics; bind with opioid receptors without causing effects of opioid binding	Opioid overdose; respiratory depression	Naloxone
Osmotic diuretics	Inhibit reabsorption of water and electrolytes to increase urinary output	Increased intracranial pressure; cerebral edema	Mannitol
Oxytocic drug	Stimulates uterine contractions to reduce bleeding after childbirth	Postpartum uterine hemorrhage	Oxytocin
Phenothiazines	Low potency	Neuroleptic; antipsychotic	Chlorpromazine, promethazine
Sedatives	CNS depression	CNS depression	Diazepam, droperidol, hydroxyzine, lorazepam, midazolam

Table 3-2 Pharmacologic Classifications by Drug (Continued)

Drug	Action	Used for	Examples
Skeletal muscle relaxants	Decrease muscle tone; inhibit voluntary movement	Neurologic disorders with muscle spasms; traumatic muscle spasms	Methocarbamol, baclofen
Sympathomimetics	Adrenergic; mimic epinephrine and norepinephrine, combining with alpha and beta receptors; stimulate alpha-1 adrenergic receptors (vasoconstriction) and beta-1 (increases cardiac output and peripheral vascular resistance) and beta-2 (broncho-constriction) adrenergic receptors	Depends on the drug used	Epinephrine, norepi-nephrine, dopamine, dobutamine, racemic epinephrine
Thrombolytics	Break up or dissolve blood clots	Ischemic strokes	Streptokinase, alteplase
Tocolytics	Used to suppress pre-mature labor; relax the smooth muscle of the uterus	Premature labor	Terbutaline
Vasodilators	Increase vessel diam-eter; coronary vessel dilators; reduce blood pressure	Hypertension; chest pain	Nitroglycerin, nitroprusside
Vasopressors	Stimulate alpha-adrenergic receptors to increase peripheral vascular resistance by contracting vessel muscles	Neurogenic shock	Dopamine, epinephrine, norepinephrine
Ventricular antiarrhythmics	Prolong action potential and refractory period; slow the sinus rate, PR and QT intervals; vasodilation; decrease peripheral vascular resistance	Ventricular arrhythmias	Lidocaine, amiodarone
Vitamin B_1	Metabolizes food into adenosine triphosphate	Alcoholism; malnutrition	Thiamine

Drug Calculations

Drug calculations begin with understanding the multiples of the metric system and their equivalents (**Table 3-3**).

Always convert the dose requested by the physician or your protocols and the dose on hand into the same measurements. (The **dose on hand (DOH)** is literally that—the dose of medication that you have on your ambulance.) As a rule of thumb, always convert into the measurement of the dosage that you will be administering to your patient. For example, if your DOH is in milligrams, and you are administering your medications in micrograms, convert everything into micrograms.

Dose on Hand and Volume on Hand

All liquid medications are packaged as a **concentration**, which is the drug's weight per volume (eg, grams, milligrams, or micrograms per milliliter). From a concentration, you can determine the DOH and the volume on hand. For example, 50% dextrose in a prefilled syringe is 25 g of the drug in 50 mL of fluid.

$$\frac{\text{Number of milligrams in container}}{\text{Number of milliliters in container}} = \text{mg/mL}$$

The following example calculates the concentration of a medication using DOH and volume on hand:

$$\frac{10 \text{ mg}}{20 \text{ mL}} = \frac{1 \text{ mg}}{2 \text{ mL}} = 0.5 \text{ mg/mL}$$

Some medication orders may require you to convert milligrams (mg) to micrograms (μg). With these orders, you need to divide a larger number (the denominator) into a smaller number (numerator). The answer will produce a decimal fraction. For example, if you are calculating a dopamine drip and the desired dose is 5 μg/min, but the DOH is in milligrams, you must convert the milligrams to micrograms by moving the decimal point three places to the right. Refer to **Table 3-3** for conversion factors.

Table 3-3 Metric Units and Their Equivalents

Units of weight (smallest to largest)
• 1 μg = 0.001 mg
• 1 mg = 1,000 μg
• 1 g = 1,000 mg
• 1 kg = 1,000 g
Units of volume (smallest to largest)
• 1 mL = 1 cc*
• 100 mL = 1 dL
• 1,000 mL = 1 L
*One milliliter (mL) of water weighs 1 g and occupies 1 cubic centimeter (cc) of volume. Thus a mL and a cc both express one one-thousandth of a liter and are, therefore, equivalent expressions.

The following problem is an example of calculating a concentration in which units need to be converted.

> *Example:* You have received an order to initiate a dopamine drip. You have one single-dose vial containing 400 mg of dopamine, one IV bag containing 250 mL of normal saline, and a 60-gtt/mL administration set. Once the vial of dopamine is added to the 250-mL bag of fluid, what will be the concentration of dopamine, in micrograms?

First, convert the units from milligrams to micrograms:

$$400 \text{ mg} \times 1{,}000 \text{ µg} = 400{,}000 \text{ µg}$$

Next calculate the concentration:

$$\frac{400{,}000 \text{ µg}}{250 \text{ mL}} = \frac{1{,}600 \text{ µg}}{1 \text{ mL}}$$

The concentration would be 1,600 µg/mL.

Calculating With the "Concentration on Hand" Formula

Example: The physician orders 80 mg of furosemide for your patient. The concentration available is 100 mg/10 mL.

$$\text{Volume to be administered } (x) = \frac{(\text{Volume on hand}) \times (\text{Ordered dose})}{(\text{Concentration on hand})}$$

Volume on hand = 10 mL
Ordered dose = 80 mg
Concentration = 100 mg
Volume to be administered = 8 mL

Calculating IV Drip Rates

Here is the formula for calculating rate-dependent doses:

$$\frac{DD}{DOH} \times \frac{gtt}{mL} = \text{Rate}$$

- **DD** represents the desired dose as ordered by protocol, the medical director, or another physician.
- **DOH** represents the dose on hand in the medication container.
- **gtt/mL** represents the number of drops per milliliter as dictated by the administration set.
- <u>Rate</u> represents the number of drops per minute to which the administration set must be set to administer the dose ordered.

Example: You are ordered to initiate a lidocaine drip for a patient being transported to a tertiary care facility. The orders require you to give 2 mg/min. After you repeat the order to the online medical control physician, you open the medication drawer in the ambulance and find that the lidocaine is stocked in 250-mL bags containing 1 g of lidocaine. A microdrip administration is already in use for the patient.

$$\frac{250 \text{ mL}}{1{,}000 \text{ mg}} \times \frac{2.0 \text{ mg}}{1.0 \text{ min}} \times \frac{600 \text{ gtt}}{1.0 \text{ mL}} = 300 \text{ gtt/min}$$

You would want to infuse the lidocaine at 300 gtt/min.

Condition and Treatment Quick Guide

This chapter concludes with **Table 3-4**, a condition and treatment quick guide.

Table 3-4 Condition and Initial Treatment Quick Guide

Condition	Treatment	Adult Dose	Pediatric Dose
Acute Psychotic Episodes/Combativeness			
Acute psychotic episodes	Haloperidol	IV: 5 mg IM: 5 mg	IV: 0.05 mg/kg IM: 0.05 mg/kg
Acute psychotic episodes	Midazolam	IV: 0.02-0.05 mg/kg IM: 5 mg	IV: 0.025-0.05 mg/kg IM: 0.1-0.15 mg/kg
Acute psychotic episodes	Droperidol	IV: 2.5 mg IM: 2.5 mg	IV: 0.1 mg/kg IM: 0.1 mg/kg
Allergic Reactions and Anaphylaxis			
Allergic reaction	Diphenhydramine	IV: 50 mg IM: 50 mg	IV: 1-2 mg/kg
Anaphylaxis	Epinephrine	SQ: 0.3 mg	SQ: 0.01 mg/kg
Anaphylaxis	Epinephrine infusion	Infusion: 2-10 µg/kg/min	Infusion: 0.1-1 µg/kg/min
Anaphylaxis	Methylpred-nisolone	IV: 1-2 mg/kg IM: 1-2 mg/kg	IV: 1-2 mg/kg
Anaphylaxis	Normal saline	Infusion: 250 mL to maintain SBP of 90 mm Hg or radial pulses	Infusion: 20 mL/kg titrated to maintain radial or brachial pulses
Bradycardias			
Bradycardia (symptomatic; 2nd degree type II and 3rd degree blocks)	Transcutaneous pacing	70 bpm beginning at 30 mA; increase by 10 mA until capture	Not indicated for pediatric use
Bradycardia (junctional, sinus, and 2nd degree type I block)	Atropine	IV: 0.5 mg	IV: 0.02 mg/kg IO: 0.02 mg/kg ETT: 0.03 mg/kg
Bradycardia	Epinephrine	Not indicated for adult use	IV: 0.01 mg/kg IO: 0.01 mg/kg ETT: 0.1 mL/kg
Bradycardia	Epinephrine infusion	Infusion: 2-10 µg/kg/min	Infusion: 0.1-1 µg/kg/min
Asystole	Normal saline	Infusion: 250 mL	Infusion: 20 mL/kg bolus
Asystole	Epinephrine	IV: 1 mg IO: 1 mg	IV: 0.01 mg/kg IO: 0.01 mg/kg ETT: 0.1 mL/kg
Asystole	Atropine	IV: 1 mg IO: 1 mg	IV: 0.02 mg/kg IO: 0.02 mg/kg ETT: 0.03 mg/kg
Pulseless electrical activity	Normal saline	Infusion: 250 mL bolus	Infusion: 20 mL/kg bolus
Pulseless electrical activity	Epinephrine	IV: 1 mg IO: 1 mg	IV: 0.01 mg/kg IO: 0.01 mg/kg ETT: 0.1 mL/kg

Table 3-4 Condition and Initial Treatment Quick Guide (Continued)

Condition	Treatment	Adult Dose	Pediatric Dose
Pulseless electrical activity	Atropine	IV: 1 mg IO: 1 mg	IV: 0.02 mg/kg IO: 0.02 mg/kg ETT: 0.03 mg/kg
Chest Pain			
Chest pain	Oxygen	15 L/min	Not indicated for pediatric use
Chest pain	Aspirin	PO: 160-325 mg	Not indicated for pediatric use
Chest pain	Nitroglycerin	SL: 0.4 mg	Not indicated for pediatric use
Chest pain	Morphine	IV: 2-4 mg	Not indicated for pediatric use
Congestive Heart Failure (CHF)/Acute Pulmonary Edema			
CHF/pulmonary edema	Nitroglycerin	SL: 0.4 mg	Not indicated for pediatric use
CHF/pulmonary edema	Furosemide	IV: 0.5-1.0 mg/kg	Not indicated for pediatric use
CHF/pulmonary edema	Morphine	IV: 2-4 mg	Not indicated for pediatric use
Diabetic Reactions			
Hyperglycemia	Normal saline	Infusion: 250 mL to maintain SBP of 90 mm Hg or radial pulses	Infusion: 20 mL/kg over 20-30 min titrated to maintain radial or brachial pulses
Hypoglycemia with alcohol intoxication	Thiamine	IV: 100 mg IM: 100 mg	Not indicated for pediatric use
Hypoglycemia	Dextrose	IV: 50% 25 g	IV: 25% 0.5-1 g/kg/dose
Hypoglycemia	Glucagon	IV: 0.5-1 mg IM: 0.5-1 mg IN: 0.5-1 mg	IV: 0.5-1 mg IM: 0.5-1 mg IN: 0.5-1 mg
Electrolyte Imbalances			
Hyperkalemia	Normal saline	Infusion: 250 mL to maintain SBP of 90 mm Hg or radial pulses	Infusion: 20 mL/kg over 20-30 min titrated to maintain radial or brachial pulses
Hyperkalemia	Calcium gluconate	IV: 10-20 mL of 10% solution	Not indicated for pediatric use
Hyperkalemia	Sodium bicarbonate	IVP: 1 mEq/kg	Not indicated for pediatric use
Heat Illness			
Fever	Acetaminophen	Not indicated for adult use	PR: 15 mg/kg
Heat cramps	Ketorolac	IV: 30 mg IM: 60 mg	Not indicated for pediatric use

Continues

Table 3-4 Condition and Initial Treatment Quick Guide (Continued)

Condition	Treatment	Adult Dose	Pediatric Dose
Hypotension			
Hypotension	Normal saline	Infusion: 250-500 mL to maintain SBP of 90 mm Hg or radial pulses	Infusion: 20 mL/kg over 20-30 min titrated to maintain radial or brachial pulses
Hypotension	Lactated Ringer's solution	Infusion: 250-500 mL to maintain SBP of 90 mm Hg or radial pulses	Infusion: 20 mL/kg over 20-30 min titrated to maintain radial or brachial pulses
Hypotension	Dopamine infusion	Infusion: 2-20 µg/kg/min	Infusion: 2-20 µg/kg/min
Hypotension	Dobutamine infusion	Infusion: 2-20 µg/kg/min	Infusion: 2-20 µg/kg/min
Nausea and Vomiting			
Nausea and vomiting	Promethazine	IV: 12.5-25.0 mg IM: 12.5-25 mg	IV: 0.25 mg/kg
Nausea and vomiting	Ondansetron	IV: 4 mg	IV: 0.1 mg/kg
Respiratory Emergencies			
Respiratory distress	Albuterol/ ipratropium	Albuterol nebulized: 1.25-2.5 mg Ipratropium: 0.5 mg	Albuterol nebulized: 1.25-2.5 mg
Respiratory distress	Albuterol	Nebulized: 1.25-2.5 mg	Nebulized: 1.25-2.5 mg
Respiratory distress	Levalbuterol	Nebulized: 1.25 mg	Nebulized: 0.63 mg
Respiratory distress	Methylprednisone	IV: 1-2 mg/kg IM: 1-2 mg/kg	IV: 1-2 mg/kg
Respiratory distress	Epinephrine	SQ: 0.3 mg Nebulized: 5 mg	SQ: 0.01 mg/kg/min Nebulized: 0.5 mg
Respiratory distress	Magnesium sulfate infusion	Infusion: 2 g	IV: 25-50 mg/kg IO: 25-50 mg/kg
Seizures			
Seizures	Diazepam	IV: 5-10 mg	PR: 0.1-0.3 mg/kg IV: 0.2 mg/kg
Seizures	Midazolam	IV: 2.5-5.0 mg IM: 5 mg IN: 5 mg	Not indicated for pediatric use
Seizures	Lorazepam	IV: 2-4 mg IM: 2-4 mg	IV: 0.05-0.2 mg/kg
Eclampsia	Magnesium sulfate infusion	Infusion: 2 g	Not indicated for pediatric use
Toxins and Poisonings			
Organophosphate poisoning	Normal saline	Infusion: 250 mL to maintain SBP of 90 mm Hg or radial pulses	Infusion: 20 mL/kg titrated to maintain radial or brachial pulses

Table 3-4 Condition and Initial Treatment Quick Guide (Continued)

Condition	Treatment	Adult Dose	Pediatric Dose
Organophosphate poisoning	Atropine	IV: 2-4 mg	IV: 0.02 mg/kg
Overdose (aspirin)	Sodium bicarbonate	IV: 1 mEq/kg	IV: 1 mEq/kg
Overdose (aspirin)	Normal saline	Infusion: 250 mL to maintain SBP of 90 mm Hg or radial pulses	Infusion: 20 mL/kg titrated to maintain radial or brachial pulses
Overdose (benzodiazepine)	Flumazenil	IV: 0.2 mg	Not indicated for pediatric use
Overdose (opioids)	Naloxone	IV: 0.4-2.0 mg IM: 0.4-2.0 mg IN: 0.4-1.0 mg	SIVP: 0.1 mg/kg
Overdose (TCAs)	Normal saline	Infusion: 250 mL to maintain SBP of 90 mm Hg or radial pulses	Infusion: 20 mL/kg titrated to maintain radial or brachial pulses
Overdose (TCAs)	Sodium bicarbonate	IV: 1 mEq/kg	IV: 1 mEq/kg
Tachycardias			
Atrial fibrillation/atrial flutter	Diltiazem	IV: 0.25 mg/kg	Not indicated for pediatric use
Narrow complex tachycardia (unstable)	Synchronized cardioversion	Monophasic: 100 J Biphasic: 75 J	0.5-1.0 J/kg
Narrow complex tachycardia (stable)	Adenosine	IV: 6 mg	IV: 0.1-0.2 mg/kg
Ventricular fibrillation/ pulseless ventricular tachycardia	Defibrillation	Monophasic: 200 J Biphasic: 120 J	2 J/kg
Ventricular fibrillation/ pulseless ventricular tachycardia	Vasopressin	IV: 40 units IO: 40 units	Not indicated for pediatric use
Ventricular fibrillation/ pulseless ventricular tachycardia	Epinephrine	IV: 1 mg IO: 1 mg	IV: 0.01 mg/kg IO: 0.01 mg/kg ETT: 0.1 mL/kg
Ventricular fibrillation/ pulseless ventricular tachycardia	Lidocaine	IV: 1-1.5 mg/kg IO: 1-1.5 mg/kg	IV: 1 mg/kg IO: 1 mg/kg ETT: 2-3 mg/kg
Ventricular fibrillation/ pulseless ventricular tachycardia	Amiodarone	IV: 300 mg IO: 300 mg	IV: 5 mg/kg IO: 5 mg/kg
Ventricular fibrillation/ pulseless polymorphic ventricular tachycardia	Magnesium sulfate	IV: 2 g IO: 2 g	IV: 25-50 mg/kg IO: 25-50 mg/kg
Wide complex tachycardia (unstable)	Synchronized cardioversion	Monophasic: 100 J Biphasic: 75 J	0.5-1.0 J/kg
Wide complex tachycardia (stable)	Lidocaine infusion	Infusion: 1-4 mg/min	Infusion: 20-50 μg/kg/min

Continues

Table 3-4 Condition and Initial Treatment Quick Guide (Continued)

Condition	Treatment	Adult Dose	Pediatric Dose
Wide complex tachycardia (stable)	Magnesium sulfate infusion	IV: 2 g	IV: 25-50 mg/kg
Trauma			
Pain management	Meperidine	IV: 50-100 mg IM: 50-100 mg	IV: 1-2 mg/kg IM: 1-2 mg/kg
Pain management	Morphine	IV: 2-4 mg	IV: 0.1-0.2 mg/kg
Pain management	Fentanyl citrate	IV: 0.5-2.0 µg/kg IM: 0.5-2.0 µg/kg IN: 0.5 µg/kg	IV/IM/IO: 1.7-3.3 µg/kg (2-12 years)
Pain management	Ketorolac	IV: 30 mg IM: 60 mg	Not indicated for pediatric use
SBP, systolic blood pressure; ETT, endotracheal tube; TCAs, tricyclic antidepressants; SIVP, slow IV push.			

Vital Vocabulary

agonists Substances that mimic the actions of a specific neurotransmitter or hormone by binding to the specific receptor of the naturally occurring substance.

antagonists Molecules that block the ability of a given chemical to bind to its receptor, preventing a biologic response.

concentration The total weight of a drug contained in a specific volume of liquid.

dose on hand (DOH) Dose of medication available to the caregiver.

metabolites Smaller chemical compounds that are produced as a result of metabolism (eg, of a drug).

rate The number of drops per minute (gtt/min) to which an IV administration must be established to administer the desired dose.

Trauma

Trauma and Energy

Trauma is the acute physiologic and structural change (injury) that occurs in a patient's body when an external source of energy dissipates faster than the body's ability to sustain and dissipate that energy. **Mechanical** energy is energy from motion (a moving vehicle); potential energy is energy stored in an object (a concrete wall).

Motor Vehicle Collisions and Motorcycle Crashes

Predict the types of injury by examining the scene. There are five types of motor vehicle collision (MVC) impact patterns: frontal (or head on), lateral (or side), rear, rotational, and rollover. Interior damage (dash, steering wheel, and windshield) may also indicate the nature of injury. Common MVC injuries include:

- Facial injuries
- Soft-tissue neck trauma
- Larynx and tracheal trauma
- Fractured/flail sternum
- Myocardial contusion
- Pericardial tamponade
- Pulmonary contusion
- Hemothorax/pneumothorax
- Rib fractures
- Flail chest
- Ruptured aorta
- Intra-abdominal injuries (eg, spleen, liver, pancreas, kidneys)
- Spine, pelvic, and extremity fractures

Injury Patterns Associated With Motor Vehicle Collisions

Frontal Impact MVC: Up and Over

In the up-and-over pathway, the lead point is the head, which takes a higher trajectory, impacting the windshield, roof, mirror, or dashboard. Depending on the point of impact, the following injuries are possible:

- Rib fracture, ruptured diaphragm, hemopneumothorax, pulmonary contusion, cardiac contusion, myocardial rupture, vascular disruption (aortic rupture)
- Abdominal impact: Kidneys, liver, and spleen subject to vascular tears; disruption of renal vessels; liver laceration; spleen rupture; ruptured diaphragm
- Head as point of impact: Injury of cervical vertebrae, cervical flexion, axial loading and/or hyperextension, severe angulation of the cervical vertebrae, brain trauma, intracranial vascular disruption

Frontal Impact MVC: Down and Under

The down-and-under pathway is traveled by an occupant who slides under the steering column, with the knees hitting the dashboard; therefore, take note of the steering column and dashboard.

Look for the following injuries:

- Knee dislocation, patellar fracture, femur fracture, fracture or posterior dislocation of the hip, fracture of the acetabulum, vascular injury, and hemorrhage

Lateral Impact MVC

- Rib fractures; compression of the torso, pelvis, and extremities; pulmonary contusion; ruptured liver or spleen; fractured clavicle; fractured pelvis; and head and neck injury

Rollover-Impact MVC

- Can be any type of injury; serious even if victim wore a seat belt; in unrestrained victims, head and neck injuries likely

Rotational Impact MVC

- Injuries similar to those of frontal and lateral impact collisions

Rear-Impact MVC

- Back and neck injuries and cervical strain or fracture caused by hyperextension; injury to cervical portion of the spine

MVC With Ejection

- One in three victims experiences a cervical spine injury

Pedestrian Injuries: Adult

- Impact occurs in three phases:
  - Legs, hips hit by bumper: Lower extremity injuries, particularly to knee and leg; tibia-fibula fractures; knee dislocations with severe multiligamentous injury common
  - Torso to automobile hood: Head, pelvis, chest, and coup-contrecoup traumatic brain injuries; lateral compression pelvic fractures are common and can cause open fractures with bony punctures to the vagina (women) and other viscera
  - Pedestrian to ground

Pedestrian Injuries: Pediatric or Short Stature

- Impact occurs in three phases:
  - Thighs, pelvis, or torso hit by bumper: Multisystem injuries involving the head, chest, abdomen, and long bones; multiple extremity and pelvic, abdominal, and thoracic crush fractures
  - Chest and abdomen to grille or low hood: Sternal and rib fractures
  - Head and face to hood and then ground: Skull and facial fractures, facial abrasions, closed head injury

Motorcycle Crashes

- **Head-on collisions:** Secondary impacts with the handlebars; head and neck trauma and compression injuries to the chest and abdomen; midshaft femur fractures; bilateral fractures to the femur and lower leg; severe perineal injuries if the groin strikes the fuel tank
- **Angular impact collisions:** Crushing-type injuries—open fractures to the femur, tibia, and fibula, and fracture and dislocation of the malleolus

Assessment

- Scene size-up
  - Ensure body substance isolation (BSI).
  - Maintain c-spine control.
- Initial/primary assessment
  - Assess level of consciousness (LOC).
  - Assess ABCs (airway, breathing, and circulation).

- Manage airway. If helmets are involved and the need for a definitive airway exists, the helmet should be removed.
- Evaluate transport considerations (position of comfort).
- *Do not remove helmet if*
  - Patient is undoubtedly dead.
  - Impaled object is piercing the head through the helmet.
  - Patient's airway and breathing can be maintained with the helmet in place.
- Focused history and physical exam/secondary assessment

Management

- Manage ABCs.
- Treat life-threatening illness/injuries.
- Suction airway as needed.
- Obtain SAMPLE history and chief complaint (OPQRST).
- Administer oxygen at 15 L/min via nonrebreathing mask or bag-mask ventilation.
- Establish two large-bore IVs.
- *Do not give anything by mouth.*
- Attach cardiac monitor and pulse oximeter.
- Apply loose dressings to cover nose and ears if fluid is present. This allows drainage and prevents tamponade of the brain.

Falls From Heights

- Severity depends on height of fall (velocity); position at impact (head first versus feet first); area of impact (greater area generates fewer peak pressures); surface (degree of plasticity, rough or smooth); and physical condition of the victim (complicating conditions, such as osteoporosis or enlarged spleen)
- Foot and lower extremity fractures; hip, pelvic ring, and sacral fractures; vertebral compression and burst fractures, particularly of T12-L1 and L2 (the result of lumbar spine axial loading); organ damage (the result of vertical deceleration pressures); forearm and wrist fractures

Penetrating Trauma

- Stab wounds
  - Laceration wounds with potential fracture and blunt soft-tissue wounds or amputation
  - Neck wounds: Potential damage to carotid arteries, subclavian vessels, apices of the lung, the upper mediastinum, trachea, esophagus, and thoracic ducts; deep neck wounds: spinal cord injury or fracture
  - Lower chest/abdominal wounds: Potential damage to thoracic or abdominal cavity, diaphragm
- Gunshot wounds
  - Severity depends on type of firearm (rifle, shotgun, or handgun), velocity of the projectile, physical design of the projectile, distance to target, and type of tissue injured
  - Skin and subcutaneous tissue puncture, laceration, abrasion, or burns (close range); infection; deformation and tissue destruction in soft tissue and bone

Blast Injuries

- **Primary:** Caused by the pressure of the blast. Injuries affect the hollow organs of the body (lungs, gastrointestinal [GI] tract). Injuries include pneumothorax, air emboli, and GI trauma.
- **Secondary:** Caused by flying debris. Injuries noted will be cuts, abrasions, and so on.

- **Tertiary:** Caused by the impact of the body being thrown against other objects, such as walls. Damage includes injury to abdominal viscera, central nervous system (CNS), and musculoskeletal system.

Triage and Patient Assessment

Table 4-1 summarizes trauma triage for mass-casualty incidents.

Table 4-1 Trauma Triage for Mass-Casualty Incidents

Priority	Condition	Color	Note
1	Immediate	Red	Airway and breathing difficulties Severe bleeding Signs of shock Severe burns Life-threatening injuries
2	Delayed	Yellow	Significant injuries with *no* signs or symptoms of shock
3	Walking wounded	Green	Minor injuries
4	Dead/dying/expectant	Black	Cardiopulmonary arrest Injuries incompatible with life

Initial/Primary Assessment
- Determine chief complaint.
- Evaluate and treat ABCs.
- Make transport decisions.
  - Determine appropriate facility. Decide whether transport to a trauma center is needed using local system criteria and the Committee on Trauma (COT) of the American College of Surgeons criteria and call into a trauma facility. Determine whether air transport is needed.

Key Elements for Trauma Centers
- Level I: A comprehensive regional resource that is a tertiary care facility. Capable of providing total care for every aspect of injury—from prevention through rehabilitation.
  - 24-hour in-house coverage by general surgeons
  - Availability of care in specialties such as orthopaedic surgery, neurosurgery, anesthesiology, emergency medicine, radiology, internal medicine, and critical care
  - Should also include cardiac, hand, pediatric, and microvascular surgery and hemodialysis
  - Must maintain a predetermined number of resuscitation areas, intensive care unit beds, and operating rooms
  - Provides leadership in prevention, public education, and continuing education of trauma team members
  - Committed to continued improvement through a comprehensive quality assessment program and organized research to help direct new innovations in trauma care
  - Must receive a predetermined number of critical trauma patients each year
- Level II: Able to initiate definitive care for most severely injured patients
  - 24-hour immediate coverage by general surgeons
  - Availability of orthopaedic surgery, neurosurgery, anesthesiology, emergency medicine, radiology, and critical care

- Tertiary care needs such as cardiac surgery, hemodialysis, and microvascular surgery may be referred to a Level I trauma center
- Committed to trauma prevention and continuing education of trauma team members
- Provides continued improvement in trauma care through a comprehensive quality assessment program
- Level III: Has demonstrated the ability to provide prompt assessment, resuscitation, and stabilization of injured patients and emergency operations
  - 24-hour immediate coverage by emergency medicine physicians and prompt availability of general surgeons and anesthesiologists
  - Lacks much of the surgical subspecialities and intensive care treatment available at larger hospitals
  - Program dedicated to continued improvement in trauma care through a comprehensive quality assessment program
  - Has developed transfer agreements for patients requiring more comprehensive care at a Level I or Level II trauma center
  - Committed to continuing education of nursing and allied health personnel or the trauma team
  - Also dedicated to improving trauma care through a comprehensive quality assessment program
- Level IV: Has demonstrated the ability to provide advanced trauma life support (ATLS) before transfer of patients to a higher-level trauma center
  - Includes basic emergency department facilities to implement ATLS protocols and 24-hour laboratory coverage
  - Transfer to higher-level trauma centers follows the guidelines outlined in formal transfer agreements
  - Committed to continued improvement of these trauma care activities through a formal quality assessment program

The COT Criteria for Referral to a Trauma Center

1. If one or more of the following is present, the patient should be referred to a trauma center:
   - Systolic blood pressure (SBP) below 90 mm Hg
   - Glasgow Coma Scale (GCS) score of less than 14
   - Respiratory compromise with a respiratory rate (RR) of less than 10 or greater than 29
   - Revised Trauma Score (RTS) of less than 11
   - Pediatric Trauma Score (PTS) of less than 9
2. Field diagnosis of one of the following:
   - Flail chest
   - Two or more proximal long bone fractures
   - Amputation proximal to the wrist or ankle
   - Any penetrating trauma to head, neck, torso, or extremities proximal to the elbow or knee
   - Any limb paralysis
   - Pelvic fractures
   - Combination of trauma with burns
   - Open and depressed skull fractures
   - Major burns
3. Evaluate the MOI or look for evidence of high-energy trauma. Refer to a trauma center if one of the following is present:
   - Ejection from automobile
   - Death in the same passenger compartment

- Pedestrian thrown when struck by vehicle or run over or auto-pedestrian injury at more than 5 mph
- High-speed auto crash (> 40 mph)
- Intrusion into passenger compartment of more than 12"
- Major auto deformity of more than 20"
- Vehicle rollover with unrestrained passenger
- Heavy extrication time of greater than 20 minutes
- Falls of more than three times the patient's height
- Motorcycle crash at greater than 20 mph or when rider and bike are separated

4. If none of the above criteria is met, consider transfer to a trauma center if one of the following is true:
- Patient younger than 5 years or older than 55 years
- Pregnant patient
- Known immunosuppressed patient
- Known cardiac disease or respiratory disease comorbidity
- Type 1 diabetes, cirrhosis, morbid obesity, or coagulopathy

Air or Ground Transport

Consider air transport if:

- Ground transport to an appropriate facility will take an extended amount of time.
- There are multiple casualities that you are unable to manage with the resources on-scene.
- The extrication time is prolonged or patients are critically injured.
- A safe takeoff and landing zone is available.

Contraindications and relative contraindications to air transport:

- Patient is in cardiac arrest.
- Weather conditions are adverse.
- Extremely combative patients and rapid-sequence intubation (RSI) is unavailable or contraindicated.
- Patient is morbidly obese.
- Patients with barotrauma may need lower flying altitudes.
- If ground transport time to the nearest appropriate facility is shorter than awaiting arrival of air transport to scene and subsequent flight transport time, use ground transport.

Focused History and Physical Exam/Secondary Assessment

- Reconsider MOI. If significant MOI:
  - Rapid trauma assessment: Head-to-toe exam (adults, adolescents, and children; unconscious infants and toddlers) or toe-to-head exam (conscious infants and toddlers)

Detailed Physical Exam

- **DCAP-BTLS:** Deformities, contusions, abrasions, punctures/penetrations, burns/bruising, tenderness, lacerations, swelling
- **Head:** Inspect and palpate the scalp, check ears for fluid, examine eyes (pupils equal, round, and reactive to light—PERRL), check nose and mouth for potential obstructions
- **Neck:** Check for jugular venous distention, tracheal deviation
- **Chest:** Inspect, palpate, auscultate, percuss; check for paradoxical movement, entrance/exit wounds
- **Abdomen:** Inspect, palpate, percuss
- **Back:** Inspect and palpate
- **Pelvis:** Inspect and palpate (check for crepitus/instability) (anterior and lateral compression)
- **Genitalia:** Check for priapism (males) and wetness (females) because this usually indicates an acute spinal cord injury
- **Extremities**: Inspect and palpate; pulse, motor function, sensation (PMS)
- **Reassess:** Unstable patients every 5 minutes; stable patients every 15 minutes
- **Altered mental status**
  - Glasgow Coma Scale score (**Table 4-2**)
    - Revised Trauma Score (**Table 4-3**)
    - Pediatric Trauma Score (**Table 4-4**)

Table 4-2 Glasgow Coma Scale Score

Children and Adults		
Eye opening	Spontaneous	4
	To voice	3
	To pain	2
	None	1
Best verbal response	Oriented	5
	Confused	4
	Inappropriate words	3
	Incomprehensible words	2
	None	1
Best motor response	Obeys commands	6
	Localizes pain	5
	Withdraws (pain)	4
	Flexion (pain)	3
	Extension (pain)	2
	None	1
Infants and Toddlers		
Eye opening	Spontaneous	4
	To voice	3
	To pain	2
	None	1
Best verbal response	Smiles, interacts	5
	Consolable	4
	Cries to pain	3
	Moans to pain	2
	None	1
Best motor response	Normal spontaneous movement	6
	Localizes pain	5
	Withdraws (pain)	4
	Abnormal flexion	3
	Abnormal extension	2
	None	1

Rapid Trauma Assessment: Head-to-Toe Examination

The rapid trauma assessment is an important tool performed on patients with a significant MOI. It is similar to the detailed physical exam, but is done much quicker—2 to 3 minutes as compared with up to 15 minutes for the detailed physical exam.

- Perform after the cervical spine (c-spine) has been controlled, your primary assessment has been performed, and all threats to airway, breathing, and circulation have been identified and corrected.

Table 4-3 Revised Trauma Score

Glascow Coma Scale Score	Systolic BP (mm Hg)	Respiratory Rate (breaths/min)	Coded Values
13-15	> 89	10-29	4
9-12	76-89	> 29	3
6-8	50-75	6-9	2
4-5	1-49	1-5	1
3	0	0	0

Table 4-4 Pediatric Trauma Score

Patient Characteristics	+2	+1	-1
Weight (kg)	> 20	10-20	< 10
Airway	Normal	Maintained	Unmaintained
Systolic BP (mm Hg)	> 90	50-90	< 50
Central nervous system	Awake	Obtunded	Coma
Open wound	None	Minor	Major
Skeletal trauma	None	Closed	Open, multiple

- If the patient is responsive, ascertain chief complaints.
- Revisit your transport decision.

Head

- **Scalp:** Inspect and palpate the skull to check for asymmetry (swelling or depressions) or bleeding.
- **Ears:** Look in and behind the ears for cerebrospinal fluid or blood.
- **Eyes:** Check PERRL; palpate eye orbits (both sides in unison).
- **Nose:** Check for presence of cerebrospinal fluid, blood, soot, and singed hair.
- **Mouth:** Check for broken or displaced teeth, vomitus, or blood (need for suctioning).

Neck

- **Cervical spine:** Palpate, feeling for deformities; watch for a groan or grimace from the patient, which may signal tenderness in the c-spine.
- Check for signs of jugular venous distention, tracheal deviation, penetration, or subcutaneous emphysema.
- On completion of the neck exam, check your gloves for signs of bleeding.
- Add rigid c-spine collar.

Chest and Back

- **Suprasternal notch:** Inspect and palpate the chest; with both thumbs on the suprasternal notch, check for fractures (fractured clavicles are common). Check rise and fall of the chest for retractions or other signs of breathing problems.
- **Sternum:** Palpate for crepitus or abnormal motion.
- **Rib cage:** Barrel hoop the rib cage under the armpits and then at the costal margin to check for fractured ribs or a flail chest. *Note*: Large bruised areas may indicate a flail chest before paradoxical movement is evident.
- **Thoracic and lumbar spine:** Log roll the patient to examine and palpate the thoracic and lumbar spine, checking for DCAP-BTLS.

Abdomen

- The four quadrants (**Figure 4-1**): Inspect and palpate all four quadrants of the abdomen, checking for rigidity, guarding, bruising, distention, and tenderness. Pay attention to a patient's moans or groans, which signal a particular sore or tender spot. Injury to one or more abdominal organs is likely in a major traumatic event, so be quick but thorough in the assessment.

The Organs in the Four Abdominal Quadrants

Right Upper Quadrant (RUQ)
- Liver
- Colon
- Right kidney
- Aorta
- Pancreas
- Gallbladder

Left Upper Quadrant (LUQ)
- Liver
- Colon
- Aorta
- Pancreas
- Spleen
- Left kidney
- Stomach

Right Lower Quadrant (RLQ)
- Right kidney
- Colon
- Small intestines
- Right iliac artery and vein
- Bladder
- Ureter
- Appendix

Left Lower Quadrant (LLQ)
- Left kidney
- Colon
- Ureter
- Small intestines
- Left iliac artery and vein
- Bladder

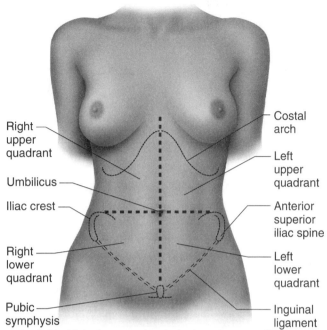

Figure 4-1 The abdomen is divided into four quadrants by imaginary vertical and horizontal lines that intersect at the umbilicus.

Pelvis

- **Pelvic girdle:** Press gently but firmly down on the iliac crest; then press inward to check for instability or pain (signs of injury to pelvic girdle).
- **Genitals:** Inspect for priapism (males) or wetness (females).

Extremities

- **Legs:** Inspect and palpate both legs from hip to ankle, looking for DCAP-BTLS; shortening or abnormal rotation of one or both legs is a sign of fracture or dislocation.
- **Feet:** Assess motor function and sensation.
  - Simultaneously assess pedal pulses, noting symmetry (suspect vascular disruption if this is the case).
  - Bilateral loss of motor function suggests spinal cord injury; unilateral loss of function suggests musculoskeletal injury (except in stroke)
- **Arms:** Inspect and palpate the arms, assessing pulse, motor function, and sensation as for the legs.

Skin

- Perfusion
- Temperature
- Diaphoresis
- Jaundice
- Pallor
- Cyanosis
- Rash
- Fever

Trauma Care

- All patients who present with an altered LOC of any type must have their glucose level checked and cardiac monitoring initiated to rule out any type of compounding medical problem.

> **Tip**
>
> Trauma is a surgical problem. The goal of trauma care is to treat, restore, and maintain stability until definitive surgical treatment can be performed. In doing so, your approach should be oriented to the patient. The priority of care is as follows:
> - Assess thoroughly.
> - Assess airway and breathing.
> - Restore your patient's perfusion.
> - Prevent further injuries.
> - Be sure to take all appropriate equipment to the patient.

- All patients who are displaying signs and symptoms of shock must be kept warm, especially patients younger than 5 years and older than 55 years.
- Endotracheal intubation: Visualize, intubate, ventilate, auscultate, confirm, and secure.
  - If orotracheal intubation is not possible, insert a rescue airway such as the Combitube or King LT. Once a rescue airway has been inserted, if able to ventilate with ease, it should remain in place until arrival at the emergency department (ED).
- Oxygenate to restore cellular perfusion.
- Fluid boluses are to be titrated to an SBP of 90 mm Hg. In adult patients, administer a fluid challenge of 250 to 500 mL. In pediatric patients, this is accomplished by administering fluid boluses of 20 mL/kg.
- Special caution should be given when giving fluid boluses to the elderly; be sure to constantly reassess lung sounds.
- All pregnant patients who are more than 20 weeks' gestation should be transported on their left side to prevent compression of the inferior vena cava (supine hypotension syndrome).
- Patients should be reassessed after *every* intervention, for positive or negative changes and for responses to treatment regimens.
- Assess breath sounds before and after any fluid boluses are administered. Prior to giving any additional boluses, these assessment findings should be documented.
- Use caution when administering fluid boluses to patients with a prior history of congestive heart failure or pulmonary edema.
- Note signs of internal bleeding: bright red blood from mouth, rectum, or other orifice; coffee ground appearance of vomitus; melena (black tarry stools); dizziness or syncope on sitting or standing.

Head and Spinal Injuries
Pathophysiology

Traumatic brain injury may be initial (occurring instantaneously at the time of impact) or secondary (occurring anywhere from minutes to days later as an aftereffect to the primary injury). There are two general types of head injury:

- **Open head injury:** Penetration of the dura mater and skull contents, exposing brain tissue to the environment (gunshot wound [GSW] is a common MOI); associated with high mortality rate or significant neurologic deficit
- **Closed head injury:** From blunt trauma; dura mater remains intact, and brain tissue is not exposed; associated with skull fractures, focal brain injuries (contusion, hemorrhage, hematomas), and diffuse brain injuries (concussion) and often complicated by increased intracranial pressure (ICP)
  - Hematomas
    - Subdural hematoma: Results from venous bleeding that occurs as a result of a head injury. Blood accumulates in the subdural space between the dura mater and the arachnoid. Your patient may experience symptoms immediately after the injury, but it could also take anywhere from several days to a week for symptoms to appear.
    - Epidural hematoma: Results from high-energy injuries that are often associated with skull fractures. The patient may experience a brief loss of consciousness and then regain consciousness. The patient may then rapidly lose consciousness again. Be sure to note any hemiplegia or hemiparalysis in the patient because the area of the head injury commonly occurs on the side **contralateral** to the side of paralysis.

- Intracerebral hematoma: Results from injury to the blood vessels in the brain. This is a result of **coup-contrecoup** injuries. Coup injuries occur when the brain actually makes contact with the skull at the point of impact. Contrecoup injuries occur on the side opposite of the point of impact. Also may be caused by hemorrhagic stroke.
- **Intracranial pressure:** When blood accumulates within the skull, or the brain begins to swell, it can lead to a rapid increase in ICP and a decrease in cerebral perfusion pressure (CPP). Normal adult ICP ranges from 0 to 15 mm Hg. As the ICP rises, the body attempts to compensate for the decline in CPP by a rise in mean (average) arterial pressure (MAP) (Cushing response). As MAP continues to rise, cerebrospinal fluid (CSF) is displaced through the foramen magnum in the skull to compensate for the expansion.

> **Tip**
>
> Cerebral perfusion pressure is the difference between mean arterial pressure and intracranial pressure:
>
> CPP = MAP − ICP

Signs and Symptoms of Increased ICP

- Altered LOC
- Paralysis
- Projectile vomiting
- Headache
- Patient is unbalanced or uncoordinated
- Upper brain stem
  - Cheyne-Stokes respirations
  - Cushing response
  - Flexion/withdrawal to pain
- Middle brain stem
  - Central neurogenic hyperventilation
  - Cushing response
  - Decerebrate posturing
- Lower brain stem
  - Ataxic respirations
  - Pupils fixed and dilated on the side opposite the injury (**anisocoria**)
  - Cushing response

> **Formulas to Remember**
>
> MAP = Diastolic pressure + 1/3 Pulse pressure

> **Cushing Response**
>
> Increased systolic blood pressure
>
> Widened pulse pressure
>
> Decreased pulse
>
> Irregular respiratory pattern

Assessment

- Scene size-up
  - Suspect in MVCs, falls from heights, assault or other direct blows to the head, sports-related injuries
  - C-spine control
- Initial/primary assessment
  - Check for altered LOC using AVPU to determine presence of brain injury.
  - Check extent of injury using Glasgow Coma Scale. The lower the score, the more serious the injury to the brain.
  - Check PERRL (recheck often).
  - Assess for signs of ICP.
  - If a helmet is compromising the airway, the helmet should be removed.
- Focused history and physical exam/secondary assessment
  - Obtain SAMPLE history and chief complaint (OPQRST).

Management

- Establish patent airway; if patient has vomited, immediately suction airway to prevent aspiration.
- Administer 100% oxygen.
  - Via nonrebreathing mask if patient is breathing adequately
  - Via bag-mask ventilation if breathing is inadequate
- Have suction ready.

- Establish two large-bore IVs.
- Attach cardiac monitor.
- Apply loose dressings to cover nose and ears if fluid is present and draining to prevent tamponading the brain.

Table 4-5 summarizes treatment of head and spinal injuries.

Table 4-5 Treatment of Head and Spinal Injuries

Treatment	Used For	Adult Dose	Pediatric Dose
Normal saline	Increase blood pressure, improve distal circulation	250-500 mL titrated to systolic blood pressure of 90 mm Hg	20 mL/kg
Methylprednisone	Decrease swelling in acute spinal cord injuries, anti-inflammatory	IV: 30 mg/kg over 30 min	IV: 30 mg/kg over 30 min

Thoracic Injuries

Pathophysiology

Traumatic thoracic injury can result in compromised ventilation, oxygenation, or circulation. Ventilation is affected when air or blood enters the pleural space, causing reduced airspace. Injuries to the chest wall or diaphragm lead to reduced movement of the thorax and inhibition of breathing; pain may also inhibit chest movement. Loss of alveolar space (as the result of alveolar collapse or incomplete chest wall expansion, hemorrhage, or airway obstruction) leads to reduced oxygenation.

Damage to cardiovascular structures in the thoracic cavity may result in systemic hypoperfusion or cardiovascular collapse. Assessing for thoracic injury is an integral part of the patient's ABCs and both the primary assessment and reassessment.

Assessment

- Scene size-up
  - Suspect in MVCs, falls from heights, assault, or other trauma.
  - Control c-spine.
- Initial/primary assessment
  - Check for LOC using AVPU to establish baseline mental status.
  - Establish and maintain ABCs.
- Focused history and physical exam/secondary assessment
  - Obtain SAMPLE history and chief complaint (OPQRST).

General Management for Thoracic Injuries

- Manage ABCs.
- Administer supplemental oxygen at 15 L/min via nonrebreathing mask or bag-mask ventilation.
- Establish and maintain airway.
- Assess for signs of shock and treat if needed.
- Transport rapidly to appropriate trauma facility.
- Monitor vital signs every 5 minutes.

Chest Wall Injuries

Flail Chest

- **Flail chest** is defined as two or more consecutive ribs broken in two or more places and is characterized by paradoxical movement of the injured area of the chest wall. May result from falls, MVCs, or assaults. Occurs in 20% of patients, with 50% associated mortality rates (higher if the patient is older than 60 years).

- Signs and symptoms
  - Tenderness
  - Paradoxical chest wall movement
  - Bruising
  - Crepitus
- Specific management
  - Stabilize flail segment with a bulky dressing.

Rib Fracture

- Most common thoracic injury, especially ribs 4 though 9.
- Signs and symptoms
  - Tenderness
  - Crepitus
- Specific management
  - Transport in a position of comfort if the patient is not c-spine immobilized.

Sternal Fracture

- Not serious in itself, but is associated with myocardial contusions, flail sternum, pulmonary contusions, head and intra-abdominal injuries, and myocardial rupture and increased mortality
- Specific management
  - Transport in a position of comfort if the patient is not c-spine immobilized.

Pulmonary Contusion

- Injury to the lung tissue as a result of blunt force trauma that inhibits the normal diffusion of oxygen and carbon dioxide; the causes are similar to those for flail chest
- Signs and symptoms
  - Hypoxia
  - Hypercarbia
  - Dyspnea
  - Tachycardia
- Specific management
  - Transport in position of comfort if the patient is not c-spine immobilized.

Lung Injuries

Simple Pneumothorax

- **Simple pneumothorax** is common in patients with thoracic trauma as a result of direct injury to the lung (rib fracture) or barotrauma (pressure such as from a steering wheel during an MVC).
- Signs and symptoms
  - Chest pain
  - Subcutaneous emphysema (distended skin that crackles on palpation)
  - Tachypnea
  - Decreased or absent breath sounds on the affected side
  - Dyspnea
  - May occur spontaneously, often in young, thin, tall men aged 20 to 40 years with narrow, long chests
- Specific management
  - Transport in a position of comfort if the patient is not c-spine immobilized.

Open Pneumothorax

- **Open pneumothorax**: Penetrating trauma (eg, GSW, stabbing) opens the pleural space to the environment, leading to negative pressure, increased air into the pleural space, pneumothorax, sucking chest wound, hypoxia, and hypercarbia.
- Signs and symptoms
  - Dyspnea
  - Pain
  - Sucking or gurgling sounds in the chest
  - Visible frothy blood on the chest
- Specific management
  - Cover the wound with an occlusive dressing. Seal an open chest wound immediately with a gloved hand, and then seal with an occlusive dressing with a flutter valve to release air that is trapped inside the chest. Assess for increasing shortness of breath or progressing pneumothorax; if present, lift one side of the occlusive dressing to release air pressure in the thoracic cavity.

Tension Pneumothorax

- **Tension pneumothorax**: Accumulation of air in the pleural space as the result of injury to the lung parenchyma (blunt injury). Barotraumas caused by positive-pressure ventilation, or tracheobronchial injuries caused by shearing, result in air being trapped (air can get in but not out), leading to increased pressure in the pleural space, lung compromise, and collapse. If severe, the heart and vascular system are also affected, leading to shock.
- Signs and symptoms
  - Anxiety
  - Cyanosis
  - Subcutaneous emphysema
  - Decreased or absent breath sounds
  - Distended neck veins
  - Hyperexpansion of one or both sides of the chest
  - Tracheal deviation to unaffected side
- Specific management
  - Cover the penetrating wound with an occlusive dressing. Seal an open chest wound immediately with a gloved hand, and then seal with an occlusive dressing with a flutter valve to release air that is trapped inside the chest. Assess for increasing shortness of breath or progressing pneumothorax; if present, lift one side of the occlusive dressing to release air pressure in the thoracic cavity.

Hemothorax

- **Hemothorax**: Results when the potential space between the parietal and visceral pleura begins to fill up with blood as a result of injury (rib fractures and injuries to lung parenchyma are most common). When both blood and air are present, the injury is called a **hemopneumothorax**.
  - **Massive hemothorax**: Accumulation of more than 1,500 mL of blood within the pleural space.
- Signs and symptoms
  - Dyspnea
  - Shock
  - Narrowing pulse pressure
  - Tracheal deviation to the unaffected side
  - Neck veins *not* distended
- Specific management
  - Cover the penetrating wound with an occlusive dressing. Seal an open chest wound immediately with a gloved hand, and then seal with an occlusive dressing with

a flutter valve to release air that is trapped inside the chest. Assess for increasing shortness of breath or progressing hemothorax; if present, lift one side of the occlusive dressing to release air pressure in the thoracic cavity.
- Perform needle decompression at the second or third intercostal space at the midclavicular line if there is a possible hemopneumothorax.

Cardiac Injuries
Pericardial Tamponade
- Excessive fluid in the pericardial sac, causing compression of the heart and decreased cardiac output. In the trauma setting, penetrating wounds are the most common cause (GSW, stabbing). Severity depends on the size of the perforation in the pericardium and the rate of hemorrhage from the cardiac wound
- Signs and symptoms
  - Beck's triad (see box)

Tip

Beck's triad is defined as jugular venous distention (JVD), muffled heart tones, and decreased blood pressure.

Myocardial Contusion
- Results when sudden deceleration forces the heart forward and into the posterior sternum, leading to local tissue contusion and hemorrhage, edema, and cellular damage within the involved myocardium. Damage to the coronary arteries and veins may compromise blood flow.
- Signs and symptoms
  - Sinus tachycardia
  - Cardiac arrhythmias, such as ventricular ectopy
  - Possible ST segment abnormalities

Other Thoracic Injuries
Diaphragmatic Rupture
- Results from rapid compression of the abdomen when there is a sharp increase in intra-abdominal pressure. This pressure causes the abdominal contents to perforate the diaphragm and herniate the chest wall. More common on the left side than the right.
- Signs and symptoms
  - Decreased ventilations
  - Decreased cardiac output
  - Decreased return of venous blood
  - Shock

Traumatic Asphyxia
- The result of severe crushing injury to the chest and abdomen resulting from intrathoracic pressure that forces blood from the right side of the heart into the veins of the upper thorax, neck, and face and ruptures the capillaries.
- Signs and symptoms
  - Discoloration to the face (cyanosis of the head, upper extremities, and torso above the level of compression)
  - Jugular venous distention
  - Ocular hemorrhage; may be mild or dramatic, leading to swelling of the conjunctiva (subconjunctival hematoma) or exophthalmos
- Specific management
  - Establish definitive airway; perform orotracheal intubation, if indicated.
  - Treat for shock.

Abdominal Injuries
Pathophysiology
Hemorrhage is a major concern in abdominal trauma and can be external or internal. Signs and symptoms will vary greatly depending on the volume of blood lost and the rate at which

the body is losing blood. Key indicators of hemorrhagic shock will become apparent with assessment of the neurologic and cardiovascular systems.

As hypovolemia increases, the patient will have initial agitation and confusion. The heart compensates early for this loss by an increase in heart rate (tachycardia) and stroke volume. As hypoperfusion continues, the coronary arteries can no longer meet the increased demands of the myocardium, which leads to ischemia and heart failure. The symptoms of cardiac dysfunction are demonstrated by the presence of chest pain, tachypnea with adventitious (abnormal) lung sounds, and dysrhythmias. If left untreated, hypoperfusion will result in anaerobic metabolism and acidosis.

Injuries to hollow or solid organs can result in the spillage of their contents into the abdominal cavity. When the enzymes, acids, or bacteria leak from hollow organs into the peritoneal or retroperitoneal space, they cause irritation of the nerve endings. These nerve ending are found in the fascia of the surrounding tissues. As the inflammation affects deeper nerve endings (such as the endings of the afferent nerves), localized pain will result. Pain is localized if the extent of the contamination is confined; pain becomes generalized if the entire peritoneal cavity is involved.

Injuries to Solid Abdominal Organs

The solid organs in the abdomen include the liver, spleen, kidneys, and pancreas. When a solid organ in the abdomen is injured during blunt or penetrating trauma, the organ releases blood into the peritoneal cavity. This can cause nonspecific signs such as tachycardia and hypotension. Because these signs may not develop until a patient has lost a significant volume of blood, normal vital signs do not rule out the possibility that there has been a significant intra-abdominal injury. Bleeding into the peritoneal cavity from solid organ injuries can also produce abdominal tenderness or distention even though the distention may not be evident until the patient has lost nearly all the blood in the abdomen. Palpation of the abdomen may reveal localized or generalized tenderness, rigidity, or rebound tenderness, all of which suggest a peritoneal injury.

Liver Injuries
- A liver injury should be suspected in all patients who have right-sided chest trauma as well as abdominal trauma.
- When injured, the liver releases blood and bile into the peritoneal cavity. The blood loss can be massive, resulting in abdominal distention, hypotension, tachycardia, shock, and even death. In addition, the release of bile into the peritoneum can produce abdominal pain and peritonitis.

Spleen Injuries
- Falls and motor vehicle crashes can injure the spleen. However, less obvious injury patterns in activities such as sports (for instance, tackling in football or checking in lacrosse) can also cause injury to the spleen.
- When the spleen ruptures, blood spills into the peritoneum, which can ultimately cause shock and death.
- Signs and symptoms
  - Usually nonspecific; as many as 40% of patients have no symptoms.
  - Some patients report only pain in the left shoulder (**Kehr's sign**) because of referred pain from diaphragmatic irritation.

Pancreas Injuries
- Pancreatic injury occurs in less than 5% of all major abdominal trauma. Because of the anatomic position of the pancreas in the retroperitoneum, it is relatively well protected. It typically takes a high-energy force to damage the pancreas. These high-energy forces are most commonly produced by penetrating trauma (for example, from a bullet) but can also be caused by blunt trauma (such as from a motor vehicle crash).

- Signs and symptoms
  - Subtle or absent signs and symptoms initially; pancreatic injury should be suspected in any rapid decelerating injury.
  - Over the course of hours to days, pancreatic injuries result in the spillage of enzymes into the retroperitoneal space, potentially damaging surrounding structures and leading to infection and retroperitoneal abscess.
  - Injury should be suspected after a localized blow to the midabdomen. These patients usually experience a vague upper and midabdominal pain that radiates to the back.

Injuries to Hollow Intraperitoneal Organs
- The hollow organs of the abdomen include the stomach, small and large intestines, and bladder.
- Signs and symptoms
  - Hollow visceral injuries produce most of their symptoms from peritoneal contamination. When a hollow organ such as the stomach or bowel is injured, it releases its contents into the abdomen. These contents may irritate the abdomen, producing symptoms.
  - When the patient has the seatbelt sign—a contusion or abrasion across the lower abdomen—this usually means that he or she also has intraperitoneal injuries.

Injuries to the Small and Large Intestines
- The intestines are commonly injured from penetrating trauma, although they can be injured from severe blunt trauma as well.
- When ruptured, the intestines spill their contents (which contain fecal matter and a large amount of bacteria) into the peritoneal or retroperitoneal cavities, resulting in peritonitis.

Stomach Injuries
- Most injuries to the stomach result from penetrating trauma; the stomach is rarely injured from blunt trauma. When rupture of the stomach does occur after blunt trauma, it is usually associated with a recent meal or inappropriate use of a seatbelt.
- Signs and symptoms
  - Spillage of acidic material into the peritoneal space can create chemical irritation that produces abdominal pain and peritoneal signs relatively quickly.
  - Patients taking antacid medications may have delayed symptoms.

Bladder Injuries
- Bladder injuries occur as a result of penetrating and blunt abdominal trauma. The likelihood of a bladder injury varies by the severity of the mechanism, but also by the degree of the bladder distention. The fuller the bladder, the greater the opportunity for injury.
- Bladder injuries are usually associated with pelvic injuries from motor vehicle crashes, falls from heights, and physical assaults to the lower abdomen. These MOI may cause a pelvic fracture to perforate the bladder.
- Signs and symptoms
  - Generally nonspecific but may present as gross hematuria, suprapubic pain and tenderness, difficulty voiding, and abdominal distention, guarding, or rebound tenderness.
  - The presence of signs of peritoneal irritation may also indicate the possibility of an intraperitoneal bladder rupture.

Management of Abdominal Injuries
- Ensure an open airway while taking spinal precautions.
- Administer high-concentration oxygen via a nonrebreathing mask.

- Establish IV access with two large-bore lines, and start replacing fluid with lactated Ringer's solution or normal saline. Do not delay transport to initiate IV therapy.
- Minimize external hemorrhage by applying pressure dressings.
- Apply a cardiac monitor.
- Transport the patient to the appropriate hospital or regional trauma center, depending on your local transport protocols.

Injuries to the Face

Pathophysiology

Injuries to the head, neck, and face are common in trauma settings. There are two general types:

- Injuries to bone
  - Nasal fractures (most common)
  - Zygomatic fractures
  - Fracture or dislocation of the mandible
  - Maxillary fractures: Fractures to the midface, characterized by severity
    - **Le Fort I:** Horizontal fracture of the maxilla involving the hard palate and inferior maxilla
    - **Le Fort II:** Pyramidal fracture involving the nasal bone and inferior maxilla
    - **Le Fort III:** Fracture of all the midfacial bones, separating the entire midface from the cranium (craniofacial disjunction)
  - Orbital fractures of the eye
  - Fractured or avulsed teeth
- Soft-tissue injuries
  - Lacerations, foreign bodies, or impaled objects to the soft tissue of the face, mouth, oropharynx, tongue

Signs and Symptoms

- Bone injuries
  - **Nasal fractures:** Swelling, tenderness, and crepitus on palpation of the nasal bone; lateral displacement of the nasal bone from the normal midline position; possible nosebleed, which can compromise the patient's airway
  - **Zygomatic fractures:** Trismus, subconjunctival hemorrhage, infraorbital anesthesia, difficulty opening the mouth, and flattening of the midface over the fracture site
  - **Fracture or dislocation of the mandible:** Suspect fracture if blunt force trauma to the lower third of the face and dental malocclusion, numbness of the chin, and inability to open mouth; swelling and ecchymosis over the fracture are likely; partially or completely avulsed teeth
    - Mandibular dislocations most often occur as the result of wide yawning or mouth opening; mouth locks in a wide-open position; muscle spasms lead to severe pain
  - **Maxillary fractures:** Massive facial swelling, instability of the midfacial bones, malocclusion, elongated appearance of the patient's face
  - **Orbital fractures of the eye:** Double vision (blowout fractures), numbness in cheeks or above the eyebrow as the result of nerve damage; inferior orbit fractures (most common) can cause paralysis of upward gaze

Assessment

- Scene size-up
  - Ensure BSI.
  - Control c-spine (always assume a c-spine injury with facial trauma).

- Initial/primary assessment
  - Evaluate LOC.
  - Assess ABCs.
  - Treat life-threatening injuries.
  - Transport patient in a position of comfort.
- Focused history and physical exam/secondary assessment
  - Apply cardiac monitoring and pulse oximeter.
  - Obtain SAMPLE history and chief complaint (OPQRST).

Management

- Apply supplemental oxygen at 15 L/min via nonrebreathing mask or bag-mask ventilation.
- Suction airway as needed.
- Establish two large-bore IVs.
- *Do not give anything by mouth.*
- Use a cold pack or ice to reduce swelling.

Eye Injuries

Eye injuries may result from blunt trauma, penetrating trauma, or burns. Because eye injuries are relatively uncommon and may result in vision loss, proper assessment and management are vital.

Pathophysiology

- Small or moderate-size foreign bodies resting on the surface of the eye may lead to extreme irritation and conjunctivitis (inflamed, red conjunctiva and heavy tearing, along with pain and light sensitivity, making it difficult for the patient to keep the eyes open). Blunt trauma to the eye can lead to swelling, ecchymosis, or rupture of the globe.
- **Hyphema** is the presence of blood behind the cornea and is a sign of severe intraocular injury.
- **Retinal detachment** is a very serious complication that can lead to permanent vision loss. Chemicals, heat, and light rays can all burn the delicate eye tissue. Exposure to extremely bright light (infrared rays, eclipse light, laser burns) can cause retinal injury; superficial burns (ultraviolet rays, prolonged sunlamp exposure, or snow blindness) may result in corneal damage and severe conjunctivitis.

Signs and Symptoms

- Visual loss that does not improve when the patient blinks (damage to the globe or optic nerve)
- Double vision (trauma involving the extraocular muscles, such as fracture of the orbit)
- Severe eye pain
- Foreign body sensation (superficial injury to the cornea, foreign body trapped behind the eyelids)
- Anisocoria (pupils are a different size)—often present in ocular injury or closed head trauma
- Hyphema—blood in the anterior chamber
- Subconjunctival hemorrhage—blood over the white of the eye

Assessment

- Scene size-up
  - Ensure BSI.
  - Determine MOI. Consider c-spine immobilization (especially if hyphema or globe rupture); perform rapid trauma assessment.
- Initial/primary assessment
  - Assess ABCs.
  - Most eye injuries are serious emergencies and require rapid transport.

- Focused history and physical exam/secondary assessment
  - Evaluate each orbital structure.
    - **Orbital rim:** For ecchymosis, swelling, lacerations, and tenderness
    - **Eyelids:** For ecchymosis, swelling, and lacerations
    - **Corneas:** For foreign bodies and hyphema
    - **Conjunctivae:** For redness, pus, inflammation, bleeding, and foreign bodies
    - **Globes:** For redness, abnormal pigmentation, and lacerations
    - **Pupils:** For size, shape, equality, and reaction to light
    - **Eye movements in all directions:** For paralysis of gaze or dysconjugate gaze
    - **Visual acuity:** Ask patient to read a newspaper or visual acuity chart; test each eye separately and document results.

Management

- **Eyelid injuries:** Use gentle manual pressure to control bleeding; lightly patch the affected eye.
- **Globe injuries:** For lacerations, abrasions, and contusions, apply aluminum eye patches (not gauze patches). For penetrating globe injuries, follow these three principles:
  - *Never exert pressure* on the eye or manipulate the globe in any way.
  - If globe is exposed, gently apply a moist, sterile dressing to prevent drying.
  - Cover both eyes with a protective eye shield, cup, or sterile dressing. ·
- **Hyphema or globe rupture:** Immobilize c-spine; elevate the head of the backboard 40° to minimize ICP.
- **Impaled objects:** Stabilize the object (do not remove) and cover both of the patient's eyes to limit eye movement.
- **Burns**
  - **From ultraviolet light exposure:** Cover affected eye with sterile, moist pad and eye shield. If pain is severe, lightly apply cool compresses.
  - **Chemical burns:** Immediately irrigate the eye with sterile water or a saline solution (**Figure 4-2**), taking care to protect the uninjured eye.
- All eye injuries require rapid transport to the hospital.

Irrigation Tips

- When irrigating the eye, *never* use any chemical antidotes, such as vinegar or baking soda!
- *Use sterile water or saline solution only.*
- Irrigate for at least 5 minutes.
- If the burn was caused by an alkali or strong acid, irrigate for at least 20 minutes.

Ear Injuries

Pathophysiology

Lacerations, avulsions, and contusions to the external ear can occur following blunt or penetrating trauma. The pinna can be contused, lacerated, or partially or completely avulsed; because of its poor blood supply, it tends to heal slowly.

Foreign bodies or pressure-related trauma (eg, barotrauma, explosions) may cause a perforation of the tympanic membrane (ruptured eardrum). The tympanic membrane tends to heal spontaneously, but careful evaluation for other serious injuries is needed.

Signs and Symptoms

- Bleeding
- CSF drainage if serious head trauma has occurred

Assessment

- Scene size-up
  - Ensure BSI.
- Initial/primary assessment
  - Assess ABCs.

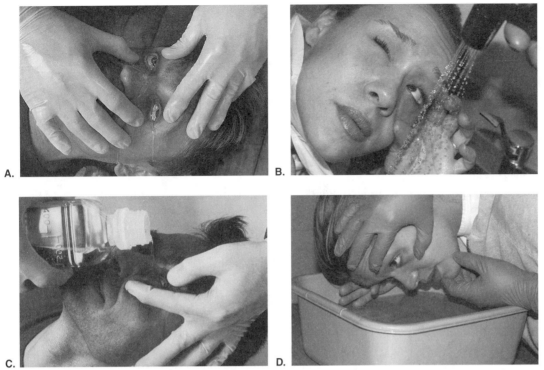

Figure 4-2 Four ways to effectively irrigate the eye. **A.** Nasal cannula. **B.** Shower. **C.** Bottle. **D.** Basin.

- Focused history and physical exam/secondary assessment
  - Evaluation of external ear drum and middle ear injuries should take place in the hospital setting.

Management
- Apply gentle manual pressure to control bleeding.
- If bleeding is heavier, apply a soft, padded dressing between the ear and scalp and cover the head with a roller bandage.
- Apply an ice pack to reduce swelling.
- Partial avulsions of the pinna: Carefully realign the pinna and cover with a soft, padded bandage that has been moistened with saline solution; treat complete avulsions as for an amputation.
- Stabilize any impaled object and prepare victim for rapid transport.

Oral and Dental Injuries

Oral and dental injuries are commonly associated with trauma to the face (eg, MVCs, direct blows to the mouth or chin). Penetrating trauma is commonly the result of GSWs.

Pathophysiology
Lacerations and avulsions in and around the mouth are associated with intraoral hemorrhage and airway compromise. Impaled objects or fractured or avulsed teeth may lacerate the tongue and cause profuse bleeding into the upper airway. Teeth fragments may become airway obstructions. The swallowing of blood may irritate the stomach lining and lead to vomiting and aspiration.

Signs and Symptoms
- Head trauma
- Bleeding (often profuse, especially with severe maxillofacial trauma)
- Vomiting (from swallowed blood)
- Soft-tissue injuries to the cheeks or other parts of the face

Assessment

- Scene size-up
  - Ensure BSI.
  - In cases of assault, evaluate the assailant, if possible, because of the high risk of infection from exposure to oral bacteria and microorganisms.
- Initial/primary assessment
  - Assess ABCs (risk of airway compromise as the result of bleeding; swallowed blood may minimize obvious bleeding).
  - Check patient's mouth and teeth in all cases of facial trauma.

Management

- Lean patient forward to facilitate the drainage of blood from the mouth, if not c-spine immobilized; if the patient is immobilized, roll the entire backboard to the side to facilitate drainage.
- Suction oropharynx as needed.
- Perform orotracheal intubation if needed to establish or protect the airway (decreased LOC).
- Remove fractured tooth fragments.
- Restrict c-spine as indicated by the injury.
- Stabilize impaled objects; remove only if they are impeding your ability to manage the airway.
- Avulsed teeth: Place in saline or Hank's solution. Consult with medical control for possible reimplantation instructions.
- Transport rapidly.

Know Your Fracture Types

- **Complete:** Fracture goes completely through all layers
- **Incomplete:** Fracture does not extend through the entire bone
- **Open:** Fracture extends through the skin
- **Closed:** Fracture that does not penetrate the skin
- **Greenstick:** Fracture in which part of the bone is broken along the length; most common in children whose bones have not fully calcified
- **Displaced:** Fracture in which broken bone ends are no longer aligned
- **Segmental:** Two complete fractures of the same bone, which results in a free-floating bone segment
- **Comminuted:** Fracture in which the bone is broken into several small pieces or fragments
- **Impacted:** Fracture in which the bone end is forced over itself
- **Transverse:** Fracture that runs across or at a 90° angle
- **Oblique:** Fracture that runs transversely at other than a 90° angle
- **Spiral:** Fracture circumferentially around the bone
- **Hairline:** Minute fracture, which is difficult to visualize on radiographs
- **Epiphyseal:** Fracture through the growth plate of a bone

Musculoskeletal Injuries

Pathophysiology

Musculoskeletal injuries send more people in the United States to a physician than almost any other complaint, and 70% to 80% of all trauma victims with multisystem injury will have one or more musculoskeletal injuries. Although these injuries are rarely fatal themselves, they can result in short- or long-term disability. By providing prompt temporary measures, such as splinting and analgesia, you can help to reduce the period of disability.

Fractures

A fracture is a break in the continuity of a bone. **Figure 4-3** shows the various directions that a fracture may travel through a bone. Fractures may also be open or closed.

- **Open:** When the bone has punctured the skin or an object has caused an opening at the fracture site. An open fracture requires prompt evaluation in the ED because of high risk of infection and possible distal circulatory compromise.
- **Closed:** No opening in the skin.

   Table 4-6 summarizes fracture classification based on displacement.

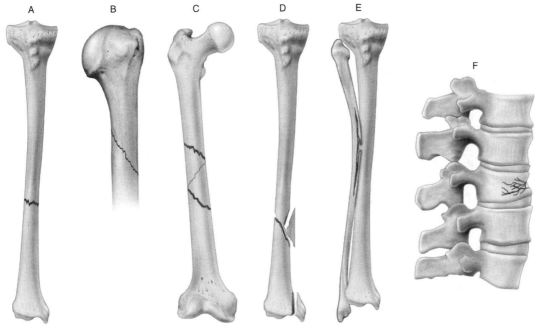

Figure 4-3 Types of fractures. **A.** Transverse fractures of the tibia. **B.** Oblique fracture of the humerus. **C.** Spiral fracture of the femur. **D.** Comminuted fracture of the tibia. **E.** Greenstick fracture of the fibula. **F.** Compression fracture of a vertebral body.

Signs and Symptoms
- General
  - Pain that is well localized to the fracture site
  - Deformity
  - Shortening (when broken ends of bone override one another)

Table 4-6 Fracture Classification Based on Displacement

Type of Fracture	Description	Common Causes
Nondisplaced fracture	Bone remains aligned in its normal position, despite the fracture.	Low-energy injury
Displaced fracture	Ends of the fracture move from their normal positions.	High-energy injury
Overriding	Muscles pull the distal fracture fragment alongside the proximal one, leading them to overlap; the limb becomes shortened.	Only occurs when a fracture is fully displaced and there is no bone contact
Distraction injury	A powerful tensile force is rapidly applied to a bone, causing it to fracture–the bone ends are pulled apart.	Industrial equipment, machinery
Impacted fracture (impaction injury)	A compressive force is applied to a bone, causing it to become wedged into another bone or compressed into itself.	More likely to happen in **cancellous bone**
Avulsion fracture	A powerful muscle contraction causes the insertion site of the muscle to be fractured off of the bone.	Sudden "jerking" of a body part
Depression fracture	Blunt trauma to a flat bone (such as the skull) causes the bone to be pushed inward.	Blunt injury

- Swelling and ecchymosis
- Guarding and loss of use
- Tenderness to palpation
- Crepitus
- Hip fractures
  - Pain and inability to move the hip. With stress fractures in young athletes and nondisplaced fractures, the patient may complain of pain in the hip or knee and may be ambulatory.
  - Possible history of other osteoporotic fractures, such as Colles or vertebral fractures.
  - Most often, femoral head fractures occur as a result of hip dislocation.
  - In femoral neck fractures, the extremity is held in a slightly shortened, abducted, and externally rotated position, unless the fracture is only a stress fracture or severely impacted. In this case, the hip is held in a natural position.
  - In intertrochanteric fractures, the extremity is held in a markedly shortened and externally rotated position.
  - In subtrochanteric fractures, the proximal femur is usually held in a flexed and externally rotated position.
- Pelvic fractures
  - Palpable instability of the pelvis on compression of the iliac wings indicates fracture.
  - If there is instability or pain while moving the hip, an acetabular fracture is possible in addition to a possible hip fracture.
  - **Grey Turner sign**: Bruising to the flanks may be noted. This is an indicator of retroperitoneal bleeding.
- Diaphyseal fractures of the femur
  - Significant pain and tenderness
  - Deformity (shortened extremity), crepitus with movement, and tenderness
  - Absent or diminished peripheral pulses
  - Swollen thigh region because of blood loss, and altered LOC due to the internal bleeding
  - Tachycardia, hypotension, and other signs and symptoms of possible shock
- Clavicular fracture
  - Shoulder shifted forward, with a palpable deformity along the clavicle
  - Pain with movement
  - Deformity, contusions
  - Swelling
  - Tenderness
  - Crepitus
  - Edema
  - Ecchymosis
  - Decreased breaths sounds on the affected side may indicate a pneumothorax
- Humerus fractures
  - Pain with palpation or movement of the shoulder or elbow
  - Ecchymosis
  - May be associated with radial nerve injury, inability to extend wrist and digits
  - Crepitus

Dislocations and Injuries to Ligaments, Muscles, and Tendons

When forced beyond their normal limit, the bones that form a joint may break or become displaced, and the supporting ligaments and joint capsule may tear. Dislocations are considered an urgent injury because of their potential to cause neurovascular compromise distal to the site of injury. Muscle and tendon injuries can result from violent muscle contractions, excessive stretching, or frequent and repetitive use.

- Dislocations: Bone is totally displaced from the joint; occur when a body part moves beyond its normal range of motion and the articular surfaces are no longer intact
- **Subluxation** is a partial dislocation; articular surfaces are no longer completely intact; part of the joint capsule and supporting ligaments may be damaged
- **Diastasis** is an increase in the distance between the two sides of a joint; occurs when the ligaments that hold two bones in a fixed position are disrupted
- Muscle and tendon injuries: Pulled muscle resulting from a violent muscle contraction or stretch (rupture of the Achilles tendon is a common athletic injury); tendinitis (inflammation of the tendon); bursitis (inflammation of the bursa); also includes sprains, strains, tendon rupture, and inflammatory processes

Signs and Symptoms

- Pain or feeling of pressure over the involved joint
- Swelling and possibly deformity
- Inability to use the limb
- Shoulder dislocations
  - **Anterior dislocation (most common):** The arm is held in slight abduction and external rotation, and the affected shoulder is boxlike with loss of deltoid contour compared to the contralateral side; the humeral head is palpable anteriorly (beneath the clavicle).
  - **Posterior dislocation:** The arm is held in adduction and internal rotation, and the anterior shoulder is boxlike and flat.
  - **Inferior dislocation:** The arm is fully abducted, with the elbow commonly flexed on or behind head, and the humeral head may be palpable on the lateral chest wall.
  - **Bilateral dislocation:** Both shoulders may appear symmetrical. Always maintain a high index of suspicion. The humeral head is palpable beneath the acromion process. The patient has difficulty with external rotation and abduction.
  - Severe pain is present.
  - Range of motion is decreased (patient cannot touch opposite shoulder).
- Hip dislocations
  - Posterior
    - Most common (90% of all hip dislocations); posterior hip dislocations occur frequently during MVCs, especially head-on collisions.
    - The patient will present with the knee flexed and the foot rotated internally.
    - Pain in the lower leg and foot may exist because of sciatic nerve injury or laceration from bony fragments.
    - Neurologic deficit ranges from pain in the sciatic nerve distribution to loss of sensation in the posterior leg and foot and loss of dorsiflexion (perineal branch) or plantar flexion (tibial branch) of the foot.
    - Hematoma from vascular injuries is possible, but relatively rare.
  - Anterior
    - Leg is externally rotated, abducted, and extended at the hip. The femoral head protrudes in the inguinal area and may be palpated anterior to the pelvis.
    - Pain is present in the hip area.
    - Patient cannot walk or adduct the leg.
    - If there is an injury to the femoral nerve, lower extremity paresis and numbness may be present.
    - If there is an injury to the femoral artery, a dull aching pain, pallor, paraesthesias, and coolness of the lower extremity may be present.

> **The Thompson Test**
>
> To determine the existence of an Achilles tendon rupture:
> - With patient in a prone position, squeeze the calf muscles of the injured leg.
> - If there is no movement of the foot, a tear to the tendon is likely. If there is flexion of the foot during the squeeze, the tendon is likely intact.

Open Injuries

General Management

- Expose the wound.
- Clean the surface of the wound by brushing away or irrigating debris with a sterile dressing.
- Use sterile dressings to cover wounds when possible.
- Cover the entire wound and surrounding area with the sterile dressing.
- Control bleeding, and then apply bandages.
- Once the bandages are in place, *do not remove.*
- *Do not bandage too tightly or too loosely.*
- Cover all edges of the dressings, excluding occlusive dressings.
- Expose fingers and toes for assessment of pulse, motor function, and sensation (PMS), if possible.
- If direct pressure and elevation fail to control bleeding, apply a tourniquet.

Amputations

- Never complete an amputation.
- Use bleeding control methods and apply a pressure dressing to the stump. Consider applying a tourniquet.
- Wrap the amputated part with sterile dressings and place it in a plastic bag on ice or ice packs.
- Do *not* immerse the part in water or saline or allow it direct contact with ice, and do not allow the amputated part to freeze.

Avulsed Teeth

Clean the socket and use pressure to stop the bleeding. Place avulsed teeth in milk.

Epistaxis (Nosebleed)

Use gauze to apply direct pressure below the nose, squeezing on both sides. For severe bleeding, lean the patient forward.

Eviscerations

- Do not touch or attempt to replace any protruding abdominal organs. Apply a sterile dressing moistened with sterile saline directly to the site.
- Cover with a large occlusive dressing.
- Place the patient on his or her back with legs flexed at the knees to reduce the pain and strain on muscles.

Impaled Objects

- As a general rule, do not remove an impaled object unless it is occluding the airway or hindering transport.
- Manually stabilize the object with a bulky dressing without putting pressure on the object itself. Splint objects impaled in the extremities.
- Place the patient on a long backboard and transport.

Impaled Object in the Cheek

Inspect the area closely. If you find perforation and can see both ends of the object, remove it in the direction it entered and suction as needed. For a conscious patient, place a sterile gauze dressing to the inside of the cheek. Only remove if the object is causing an airway obstruction. The patient will usually still be bleeding inside the mouth. Keep the patient's head up and allow him or her to use the Yankauer suction to clean out the blood.

Assessment and Treatment Procedures for Open Injuries

- Initial/primary assessment
  - Ensure BSI.
  - Immobilize the c-spine.

- Assess LOC.
- Assess ABCs.
- Treat life-threatening illness/injuries.
- Transport in left lateral recumbent/coma position.
- Focused history and physical exam/secondary assessment
  - Administer supplemental oxygen as needed, 15 L/min via nonrebreathing mask or bag-mask ventilation.
  - Obtain SAMPLE history and chief complaint (OPQRST).
  - Establish IV.
  - Splint.
  - Use a scoop stretcher for pelvic instability or apply a pelvic sling.
  - Assess distal PMS.

Vital Vocabulary

anisocoria A condition in which the pupils are not of equal size.

cancellous bone Trabecular or spongy bone.

contralateral The opposite side.

coup-contrecoup Dual impacting of the brain into the skull.

depression fracture A fracture in which the broken region of the bone is pushed deeper into the body than the remaining intact bone.

diastasis An increase in the distance between the two sides of a joint.

distraction injury An injury that results from a force that tries to increase the length of a body part or separate one body part from another.

flail chest An injury that involves two or more adjacent ribs fractured in two or more places, allowing the segment between the fractures to move independently of the rest of the thoracic cage.

Grey Turner sign Ecchymosis of the flanks.

hemopneumothorax A collection of blood and air in the pleural cavity.

hemothorax The collection of blood within the normally closed pleural space.

hyphema Bleeding into the anterior chamber of the eye; results from direct ocular trauma.

Kehr's sign Left shoulder pain that may indicate a ruptured spleen.

nondisplaced fracture A break in which the bone remains aligned in its normal position.

open pneumothorax The result of a defect in the chest wall that allows air to enter the thoracic space.

overriding The overlap of a bone that occurs from the muscle spasm that follows a fracture, leading to a decrease in the length of the bone.

retinal detachment Separation of the inner layers of the retina from the underlying choroid, the vascular membrane that nourishes the retina.

simple pneumothorax The collection of air within the normally closed pleural space.

subluxation A partial or incomplete dislocation.

tension pneumothorax A life-threatening collection of air within the pleural space; the volume and pressure have both collapsed the involved lung and caused a shift of the mediastinal structures to the opposite side.

Bleeding and Shock

Bleeding

Pathophysiology

Hemorrhage, or bleeding, can be categorized as follows:

- External (visible), due to a break in the skin (eg, gunshot wound, fracture)
- Internal (not visible outside the body), due to:
  - Trauma (eg, injury to the thorax, abdomen, pelvis)
  - Rupture (eg, gastrointestinal bleeds, ruptured aneurysm, ruptured ectopic pregnancy)

Hemorrhage can be mild, moderate, or severe. Excessive bleeding decreases **perfusion** and must be controlled immediately. Severe blood loss leads to shock, and, if untreated or uncontrollable, death.

Significant symptoms may occur once 20% of total blood volume has been lost:

- **Adult:** 1,000 mL
- **Child:** 500 mL
- **Infant:** 100 to 200 mL

Signs and Symptoms

External Bleeding

Bleeding patterns depend on the type of blood vessel injured.

- **Arterial:** Oxygen-rich blood, bright red, initially spurts from wound in time with pulse (as blood pressure drops, spurting stops and blood flows)
- **Venous:** Low oxygen content, dark red, flows from wound
- **Capillary:** Oxygen deficient, dark red, oozing

Internal Bleeding

- Pain, tenderness, swelling, or discoloration of suspected site of injury
- Bleeding from the mouth, rectum, vagina, or other body orifice
- Vomiting bright red blood or dark, coffee grounds–colored blood
- Dark, tarry stools or stools with bright red blood
- Tender, rigid, and/or distended abdomen
- Anxiety, restlessness, combativeness, or altered mental status
- Weakness, faintness, or dizziness
- Thirst
- Shallow, rapid breathing
- Rapid, weak pulse
- Pale, cool, clammy skin
- Capillary refill time greater than 2 seconds
- Dilated pupils that are sluggish to respond
- Decreasing blood pressure (late sign of shock)
- Signs and symptoms of hypovolemic shock (hypoperfusion)

Assessment

- Scene size-up
  - Ensure appropriate level of body substance isolation (BSI) precautions. Depending on the severity of bleeding and your general impression, this will entail gloves, mask, eye shield, or gown.
- Initial/primary assessment
  - Assess level of consciousness (LOC).
  - Ensure that the airway is patent and clear.
  - Ensure adequate respirations.
  - Assess pulse rate, quality, and rhythm.
  - Assess skin temperature, condition, and capillary refill.
  - Control major bleeding or significant fluid losses *now.*
    - Significant internal or external bleeding requires rapid transport to the hospital.
    - Consider immediate transport for patients exhibiting signs of hypovolemic shock.
    - Internal hemorrhage: Because it is not visible, rely on signs and symptoms and mechanism of injury to determine possible internal bleeding.
- Focused history and physical exam/secondary assessment
  - Ensuring that the patient's cervical spine is manually immobilized in the neutral in-line position, perform a rapid trauma assessment on all trauma patients with a significant mechanism of injury, quickly inspecting each part of the body and using the patient's chief complaint and symptoms to guide your assessment.
  - Obtain SAMPLE history and chief complaint (OPQRST).
- Detailed physical exam
  - Perform the detailed physical exam when time allows, usually en route if there is an extended transport time.
    - Assess the patient's mental status.
    - Assess the patient's LOC.
    - Inspect and palpate each part of the body.
    - Reevaluate the patient's vital signs and assess trends in any changes.
- Ongoing assessment/reassessment
  - Perform every 5 minutes for unstable patients; every 15 minutes for stable patients.
    - Repeat the initial/primary assessment.
    - Reassess and record vital signs.
    - Repeat the focused physical exam/secondary assessment.
    - Recheck interventions.

Management

External Bleeding

It is important to stop external bleeding for the purpose of cellular perfusion. If the patient loses too much blood, he or she can go into shock.

The following are steps for managing external bleeding, except when it is from the nose, ears, or mouth, which may indicate a basal skull fracture.

- Apply direct pressure to the wound.
- Elevate the injury above the level of the heart if no fracture is suspected.
- Consider applying a tourniquet.

Tourniquet Usage and Technique

Battlefield update: As the global war on terror continues, several important advances in the treatment of severe trauma have emerged. One of the most important advances is in the control of significant external hemorrhage, specifically with the use of tourniquets. Multiple US and foreign military reports confirm the importance of tourniquets in controlling significant external hemorrhage on the battlefield, and these practices can, and should, be utilized in the prehospital arena as well.

If direct pressure and elevation fail to control bleeding, application of a tourniquet should be considered. The most critical point in the application of any tourniquet is to ensure that it is tightened with enough pressure to impede both arterial inflow and venous outflow. The lower leg usually does not provide a good location for tourniquet application because the tibia and fibula preclude adequate arterial compression; therefore, a distal thigh tourniquet is typically required for popliteal and more distal injuries.

A few points to remember when applying a tourniquet:

- Do not apply directly over a joint.
- Use the widest device possible. Never use wire, rope, or a belt, which may cut into the skin.
- Never cover a tourniquet. Always leave it exposed, in plain view.
- Do not loosen the tourniquet once it is applied.

Internal Bleeding

If you suspect internal bleeding, treat for shock and splint injured extremities. Provide rapid transport.

Shock

Pathophysiology

Shock results from the body not receiving enough blood flow. The causes include hypovolemia, pump failure, and vessel failure. Hypoperfusion leads to diminished blood flow through the capillaries. The body shifts from aerobic to anaerobic metabolism, causing a buildup in the cells of lactic acid and other toxic waste products as well as acidosis. All are leading causes of shock. If left uncorrected, the cells will die. Tissue death, organ failure, and, eventually, patient death can result when a patient continues to lack adequate perfusion. To maintain homeostasis, the body compensates by shunting blood to the vital organs from the peripheral vascular system, leading to a state of shock.

> **Formulas to Remember**
>
> Heart rate x Stroke volume = Cardiac output
> Cardiac output x Systemic vascular resistance = Blood pressure

Phases of Shock

Compensated Shock The first stage of shock is **compensated shock**. It generally occurs in hypovolemia, when the body's compensatory responses are sufficient to overcome the decreased available fluid. The body increases catecholamine production to maintain **cardiac output (CO)** and sustain a normal systolic blood pressure (BP). The body increases its pulse rate, strength, and respirations to offset the fluid loss, which helps to reduce acidosis, and meet critical metabolic needs. The patient will present with narrowing of pulse pressure, weakening pulse, and cool and clammy skin as a result of the body shunting blood to the vital organs (heart, brain, lungs) in order to keep going. With proper treatment, recovery is likely.

Decompensated Shock The second stage of shock, **decompensated shock**, occurs when the blood volume drops by more than 30%. As the body's compensatory mechanisms begin to fail, it is no longer able to maintain systemic BP. Both systolic and diastolic pressures drop and cerebral blood flow decreases. Falling BP is the telltale sign that the patient's condition

> **Tip**
>
> Note that the body's compensatory mechanism can mask shock initially. This is especially true in children and pregnant women, who can lose 20% to 30% of their blood before showing signs of shock, and then rapidly deteriorate.

Children descend very rapidly into irreversible shock. Time is of the essence. Diligently monitor their vital signs and appearance. Provide prompt treatment and rapid transport.

has just declined into the decompensation mode. Peripheral pulses may not be palpable, and the patient's mental status becomes altered. You will also note a drop in respiratory rate. With appropriate treatment, recovery is possible.

Irreversible Shock The third and terminal stage of shock, **irreversible shock**, occurs when cellular, tissue, and organ ischemia and necrosis progress to a point where they cannot be reversed, even with the administration of fluid and restoration of perfusion. The organs have become so badly damaged from inadequate perfusion that organ failure and death are the inevitable result. **Table 5-1** lists the signs and symptoms of the different phases of shock.

Table 5-1 Pathophysiologic Changes at Each Phase of Shock

	Compensated	Decompensated	Irreversible
Mental status	No change	Altered	Unresponsive
Heart rate	Increased	Increased	Bradycardia
Respirations	Increased	Labored or irregular	Decreased
Blood pressure	No change	Hypotension narrows pulse pressure	Profound hypotension
Skin	Clammy, pale, and cool	Diaphoresis	Cold

Assessment

- Scene size-up
- Initial/primary assessment
  - Ensure BSI.
  - Monitor the patient's LOC.
  - Manage ABCs.
  - Provide high-flow supplemental oxygen.
  - Treat life-threatening illness/injury.
  - Transport considerations: Place patient in shock position (**Figure 5-1**) and rapidly transport to appropriate hospital with timely communication.
- Focused history and physical exam/secondary assessment
  - Monitor pulse oximetry.
  - Obtain SAMPLE history and chief complaint (OPQRST).
  - Monitor vital signs.
  - Perform cardiac monitoring.
- Detailed physical exam
  - Perform the detailed physical exam when time allows, usually en route if there is an extended transport time.
    - Assess the patient's mental status.
    - Assess the patient's LOC.
    - Inspect and palpate each part of the body.
    - Reevaluate the patient's vital signs and assess trends in any changes.
- Ongoing assessment/reassessment
  - Perform every 5 minutes for patients in shock.
    - Repeat the initial/primary assessment.
    - Reassess and record vital signs.
    - Repeat the focused physical exam/secondary assessment.
    - Recheck interventions.

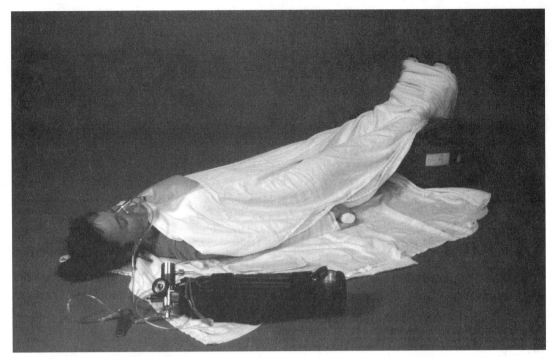

Figure 5-1 The shock position.

Management

- Administer 100% oxygen to increase patient's oxygenation (check that patient's skin is becoming pink and LOC is improving).
- Establish intravenous (IV) line and administer volume expanders.
- Elevate the legs to help shunt blood to the core (shock position).
- *Give nothing by mouth.*

Specific Types of Shock

The different types of shock can be categorized according to their mechanism. The three major types of shock and three subtypes are as follows.

- Obstructive shock
  - Caused by conditions that obstruct blood flow
- Cardiogenic shock
  - Caused by pump failure
- Hypovolemic shock
  - Caused by fluid loss (blood, fluid, electrolytes)
- Distributive shock
  - Caused by vasodilation and includes three subtypes:
    - Septic shock, caused by vasodilation resulting from a widespread infection
    - Neurogenic shock, caused by vasodilation resulting from failure of the nervous system; usually associated with spinal cord injury
    - Anaphylactic shock, caused by vasodilation from an allergic reaction

Cardiogenic Shock

Pathophysiology of Cardiogenic Shock <u>Cardiogenic shock</u> results when the heart cannot pump enough blood to maintain adequate peripheral oxygen delivery. Systemic circulation cannot be maintained if there is damage to 40% or more of the left ventricular myocardium. Initial insult leads to decreased myocardial contractility, which leads to decreased stroke volume. The mechanism is as follows:

1. Decreased left ventricular emptying leads to left ventricular dilation and backup of blood into the lungs, which leads to pulmonary congestion. Breath sounds have rales.

2. Increased heart rate leads to increased myocardial O_2 demand. If myocardial perfusion cannot keep up with demand due to shock or blockage, myocardial hypoxia occurs, leading to further pump failure, worsening of CO, decompensation, and death. Therefore, increased heart rate cannot compensate indefinitely.

3. Decreased right ventricular emptying leads to right ventricular dilation and backup of blood to peripheral system, which leads to jugular venous distension (JVD). Decreased blood flow to the lungs decreases oxygenation. In right ventricular failure, lung sounds are clear because the lungs are not congested. Increased respiratory rate occurs to compensate for decreased oxygenation.

Signs and Symptoms of Cardiogenic Shock
- Altered mental status (hypoxia)
- Respiratory distress
- Chest pain
- Reduced urine output (vasoconstriction)
- Hypotension (failure of compensatory mechanism)
- Cyanosis (hypoxia)
- Unconsciousness, absent reflexes (electrolyte imbalance, acid-base imbalance)
- Slow, shallow, or Cheyne-Stokes respirations (respiratory center depression)
- Peripheral venous collapse
- Cold, clammy skin (shunting of peripheral vascular system)
- Rapid, shallow respirations
- Low oxygen saturation (decreased perfusion)

Assessment of Cardiogenic Shock
- Scene size-up
  - Ensure BSI.
- Initial/primary assessment
  - Monitor the patient's LOC.
  - Manage ABCs.
  - Treat life-threatening illness/injury.
  - Transport considerations: Consider immediate transport if unstable.
- Focused history and physical exam/secondary assessment
  - Monitor vital signs.
  - Perform cardiac monitoring
- Detailed physical exam
  - Perform the detailed physical exam when time allows, usually en route if there is an extended transport time.
    - Assess the patient's mental status.
    - Assess the patient's LOC.
    - Inspect and palpate each part of the body.
    - Reevaluate the patient's vital signs and assess trends in any changes.
- Ongoing assessment/reassessment
  - Perform every 5 minutes.
    - Repeat the initial/primary assessment.
    - Reassess and record vital signs.
    - Repeat the focused physical exam/secondary assessment.
    - Recheck interventions.

Management of Cardiogenic Shock
- Administer supplemental oxygen to ensure end-organ perfusion.
- Establish IV and administer volume expanders such as normal saline or lactated Ringer's solution.
- Administer 250 to 500 mL fluid challenge, if lung sounds are clear.
- If rales are present, administer vasopressor support.
- Perform cardiac monitoring.
- Keep the patient warm.
- Transport in a positon of comfort, preferably a high-Fowler's position, to help decrease pulmonary edema.

Table 5-2 summarizes the treatment of cardiogenic shock.

Table 5-2 Treatment of Cardiogenic Shock

Treatment	Used For	Adult Dose	Pediatric Dose
Nitroglycerin	Chest pain Increased heart rate Decreased blood pressure	SL: 0.3-0.4 mg	Not indicated for pediatric use
Aspirin	Helps prevent clot formation to limit coronary blockage	PO: 160-325 mg	Not indicated for pediatric use
Furosemide	Reduces cardiac preload by increasing venous capacitance (diuretic)	SIVP: 0.5-1.0 mg/kg	IV/IO: 1 mg/kg
Inotropic drugs Epinephrine	Increases contractility Causes vasoconstriction	Not indicated for adult patients	IV: 0.01 mg/kg IO: 0.01 mg/kg ETT: 0.1 mg/kg
Dopamine	Increases cardiac output	2-20 µg/kg/min IV/IO	2-20 µg/kg/min IV/IO
SL, sublingual; PO, by mouth; SIVP, slow intravenous push; IV/IO, intravenous or intraosseus; ETT, endotracheal tube.			

Obstructive Shock
Pathophysiology of Obstructive Shock **Obstructive shock** is caused by conditions that obstruct blood flow and lead to reduced perfusion and shock. Common causes of obstructive shock include tension pneumothorax, cardiac tamponade, and pulmonary embolus.

Signs and Symptoms of Obstructive Shock
- Low blood pressure
- Cool, clammy skin
- Rapid, shallow respirations
- Altered mental status
- Hypothermia
- Tension pneumothorax: Drop in blood pressure and jugular venous distension
- Cardiac tamponade: Muffled heart sounds and systolic and diastolic blood pressures starting to merge
- Pulmonary embolus: Sharp, stabbing chest pain
- Dyspnea, anxiety

Assessment of Obstructive Shock
- Scene size-up
- Ensure BSI.

- Initial/primary assessment
  - Monitor the patient's LOC.
  - Manage ABCs.
  - Treat life-threatening illness/injury.
  - Transport considerations: Consider immediate transport if unstable.
- Focused history and physical exam/secondary assessment
  - Obtain SAMPLE history and chief complaint (OPQRST).
  - Monitor vital signs.
  - Perform cardiac monitoring
- Detailed physical exam
  - Perform the detailed physical exam when time allows, usually en route if there is an extended transport time.
    - Assess the patient's mental status.
    - Assess the patient's LOC.
    - Inspect and palpate each part of the body.
    - Reevaluate the patient's vital signs and assess trends in any changes.
- Ongoing assessment/reassessment
  - Perform every 5 minutes.
    - Repeat the initial/primary assessment.
    - Reassess and record vital signs.
    - Repeat the focused physical exam/secondary assessment.
    - Recheck interventions.

Management of Obstructive Shock
- Administer supplemental oxygen to ensure end-organ perfusion.
- Perform cardiac monitoring.
- Keep the patient warm.
- If patient exhibits signs of a tension pneumothorax, perform needle decompression to improve CO.
- In cases of suspected cardiac tamponade, the patient will need pericardiocentesis at the emergency department (ED); transport rapidly.

Hypovolemic Shock
Pathophysiology of Hypovolemic Shock <u>Hypovolemic shock</u>, also called hypovolemia, is characterized by internal or external fluid loss, or both. It is the most common form of shock in the prehospital setting. In hypovolemic shock, decreased intravascular volume leads to low venous return, which leads to decreased tissue perfusion. Reduced oxygenation and transport of nutrients to cells results in multiple organ dysfunction.

Signs and Symptoms of Hypovolemic Shock
- Internal or external hemorrhage from any source—blood loss is most common cause
- Dehydration (leads to acidosis)
- Diarrhea (leads to acidosis)
- Sweating
- Burns (result in loss of plasma)
- Confusion, anxiety
- Lightheadedness
- Nausea
- Tachycardia (sympathetic stimulation, hypoxia)
- Weak, thready, rapid pulse (caused by reduced stroke volume; vasoconstriction)

- Tachypnea
- Cold, clammy, pale skin (caused by vasoconstriction)
- Low urine output (caused by vasoconstriction, low fluid volume)
- Altered mental status
- Orthostatic hypotension/postural hypotension (decompensation)

Table 5-3 summarizes the treatment of hypovolemic shock.

Table 5-3 Treatment of Hypovolemic Shock

Treatment	Used For	Adult Dose	Pediatric Dose
Normal saline	Fluid replacement	250-500 mL	10-20 mL/kg
Sodium bicarbonate	Management of metabolic acidosis	IV: 1 mEq/kg	IV: 1 mEq/kg

Assessment of Hypovolemic Shock
- Scene size-up
  - Ensure BSI.
- Initial/primary assessment
  - Monitor the patient's LOC.
  - Manage ABCs.
  - Treat life-threatening illness/injury.
  - Transport considerations: Use shock position.
- Focused history and physical exam/secondary assessment
  - Obtain SAMPLE history and chief complaint (OPQRST).
  - Monitor vital signs.
  - Perform cardiac monitoring.
- Detailed physical exam
  - Perform the detailed physical exam when time allows, usually en route if there is an extended transport time.
    - Assess the patient's mental status.
    - Assess the patient's LOC.
    - Inspect and palpate each part of the body.
    - Reevaluate the patient's vital signs and assess trends in any changes.
- Ongoing assessment/reassessment
  - Perform every 5 minutes.
    - Repeat the initial/primary assessment.
    - Reassess and record vital signs.
    - Repeat the focused physical exam/secondary assessment.
    - Recheck interventions.

Management of Hypovolemic Shock
- Administer oxygen at 15 L/min via nonrebreathing mask.
- Keep the patient warm.
- Maintain systolic blood pressure of 90 mm Hg or until radial pulses are present.

Distributive Shock: Septic Shock, Neurogenic Shock, and Anaphylactic Shock

Distributive shock occurs when there is widespread dilation of the resistance vessels (small arterioles), the capacitance vessels (small venules), or both. As a result, the circulating blood volume pools in the expanded vascular beds and tissue perfusion decreases. The three most common types of distributive shock are septic shock, neurogenic shock, and anaphylactic shock.

Pathophysiology of Septic Shock <u>Septic shock</u> is caused by the release of toxins into the bloodstream from an infection. In the initial stage, CO is increased because toxins in the bloodstream cause vasodilation, preventing an increase in blood pressure. In the final stage of septic shock, toxins have built up to the point of causing an increased cell permeability and capillary leak, which can lead to hypovolemia as well.

Signs and Symptoms of Septic Shock
- Possible fever (caused by infection)
- Reduced urine output (caused by decreased blood flow to the kidneys)
- Hypotension (caused by failure of compensatory mechanism)
- Cyanosis (caused by hypoxia)
- Altered mental status
- Increased heart rate
- Edema

Assessment of Septic Shock
- Scene size-up
  - Ensure BSI.
- Initial/primary assessment
  - Monitor the patient's LOC.
  - Manage ABCs.
  - Treat life-threatening illness/injury.
  - Transport considerations: Load and go, using a position of comfort.
- Focused history and physical exam/secondary assessment
  - Administer oxygen at 15 L/min via nonrebreathing mask.
  - Monitor pulse oximetry.
  - Obtain SAMPLE history and chief complaint (OPQRST). Patient may have a history of recent infection, abdominal pain, or urinary symptoms.
  - Monitor vital signs.
- Detailed physical exam
  - Perform the detailed physical exam when time allows, usually en route if there is an extended transport time.
    - Assess the patient's mental status.
    - Assess the patient's LOC.
    - Inspect and palpate each part of the body.
    - Reevaluate the patient's vital signs and assess trends in any changes.
- Ongoing assessment/reassessment
  - Perform every 5 minutes.
    - Repeat the initial/primary assessment.
    - Reassess and record vital signs.
    - Repeat the focused physical exam.
    - Recheck interventions.

Management of Septic Shock
- Establish IV.
- Perform cardiac monitoring.
- Administer inotropic and vasopressor drugs (dopamine) to improve perfusion.
- *Give nothing by mouth.*

- Prepare to suction.
- Keep the patient warm.

Table 5-4 summarizes the treatment of septic shock.

Table 5-4 Treatment of Septic Shock

Treatment	Purpose	Adult Dose	Pediatric Dose
Normal saline	Perfusion	500 mL to maintain SBP of 90 mm Hg or radial pulses	10-20 mL/kg titrated to maintain radial or brachial pulses
Lactated Ringer's solution	Perfusion	500 mL to maintain SBP of 90 mm Hg or radial pulses	10-20 mL/kg titrated to maintain radial or brachial pulses
Dopamine	Stimulate alpha-adrenergic receptors to increase peripheral vascular resistance by contracting vessels	2-20 µg/kg/min	2-20 µg/kg/min
SBP, Systolic blood pressure.			

Pathophysiology of Neurogenic Shock **Neurogenic shock**, also called spinal shock or vasogenic shock, occurs when the nervous system fails to control the diameter of the blood vessels. This leads to an increase in the volume of the cardiovascular system. Blood pools in certain areas of the body, causing a decrease in venous return to the heart. It is usually caused by damage to the spinal cord, causing the sympathetic nervous system to stop secreting epinephrine.

Signs and Symptoms of Neurogenic Shock
- Symptoms related to spinal cord injury (tingling, numbness, loss of sensation, pain, paralysis)
- Inability to feel or move significant area/loss of sympathetic tone
- Altered mental status
- Hypoperfusion
- Warm, dry skin
- Priapism
- Incontinence

Assessment of Neurogenic Shock
- Scene size-up
  - Ensure BSI.
- Initial/primary assessment
  - Monitor the patient's LOC.
  - Manage ABCs.
  - Treat life-threatening illness/injury.
  - Transport considerations: Immobilize patient to long backboard.
- Focused history and physical exam/secondary assessment
  - Monitor pulse oximetry.
  - Obtain SAMPLE history and chief complaint (OPQRST).
  - Monitor vital signs.
- Detailed physical exam
  - Perform the detailed physical exam when time allows, usually en route if there is an extended transport time.

- Assess the patient's mental status.
- Assess the patient's LOC.
- Inspect and palpate each part of the body.
- Reevaluate the patient's vital signs and assess trends in any changes.
- Ongoing assessment/reassessment
  - Perform every 5 minutes.
    - Repeat the initial/primary assessment.
    - Reassess and record vital signs.
    - Repeat the focused physical exam/secondary assessment.
    - Recheck interventions.

Management of Neurogenic Shock
- Administer oxygen at 15 L/min via nonrebreathing mask.
- Establish IV; administer volume expanders.
- Perform cardiac monitoring.
- *Give nothing by mouth.*
- Keep the patient warm.

Table 5-5 summarizes the treatment of neurogenic shock.

Table 5-5 Treatment of Neurogenic Shock

Treatment	Used For	Adult Dose	Pediatric Dose
Oxygen	Increases perfusion	15 L/min via non-rebreathing mask	15 L/min via nonrebreathing mask
Normal saline	Increases perfusion, hydration, BP	250-500 mL	10-20 mL/kg
Methylprednisolone	Anti-inflammatory for reduction of post-traumatic spinal cord edema	30 mg/kg IV over first 30 min followed by infusion of 5.4 mg/kg/h × 23-47 hours	IV: 30 mg/kg over 30 min Infusion: 5.4 mg/kg/h
Dopamine IV drip	Stimulate alpha-adrenergic receptors to increase peripheral vascular resistance by contracting vessels	Infusion: 2-20 µg/kg/min	Infusion: 2-20 µg/kg/min

Pathophysiology of Anaphylactic Shock Anaphylaxis occurs when the immune system has become hypersensitive to one or more substances. Mast cells recognize the substance as potentially harmful and begin releasing chemical mediators. Histamine and leukotrienes cause immediate vasodilation, smooth muscle dilation, and decreased contractility of the heart, leading to hypotension. **Anaphylactic shock** occurs when anaphylactic reactions are not treated immediately.

Signs and Symptoms of Anaphylactic Shock
- Swelling of soft tissue, tongue, pharynx
- Headache
- Coughing, sneezing, wheezing
- Hives
- Itchy, watery eyes
- Tachypnea
- Runny nose

- Tachycardia
- Urticaria

Assessment of Anaphylactic Shock
- Scene size-up
  - Ensure BSI.
- Initial/primary assessment
  - Monitor patient's LOC.
  - Manage ABCs.
  - Treat life-threatening illness/injury.
  - Transport considerations: Transport patient in position of comfort.
- Focused history and physical exam/secondary assessment
  - Obtain SAMPLE history and chief complaint (OPQRST). Patient may have a history of allergies or a bee sting.
  - Monitor vital signs.
  - Perform cardiac monitoring.
- Detailed physical exam
  - Perform the detailed physical exam when time allows, usually en route if there is an extended transport time.
    - Assess the patient's mental status.
    - Assess the patient's LOC.
    - Inspect and palpate each part of the body.
    - Reevaluate the patient's vital signs and assess trends in any changes.
- Ongoing assessment/reassessment
  - Perform every 5 minutes.
    - Repeat the initial/primary assessment.
    - Reassess and record vital signs.
    - Repeat the focused physical exam/secondary assessment.
    - Recheck interventions.

Management of Anaphylactic Shock
- Administer oxygen at 15 L/min via nonrebreathing mask.
- Establish an IV.

Table 5-6 summarizes the treatment of anaphylactic shock.

Table 5-6 Treatment of Anaphylactic Shock

Treatment	Used For	Adult Dose	Pediatric Dose
Epinephrine Epinephrine drip	Stimulates both alpha- and beta-adrenergic receptors in order to produce a rapid increase in blood pressure, ventricular contractility, and heart rate	IV: 0.3-0.5 mg SQ: 0.3-0.5 mg Infusion: 2-10 µg/kg/min	SQ: 0.01 mg/kg 0.1-1 µg/kg/min
Diphenhydramine	Antihistamine—prevents the physiologic actions of histamine by blocking H_1 and H_2 receptors	IV: 25-50 mg IM: 25-50 mg	IV/IO: 1-2 mg/kg
Albuterol	Bronchodilation	Nebulizer: 1.25-2.5 mg	Nebulizer: 2.5 mg (0.5 mL of the 0.083% solution) added to 2 mL of normal saline

Continues

Table 5-6 Treatment of Anaphylactic Shock (Continued)

Treatment	Used For	Adult Dose	Pediatric Dose
Corticosteroids	Anti-inflammatory–suppresses acute and chronic inflammation, potentiates vascular smooth muscle from relaxation by beta-adrenergic agonists, and may alter airway hyperactivity	IV: Methylprednisolone 125 mg	IV: 0.25-1.0 mg/kg
Dopamine	Stimulates alpha-adrenergic receptors to increase peripheral vascular resistance by contracting vessels	Infusion: 2-20 µg/kg/min	Infusion: 2-20 µg/kg/min

Vital Vocabulary

__anaphylactic shock__ A severe hypersensitivity reaction that involves bronchoconstriction and cardiovascular collapse.

__cardiac output (CO)__ Amount of blood pumped by the heart per minute, calculated by multiplying the stroke volume by the heart rate per minute.

__cardiogenic shock__ A condition caused by loss of 40% or more of the functioning myocardium; the heart is no longer able to circulate sufficient blood to maintain adequate oxygen delivery.

__compensated shock__ The early stage of shock, in which the body can still compensate for blood loss.

__decompensated shock__ The late stage of shock, when blood pressure is falling.

__distributive shock__ A condition that occurs when there is widespread dilation of the resistance vessels (small arterioles), the capacitance vessels (small venules), or both.

__hypovolemic shock__ Hypovolemic shock is an emergency condition in which severe blood and fluid loss makes the heart unable to pump enough blood to the rest of the body.

__irreversible shock__ The final stage of shock, resulting in death.

__neurogenic shock__ Circulatory failure caused by paralysis of the nerves that control the size of the blood vessels, leading to widespread dilation; seen in spinal cord injuries.

__obstructive shock__ Shock that occurs when blood flow in the heart or great vessels becomes blocked.

__perfusion__ The circulation of blood within an organ or tissue in adequate amounts to meet the cells' needs.

__septic shock__ Shock that occurs as a result of widespread infection, usually bacterial. Untreated, the result is multiple organ dysfunction syndrome (MODS) and often death.

CHAPTER

6 Burns

Pathophysiology

Burns are soft-tissue injuries created by destructive energy transfer via radiation, thermal, chemical, or electrical energy. Significant damage to the skin and soft tissues may make the body vulnerable to bacterial invasion, temperature instability, and major disturbances of fluid balance. Burn severity is determined by *depth* (superficial, partial thickness, or full thickness), *length of exposure*, *what the patient was exposed to*, and the *body surface area* (BSA) affected. Severity is also determined by the age of the patient, area of the body involved, and any underlying comorbidities. Finally, these additional factors also have an effect on the severity of the burn:

- Skin and underlying tissue thickness (patients with thinner skin and underlying tissues, such as older or chronically ill patients, may receive a partial-thickness burn from an exposure that would cause only a superficial burn in a patient with thicker skin and soft tissues)
- Presence of conductive or insulating substances (eg, oils and hair hold heat and are great conductors)
- Peripheral circulation (assists in dissipation of heat)
- Water content of skin

Depending on the extent of the burn, the patient can have an isolated local response or a combined local and systemic response, described in **Table 6-1**.

As a result of these generalized systemic effects, end-organ failure can occur or be worsened. The common end organs affected include the kidneys. As a result of hypovolemia, vasoconstriction, increased blood viscosity (as a result of plasma loss), and the increased amount of large molecules that need to be filtered (such as myoglobin), the kidneys are subjected to multiple insults that affect their function. Early signs of renal function changes include decreased urine output and changes in urine color. Dark or port wine–colored urine can suggest **rhabdomyolysis**, or significant damage to underlying muscles and tissue.

Burn Shock

Burn shock is essentially hypovolemic shock resulting from burns, specifically from either fluid loss across burned skin or volume shifts in the rest of the body due to capillary leakage, which increases extracellular volume and decreases intravascular volume, eventually leading to shock. Hemodynamic effects include increased cardiac output early, then later decreased cardiac output as shock becomes decompensated. Other points regarding burn shock include the following:

- Develops within 6 to 8 hours. Not usually seen in the field. If the acute burn patient displays evidence of shock, look for another injury as the cause.
- Emergent phase: Initial decrease in blood flow to the affected area.
- Fluid shift phase: Occurs when the release of vasoactive substances from the burned tissues increases capillary permeability, producing intravascular fluid loss and wound edema.
- Chills and nausea can indicate a mild form of burn shock, as a result of the fluid shifts and electrolyte disturbances altering end-organ perfusion.

Table 6-1 Local Response Versus Systemic Response to Burns

Local Response
Tissues are either destroyed at the time the injury occurs or have their metabolic functions disrupted so that cellular death eventually results.

Systemic Response

In cases of major burn severity, changes in circulation and perfusion can occur. These are as a result of:
1. Massive fluid shift resulting in decreased circulatory volume (hypovolemia)
2. Vascular changes
   a. Decreased circulation in areas of injury as a result of vascular damage
   b. Early generalized vasoconstriction as a result of catecholamine release
   c. Late vasodilation as a result of loss of vasomotor control due to decreased perfusion and loss of catecholamine secretion
   d. Increased capillary permeability resulting in fluid shifts and subsequent hypovolemia
3. Decreased cardiac output (changes in cardiac output can be increased or decreased depending on severity of volume changes and time since burn)
   a. Patients may become hyperdynamic in early stages as a result of catecholamine release.
   b. In later stages or with more significant injury, hypovolemia and hypoperfusion can result in decreased cardiac output and begin the downward spiral of irreversible shock.

Types of Burns

Thermal Burns

Thermal burns can occur when the skin is exposed to temperatures greater than 111°F (44°C).

- **Flame burns:** Caused by an open flame. May be superficial or deep, especially if clothing catches fire. Flame burns are often associated with inhalation injuries.
- **Scald burns:** Produced by contact with hot liquids. Can often cover large surface areas or irregularly shaped areas. Injuries and burn severity may be increased if hot liquid soaks into clothing or adheres to skin (eg, oil, grease). Scald burns may not fully present themselves initially. Burns that may initially appear minor may progress to full-thickness burns over the first 12 to 24 hours.
- **Contact burns:** Produced by contact with a hot object. Generally superficial (first or second degree) because the victim reflexively pulls away from the source of heat. In patients who are unconscious, intoxicated, restrained, or impaired (eg, a stroke victim who falls against a household radiator), injuries may be severe.
- **Steam burns:** Caused by direct exposure to hot steam, as from a broken pipe. Common household burn caused by microwave ovens. Strongly associated with upper airway trauma.
- **Radiation burns:** Relatively rare, caused by exposure to heat (eg, a lightning strike, welding, explosion, sunburns) and exposure to medical radiation treatment.

Burn Injury Zones

Burn injury is described by three pathologic progressions (zones) radiating out from the central area of most damage.

- **Zone of coagulation:** Central area of the burn that has sustained the worst of the injury. Cell membranes rupture and blood coagulates. No viable tissue; little or no blood flow.
- **Zone of stasis:** Potentially viable tissue; ischemic as a result of clotting and vasoconstriction. Tissue necrosis may occur within 24 to 48 hours.
- **Zone of hyperemia:** Outer area of burn, least affected by thermal injury. Increased blood flow as a result of normal inflammatory responses. This occurs within 7 to 10 days.

Potential Physical Abuse

Burns can be a sign of potential physical abuse. Burns that are in distinguishable shapes, unusual patterns, or in atypical places (genitalia, buttocks, and thighs) may be signs of abuse in children, the elderly, and disabled persons. Examples include "stocking burns," in which both feet have been immersed in hot water; cigarette or cigar burns; and cases in which the story regarding the burn does not match your assessment of the patient or the scene, or both.

Chemical Burns

Chemical burns occur when skin comes in contact with strong acids, alkalis (also known as *bases*), oxidizers, or other corrosive materials. Although all tissues are at risk when they are exposed to these chemicals, the eyes and the mucous membranes are at the greatest risk for injury. Because of the unique nature of chemical burns, a thorough assessment of severity must be done, because limiting the criteria to only BSA or location does not always accurately indicate the extent of the burn; even small amounts of phenols and highly corrosive acids can penetrate the skin quickly and deeply. **Table 6-2** lists examples of chemical burns.

Table 6-2 Chemical Burns

Chemical Type	Examples	Injury
Acids	Muriatic acid, hydrochloric acid, hydrofluoric acid	Coagulative necrosis
Bases and alkalis	Hydroxides, lime, drain cleaner, oven cleaner, lye	Liquefactive necrosis and protein denaturation
Oxidizing agents	Hydrogen peroxide, sodium chlorate	Exothermic (heat) reaction in addition to tissue destruction; can cause systemic poisoning
Phosphorus	White phosphorus, tracer ammunition, fireworks	Burns when exposed to air; can cause systemic poisoning
Vesicants	Lewisite, sulfur mustard (mustard gas), phosgene oxime	Blister agents; respiratory compromise if inhaled

Electrical Burns

There are three types of electrical burns:

- **Type I:** Direct contact with electrical current. External signs of burning are most significant at entrance and exit sites (**Figure 6-1**). Internal damage may be severe.
- **Type II:** Flash burn from proximity to the source of a high-voltage current.
- **Type III:** Flame burn that occurs when electricity ignites clothing or objects.

Non-burn-related complications of electrical injuries can be severe:

- Neurologic complications
  - Central nervous system (CNS)
    - Seizures, coma, temporary or permanent quadriplegia
    - Asphyxia and cardiac arrest leading to death
  - Peripheral nervous system
    - Muscle spasms resulting in bone dislocation or fracture

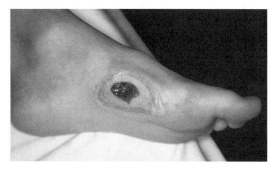
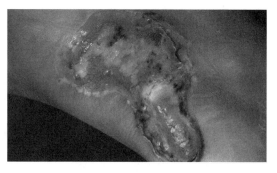

A. **B.**

Figure 6-1 Electrical burns have entrance and exit wounds. **A.** The entrance wound is often quite small. **B.** The exit wound can be extensive and deep.

- Cardiac arrhythmias
  - Occur as a result of current passing through heart.
    - Damage to conduction system
    - Damage to heart muscle tissue
  - Ventricular fibrillation (VF) and ventricular tachycardia (VT) are common in electrical burns.
    - Any patient who has been exposed to an electrical injury needs to be treated with a high index of suspicion and closely monitored.

Radiation Burns

Radiation burns are a result of being exposed to a radioactive source or substance. There are three types of ionizing radiation: alpha (α) (travels only inches through the air, has little penetrating energy, and is easily stopped by skin); beta (β) (can travel up to 10 feet in the air, is able to penetrate several layers of clothing and to penetrate the first few millimeters of skin, but can be stopped by specially designed protective clothing); and gamma (γ) (very penetrating; can pass through the body and solid materials).

Radiation tends to affect rapidly dividing or rapidly reproducing cells first. The most common of these are cells such as erythrocytes, leukocytes, and bone marrow, as well as the mucous membranes, the hair, the blood, many cancerous cells (hence radiation treatment), and fetuses. When assessing these patients, watch for symptoms associated with these systems because they are the earliest signs of injury. Acute radiation syndrome is manifested by hematologic, CNS, and gastrointestinal changes (eg, nausea and vomiting) over time. Signs such as vomiting or an altered mental status soon after an exposure are often predictors of poor patient outcomes.

Airway Burns and Inhalation Poisoning

Airway burns, or inhalation burns, can cause serious and rapid airway compromise.

- Thermal heat inhalation can irritate the lungs and airway, causing coughing, wheezing, and swelling of upper airway tissues (may hear **stridor**).
- Steam and chemical inhalation is associated with **subglottic** (vocal cords and larynx) and lower airway damage.
- Smoke inhalation, a major cause of death from fire, results from breathing the by-products of combustion, leading to upper airway compromise, pulmonary injury, and potentially asphyxia.

Carbon Monoxide Poisoning

Although not a burn injury, carbon monoxide poisoning is a common complication associated with burn injury or exposure to a smoke/fire environment. Carbon monoxide is a tasteless, colorless, odorless gas that can result from combustion. Exposure to carbon monoxide can result in hypoxia as a result of its natural affinity for hemoglobin (approximately 200 times greater affinity than oxygen) and asphyxia.

Depth of Burns

- **Superficial burn** (first degree) involves only the epidermis. Such a burn is typically secondary to exposure to low-intensity heat or to a short-duration flash exposure to heat.
- **Partial-thickness burn** (second degree) affects the epidermis and varying degrees of the dermis. There are two types:
  - **Superficial partial-thickness burn:** Affects the epidermis and upper half of the dermis, leaving the basal layers of the skin intact. Hair follicles remain intact. Edema

fluid infiltrates the dermal-epidermal junction, which causes the creation of the blisters that are characteristic of partial-thickness burns.

– **Deep partial-thickness burn:** Extends into the lower half of the dermis, damaging hair follicles and sweat and sebaceous glands. Often caused by hot liquids, steam, or grease.

- **Full-thickness burn** (third degree) destroys epidermis and dermis, and possibly subcutaneous tissues, bone, muscle, and/or organs. Capillaries and sensory nerves are destroyed. The skin can no longer generate new skin cells, so skin grafting is needed.

Figure 6-2 illustrates the appearance of superficial, partial-thickness, and full-thickness burns.

Signs and Symptoms

- Superficial burns (first degree)
  - Reddened, inflamed skin (sunburn)
  - Pain
  - Peeling as the burn heals (from sloughing off the dead epidermal cells)
- Partial-thickness burns (second degree)
  - Red, wet tissue
  - Blanched skin surrounding injury (mottled effect)
  - Blisters
  - Extreme pain
  - Hypovolemic shock as a result of significant fluid loss
- Full-thickness burns (third degree)
  - **Eschar** (dry, leathery skin)
  - White, dark brown, or charred skin
  - Absence of pain as a result of loss of sensory nerves (however, patients often experience extreme pain in the surrounding areas, which are partial-thickness burns)
- **Inhalation injury**
  - Burns around the nose or mouth
  - Soot in the mouth or nose

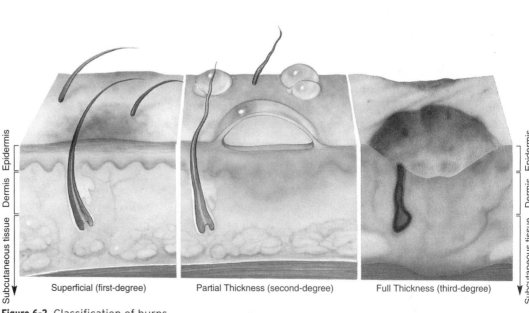

Figure 6-2 Classification of burns.

- Singed nose or facial hair
- Difficulty speaking
- Inspiratory stridor
- Edema of lips and mouth
- Coughing/wheezing
- Decreased ability to swallow
- Circumferential burns around the neck

Assessment

- Scene size-up
  - Scene safety: Beware of burning-building hazards (toxic gases, structural damage) and sources of electrical hazards, radiation, or chemicals.
  - Ensure body substance isolation (BSI): Wear gloves and a face mask or eye shield to protect against leaking body fluids.
  - Remove victim's clothing and other articles that may become restrictive as a result of swelling (eg, watches, rings).
  - Transport considerations: Circumferential burns will possibly require an escharotomy and thus require rapid transport. Place patient in a position of comfort.
- Initial/primary assessment
  - Manage ABCs (airway, breathing, circulation).
  - Look for locations/functions affected.
  - Determine burn depth (partial- and full-thickness burns only).
  - Estimate total body surface area (TBSA) using the **rule of nines** or the **rule of palms**.
  - Electrical burns: Perform rapid head-to-toe assessment; look for entry and exit wounds.
  - Evaluate degree of burn injury (zone of coagulation, zone of stasis, zone of hyperemia).
  - Evaluate the severity of the burn. **Table 6-3** describes three categories: critical/major, moderate, and minor.
  - In your initial assessment, evaluate for:
    - Bleeding
    - Circulatory inadequacy
    - Presence or absence of pain
    - Swelling
    - Skin color
    - Capillary refill time
    - Moisture/blisters
    - Appearance of wound edges
    - Presence of foreign bodies or contaminants
- Focused history and physical exam/secondary assessment
  - Monitor vital signs.
  - Observe for burn shock.
  - Perform rapid trauma assessment to assess for other life-threatening injuries.
  - Check for **circumferential burns** (which require rapid transport).
- Detailed physical exam and ongoing assessment/reassessment
  - Perform the detailed physical exam en route to the emergency department if the mechanism of injury is significant.

> **Rule of Nines**
>
> The rule of nines (**Figure 6-3**) is a guide that divides the body into regions, each of which has the value of 9, or 18% of the body surface area. This provides a quick and easy method to estimate large burns or burns isolated to specific areas of the body.

> **Rule of Palms**
>
> Use the rule of palms when the burn area is small. The patient's palm is equal to approximately 1% of the TBSA. This is useful for small or irregularly shaped burns.

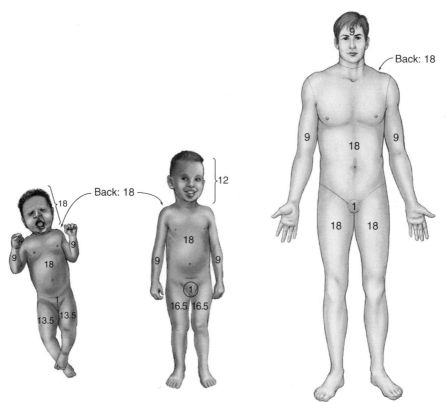

Figure 6-3 The rule of nines.

Table 6-3 Classification of Burns

Classification	Characteristics
Critical/Major	• Any partial-thickness burn of 30% or more of BSA • Any full-thickness burn of 10% or more of BSA • Inhalation injury or any burn involving the respiratory tract • Electrical injury • Full- or partial-thickness burn involving the face, eyes, ears, hands, feet, joints, or genitalia • Any circumferential burn
Moderate	• Superficial burns of 50% or more of BSA • Partial-thickness burns of 30% or less of BSA • Full-thickness burns of 10% or less of BSA
Minor	• Superficial burns of 50% or less of BSA • Partial-thickness burns of 15% or less of BSA • Full-thickness burns involving less than 2% of BSA

Management

General Management

- ABC management for respiratory or cardiac arrest
- Burns are complex, multisystem injuries. Do not allow yourself to become distracted!

- Management begins during your scene size-up and initial/primary assessment.
- Immediate management: Stop the burning process, if safe to do so. Remove the patient from the hazardous environment, smother flames, remove hot items from contact with the patient (eg, jewelry, zippers, metal buttons), flush chemicals, or remove the patient from electrical contact. Once the burning has been stopped, keep the patient warm to prevent hypothermia
- Airway management:
  1. Early and definitive airway management is paramount for patients with airway burns. Early intubation, when possible, results in an easier intubation and a better-controlled airway. This may require using rapid-sequence intubation or mediation-assisted intubation, if available.
  2. If intubation is not possible due to airway injury or edema, a surgical airway is the appropriate alternative. Nonsurgical rescue devices such as laryngeal mask airways (LMAs) and Combitubes may be ineffective in managing a patient with an airway burn and provide a false sense of security to providers.
  3. Administer oxygen at 15 L/min for all burn patients via nonrebreathing mask or bag-mask ventilation. Oxygen should be humidified, when possible, for these patients.
- Circulatory support
  – Fluid resuscitation
    - Establish at least one large-bore intravenous (IV) line, preferably two, into a large vein; an upper extremity, even if burned, is preferable to a lower extremity. Use a crystalloid solution such as lactated Ringer's solution or normal saline for initial resuscitation, per local protocols. If unable to establish IV access, or access will be delayed, intraosseous access is appropriate.

Lund and Browder Chart

The **Lund and Browder chart** (**Figure 6-4**) is a more specific method used to estimate the burned area by dividing the body into even smaller and more specific regions, as well as allowing for developmental changes in percentage of TBSA due to age. Because of the time it takes to calculate TBSA, the Lund and Browder chart is usually not used in prehospital settings; it is generally used only in the intensive care unit or burn center settings. Because of the detailed breakdown it provides, the Lund and Browder chart is considered the gold standard for documenting the body surface area involved in a burn injury.

Calculating the Mortality of a Burn Patient

A formula to calculate the mortality of a burn patient is:

Patient's age (in years) + Percentage TBSA burned = Probability of mortality

Region	%
Head	
Neck	
Ant. Trunk	
Post. Trunk	
Right arm	
Left arm	
Buttocks	
Genitalia	
Right leg	
Left leg	
Total burn	

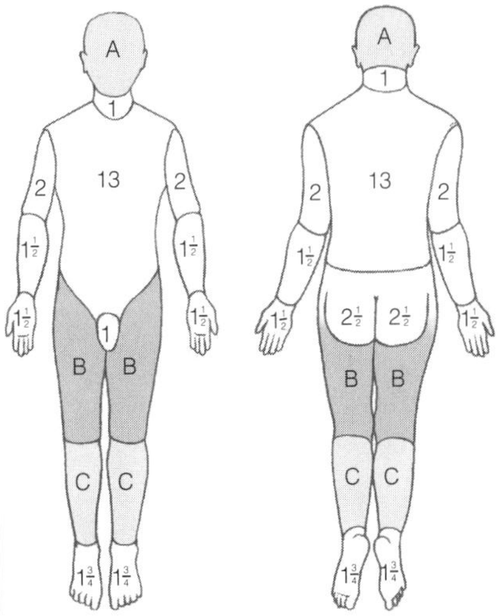

Relative percentages of body surface area affected by growth

Age (years)	A ($\frac{1}{2}$ of head)	B ($\frac{1}{2}$ of one thigh)	C ($\frac{1}{2}$ of one leg)
0	$9\frac{1}{2}$	$2\frac{3}{4}$	$2\frac{1}{2}$
1	$8\frac{1}{2}$	$3\frac{1}{4}$	$2\frac{1}{2}$
5	$6\frac{1}{2}$	4	$2\frac{3}{4}$
10	$5\frac{1}{2}$	$4\frac{1}{4}$	3
15	$4\frac{1}{2}$	$4\frac{1}{2}$	$3\frac{1}{4}$
Adult	$3\frac{1}{2}$	$4\frac{3}{4}$	3

Figure 6-4 The Lund and Browder chart.
Adapted from Lund, C. C., and Browder, N. C., *Surg. Gynecol. Obstet.* 79 (1944): 352-358.

The standard fluid replacement formula is the **Parkland formula**. The Parkland formula takes into consideration the patient's weight, percentage of TBSA burned (partial- and full-thickness burns only) and a standard fluid replacement amount.

The Parkland formula is as follows. During the first 24 hours, the burned patient will need:

4 mL × Body weight (kg) × Percentage of total body surface burned

Example:

4 mL × 125 kg × 32% = 16,000 mL of fluid

Half of the total amount, in this case 8,000 mL, should be given to the patient in the first 8 hours from the time of burn. The remaining 8,000 mL should be given in the following 16 hours.

- Fluid resuscitation should be in accordance with established guidelines, such as the Parkland formula.
- Other important concerns
  - Aggressive pain management may be required for burn patients.
  - Burned areas should be protected and covered with sterile dressings to minimize contamination by pathogenic organisms. Because of the nature of burn injuries, they can often distract providers from other injuries. Be sure to fully assess burn patients for other injuries.

Thermal burns

- Superficial burns
  - Cool with tepid water for 1 minute.
  - Do not use salves, butter, ointments, or ice.
- Partial-thickness burns
  - Cool burn area.
  - Protect burned areas with dry sterile dressings.
  - Do not rupture blisters.
  - Protect from hypothermia.
- Full-thickness burns
  - Apply sterile dry dressings.
  - Protect from hypothermia.

Burn Shock

- Ensure BSI.
- Monitor the patient's level of consciousness (LOC).
- Manage ABCs.
- Transport considerations: Once life-threatening injuries have been addressed, load and go.
- Establish a minimum of one IV, preferably two. Use a crystalloid solution such as lactated Ringer's solution or normal saline for initial resuscitation.

Chemical Burns

- Protect yourself from exposure to chemicals.
- Brush dry chemicals off patient, but be sure to protect yourself with gloves and other PPE as appropriate.
- Quickly remove patient's clothes, especially shoes and socks.
- Flush with copious amounts of water, for at least 20 minutes, before moving patient.

Electrical Burns

- Protect self and rescuers.
- Manage ABCs (open airway; perform CPR as indicated).
- Immobilize, if indicated.
- Monitor LOC.

- Check for possible internal damage (look for entrance and exit wounds; palpate skin and soft tissues).
- Establish cardiac monitoring.
- Treat wounds and injuries.
- Reassess.

Radiation Burns

- Protect self and rescuers.
- Decontaminate before transport.
  - Remove patient's clothing.
  - Gently irrigate open wounds.
- Notify the receiving facility as soon as practical.
- Keep away from the source of exposure.
- In case of sunburns (most common), remove the patient from the environment.

Vital Vocabulary

burn shock Hypovolemic shock resulting from burns, caused by fluid loss across burned skin and volume shifts in the body.

circumferential burns Burns on the neck or chest that may compress the airway or on an extremity that might act like a tourniquet.

eschar The damaged tissue that forms on the skin over a burn injury.

full-thickness burn A burn that extends through the epidermis and dermis into the subcutaneous tissues beneath; previously called a third-degree burn.

inhalation injury Injury to the airway or lungs that results from inhaling toxic or superheated gases.

Lund and Browder chart A detailed version of the rule of nines chart that takes into consideration the changes in body surface area brought on by growth.

Parkland formula A formula that recommends giving 4 mL of normal saline for each kilogram of body weight, multiplied by the percentage of total body surface area burned; sometimes used to calculate fluid needs during lengthy transport times.

partial-thickness burn A burn that involves the epidermis and part of the dermis, characterized by pain and blistering; previously called a second-degree burn.

rhabdomyolysis Caused by injury to skeletal muscle; myoglobin (a toxin) is released into plasma, often resulting in damage to the kidneys as they attempt to filter the myoglobin out of the bloodstream.

rule of nines A system that assigns percentages to sections of the body, allowing calculation of the amount of skin surface involved in the burn area.

rule of palms A system that estimates total body surface area burned by comparing the affected area with the size of the patient's palm, which is roughly equal to 1% of the patient's total body surface area.

stridor A harsh, high-pitched, crowing inspiratory sound, such as the sound often heard in acute laryngeal obstruction.

subglottic Vocal cords and laryngeal portions of the airway structure.

superficial burn A burn involving only the epidermis, producing very red, painful skin; previously called a first-degree burn.

Medical Emergencies

CHAPTER 7

Airway Management and Respiratory Emergencies

Respiratory Anatomy

The pathway of air as it enters the upper airway through the nares (nostrils) is as follows (**Figure 7-1**):

- nasopharynx
- pharynx
- trachea
- primary bronchi (right and left)
- secondary bronchi
- tertiary bronchi
- bronchioles
- alveoli

The Upper Airway

- The upper airway consists of all structures above the vocal cords. The major components are the nasopharynx, oropharynx, and larynx.
  - The nasopharynx is where inspired air is filtered, warmed, and humidified as it passes over the nasal **turbinates** en route to the lungs.
  - The oropharynx is bordered by the palates (hard and soft), cheeks, and tongue. It contains 32 teeth (in the average adult), the **adenoids**, **uvula**, and **vallecula**.
  - The **larynx** (voicebox) and the **glottis** (opening at the top of the trachea) divide the unsterile upper airway from the sterile lower airway (**Figure 7-2**). The larynx comprises the thyroid cartilage, cricoid cartridge, cricothyroid membrane, and the glottis. The thyroid cartilage is composed of two platelike structures that form the laryngeal prominence, or Adam's apple. The thyroid cartilage forms the bulk of the anterior wall of the larynx and serves to protect the vocal cords, which are located posterior to it.
  - The cricoid cartilage forms the lower part of the larynx. The function of the cricoid cartilage is to provide attachments for the various muscles, cartilages, and ligaments involved in opening and closing the airway.
  - The cricothyroid membrane lies between the thyroid and cricoid cartilages. Used when inserting surgical airways, it is important to be able to locate this landmark in an emergency.
  - The epiglottis is a leaf-shaped structure that directs substances around the glottis and into the esophagus. The glottis is the structure that occludes the trachea during swallowing or eating. It consists of two flaps that can close off the trachea. The free edges of the glottis are the vocal cords.

The Lower Airway

- The function of the lower airway is to exchange oxygen (O_2) and carbon dioxide (CO_2).
  - The trachea allows for air entry into the lungs. Consisting of many cartilaginous rings, the trachea begins immediately inferior to the glottis, extending to the level of the fifth intercostal space. From here, it branches off into both the left and right mainstem bronchi at the **carina**. It is important to note that the right mainstem bronchus is shorter and straighter, thus making it easier to accidentally intubate

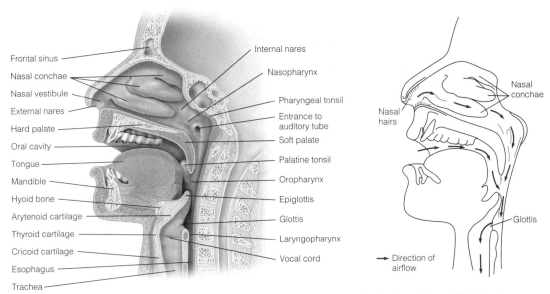

Figure 7-1 The upper airway contains many blood vessels and serves to heat and humidify the air we breathe.

the right mainstem, instead of placing the endotracheal (ET) tube at the level of the carina.

- The main component of the lower airway is the lungs. The right lung has three lobes, whereas the left lung has only two, allowing room for the heart. As the bronchi enter the lungs at the **hilum**, they branch out into smaller passages called bronchioles, which are lined with smooth muscles that dilate or contract in response to different stimuli.
- At the terminal end of the bronchioles are alveoli, which are single-layer air sacs. Alveoli are the functional units where the exchange of O_2 and CO_2 occurs.

Ventilation

There are two phases of breathing: inhalation (which is active) and exhalation (which is passive).

During the inhalation process, the intercostal muscles and the diaphragm contract and the lungs expand. This expansion causes a negative pressure in the thoracic cavity in comparison with the atmospheric pressure. Oxygen diffuses from the alveolus to the capillaries

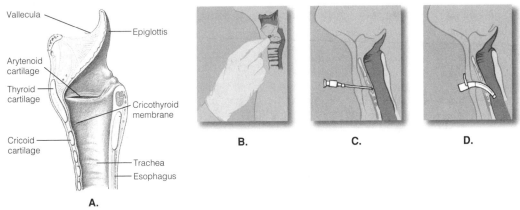

Figure 7-2 An understanding of the larynx is imperative when performing a number of airway management skills. **A.** Anatomy of the larynx. **B.** Applying pressure to the cricoid cartilage, which compresses the esophagus while keeping the trachea open (Sellick maneuver). **C.** An IV cannula is inserted into the cricothyroid membrane. **D.** A tracheostomy tube is inserted below the cricoid cartilage.

until the partial pressure of oxygen (Po_2) in the capillary is equal to that in the alveolus. On exhalation, the opposite occurs: the diaphragm relaxes (moves upward) the intercostal muscles relax, and the pressure within the thoracic cavity becomes positive, forcing air back out of the lungs.

Control centers for ventilation are located in both the **medulla** and the **pons** of the brainstem. The medulla controls automatic breathing by specific neurons that stimulate and inhibit inhalation and exhalation. The pons houses the **apneustic center**, which stimulates inspiratory neurons, and the **pneumotaxic center**, which inhibits the apneustic center, thus inhibiting inhalation and promoting exhalation. Chemoreceptors detect the amount of O_2 or CO_2 in the blood. The chemoreceptors located in the aortic arch and carotid arteries are called *peripheral chemoreceptors*; those in the medulla are called the *central chemoreceptors*.

The peripheral chemoreceptors are sensitive to the levels of O_2 in the blood. The central chemoreceptors are sensitive to blood CO_2 levels. If either O_2 or CO_2 levels vary too greatly from a set point, the negative feedback mechanism makes the proper adjustment. For example, if CO_2 levels increase, the negative feedback mechanism will increase respirations in order to expel the CO_2.

Other factors that influence ventilation include:

- Increase in body temperature
- Epinephrine release (during stress)
- Impulses from the cerebral cortex (may simultaneously stimulate **rhythmicity area** and motor neurons)

The Fick Principle

The Fick method is based on the principle that the volume of O_2 entering the pulmonary capillaries equals the volume of O_2 gained by the flowing blood. The four components of the Fick principle are:

- Ability to bring in an adequate amount of O_2
- A closed container
- An efficient pump
- Adequate on-loading and off-loading of O_2 and CO_2 at the cellular level

---

Partial Pressure

Partial pressure refers to the individual pressure exerted independently by a particular gas within a mixture of gases. The air we inhale contains a mixture of gases: 78% nitrogen, 21% O_2, and less than 1% of CO_2, argon, and helium. For example, at sea level, total atmospheric pressure is about 760 mm Hg, and air is composed of about 21% oxygen. The Po_2 in the air in this case (at sea level) is 0.21 × 760 mm Hg, or 160 mm Hg.

However, by the time the inspired air reaches the trachea, it has been warmed and humidified by the upper airway. The humidity is formed by water vapor, which, as a gas, exerts a pressure. At 99°F the water vapor pressure in the trachea is 47 mm Hg. Taking the water vapor pressure into account, the Po_2 in the trachea when breathing air is

$$(760 - 47) \times 21/100 = 150 \text{ mm Hg}$$

By the time the oxygen reaches the alveoli, the Po_2 has fallen to about 100 mm Hg. This is because the Po_2 of the gas in the alveoli (Pao_2) is a balance between two processes: the removal of O_2 by the pulmonary capillaries and its continual supply by alveolar ventilation (breathing).

Lung Sounds

Is your patient making unusual sounds during respiration? The following are important lung sounds to know.

- **Stridor:** Abnormal, high-pitched, musical breathing sound caused by a serious blockage in the upper airway. It is usually heard during inspiration. Stridor indicates a potentially life-threatening upper airway obstruction.

- **Wheezing:** A high-pitched whistling or buzzing in the lungs heard during breathing, more obvious on exhalation than inhalation; occurs when there is a narrowing or obstruction of the bronchioles.
- **Snoring:** Indicates the tongue is partially blocking the upper airway.
- **Crackles** (formerly called *rales*): Abnormal breath sounds that have a fine crackling quality. Occurs when there is an accumulation of fluid in the alveoli.
- **Gurgling:** An indication that fluid is blocking the upper airway.
- **Rhonchi:** Low-pitched sounds (like bubbling, due to fluid accumulation in the larger airways). Sometimes refers to a low-pitched crackle.

Assessing Respiratory Problems

It is important to remember that the functioning of the lungs dramatically affects other body systems, and vice versa. Therefore, when assessing respiratory problems, remember to also assess the following:

- **Neurologic status:** An altered level of consciousness (LOC) may result in respiratory compromise because of decreased respiratory drive.
- **Cardiovascular status:** Severe hypoxia often leads to tachycardia while the body compensates; at the point at which the body is unable to compensate any longer, hypoxia causes bradycardia. If untreated, hypoxia may lead to ventricular fibrillation, ventricular tachycardia, or asystole.
- **Muscles and mechanics:** Respiratory compromise means that the lungs have to work harder to maintain appropriate O_2 and CO_2 levels. The large workload causes them to use tremendous amounts of energy, which requires even more oxygen and ventilation.

Dyspnea

Signs and Symptoms

Dyspnea may include any of the abnormal breathing patterns or sounds described in **Table 7-1**. The goal in respiratory emergencies is correction of the problem, or definitive airway management, such as with an ET tube.

Table 7-1 Breathing Patterns

Pattern	Description
Agonal	Irregular gasps that are few and far between. Usually represent stray neurologic impulses in the dying patient. It is not unusual for patients who are pulseless to have an occasional agonal gasp.
Apneustic	When the pneumotaxic center in the brain is damaged, the apneustic center causes a prolonged inspiratory hold. This ominous sign indicates severe brain injury.
Biot respirations/ataxic respirations	Respirations with an irregular pattern, rate, and depth with intermittent patterns of apnea. Indicates severe brain injury or brainstem herniation.
Bradypnea	Unusually slow respirations.
Central neurogenic hyperventilation	Tachypneic hyperpnea; rapid and deep respirations caused by increased intracranial pressure or direct brain injury. Drives CO_2 levels down and pH levels up, resulting in respiratory alkalosis.

Continues

Table 7-1 Breathing Patterns (Continued)

Pattern	Description
Cheyne-Stokes respirations	Crescendo-decrescendo breathing with a period of apnea between each cycle. It is not considered ominous unless grossly exaggerated or in the context of a patient who has brain trauma.
Cough	Forced exhalation against a closed glottis; an airway-clearing maneuver. Also seen when foreign substances irritate the airways. Controlled by the cough center in the brain. Antitussive medications work on the cough center to reduce this sometimes-annoying physiologic response.
Eupnea	Normal breathing.
Hiccup	Spasmodic contraction of the diaphragm causing short inhalations with a characteristic sound. Sometimes seen in cases of diaphragmatic (or phrenic nerve) irritation from acute myocardial infarction, ulcer disease, or endotracheal intubation.
Hyperpnea	Unusually deep breathing. Seen in various neurologic or chemical disorders. Certain drugs may stimulate this type of breathing in patients who have overdosed. It does not reflect respiratory rate—only respiratory depth.
Hypopnea	Unusually shallow respirations.
Kussmaul respirations	The same pattern as central neurogenic hyperventilation, but caused by the body's response to metabolic acidosis; the body is trying to rid itself of blood acetone via the lungs. Kussmaul respirations are seen in patients who have diabetic ketoacidosis and are accompanied by a fruity (acetone) breath odor. The mouth and lips are usually cracked and dry.
Sighing	Periodically taking a very deep breath (about twice the normal volume). Sighing forces open alveoli that close in the course of day-to-day events.
Tachypnea	Unusually rapid breathing. This term does not reflect depth of respiration, nor does it mean that the patient is hyperventilating (lowering the carbon dioxide level by breathing too fast and too deep). In fact, patients who breathe very rapidly frequently move only small volumes of air and are *hypoven*tilating (much like a panting dog).
Yawning	Yawning seems to be beneficial in the same manner that sighing is. It also appears to be contagious!

Assessment

- Scene size-up
  - Ensure body substance isolation (BSI).
- Initial/primary assessment
  - Assess LOC.
  - Manage ABCs (airway, breathing, circulation).
  - Treat life-threatening illnesses/injuries.
  - Transport considerations: Transport patient in a position of comfort.
- Focused history and physical exam/secondary assessment
  - Obtain SAMPLE history and chief complaint (OPQRST).
  - Look for physical signs of chronic respiratory disease, such as barrel chest (emphysema), pursed-lip breathing (chronic bronchitis), and digital clubbing (chronic hypoxia) (**Figure 7-3**).

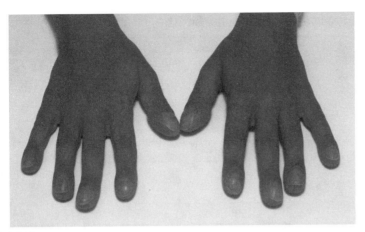

Figure 7-3 Digital clubbing.

- The tripod position (hands on knees with elbows facing outward) is often assumed by patients in respiratory distress.
  - Skin color: Cyanosis indicates desaturation or chronic obstructive disease.
- Jugular venous distention indicates heart failure, cardiac tamponade, pressure on the thorax, pneumothorax (especially tension pneumothorax), or chronic obstructive pulmonary disease (COPD).
- Distended liver indicates right-sided heart failure.
- Check for peripheral edema.

Positive Pressure Ventilation

- Methods of positive-pressure ventilation
  - Mouth-to-mask
  - Two-person bag-mask ventilation
  - Flow-restricted, oxygen-powered ventilation device
  - One-person bag-mask ventilation

Note: The methods are listed in order of preference, because research has demonstrated that personnel who ventilate patients infrequently have great difficulty maintaining an adequate seal between the mask and the patient's face.

Tip

Pathologic signs that a patient is using accessory muscles to assist breathing include the following:

- Bony retraction of the sternum or ribs with each breath (pediatric)
- Soft-tissue retractions around the ribs (adult)
- Nasal flaring on inhalation
- Tracheal tugging
- Asymmetric chest wall movement
- **Pulsus paradoxus**

Intubation

Endotracheal Tubes

- Cuffed tubes may be used in infants and children. However, as a general rule in the prehospital setting, uncuffed ET tubes are recommended in the emergent setting in patients younger than 8 years.

Endotracheal Tube Measurements

Table 7-2 lists ET tube measurements.

Table 7-2 Recommended Endotracheal Tube Sizes, by Age

Person	ET Tube Size	Suction Catheter Size (French)
Premature infant (< 1 kg)	2.5	5
Premature infant (1-2 kg)	3.0	5 or 6
Premature infant (2-3 kg)	3.0-3.5	6 or 8
0 months to 1 year (3-10 kg)	3.5-4.0	8

Continues

Table 7-2 Recommended Endotracheal Tube Sizes, by Age (Continued)

Person	ET Tube Size	Suction Catheter Size (French)
1 year (10-13 kg)	4.0	8
3 years (14-16 kg)	4.5	8-10
5 years (16-20 kg)	5.0	10
6 years (18-25 kg)	5.5	10
8 years (24-32 kg)	6.0 cuffed	10-12
12 years (32-54 kg)	6.5 cuffed	12
16 years (≥ 50 kg)	7.0 cuffed	12
Adult female	7.0 cuffed	12-14
Adult male	7.0-8.0 cuffed	14

Endotracheal Intubation Procedures

When you are unable to ventilate an unresponsive patient with basic life support methods, intubation is required. Intubation is the most definitive means of securing a patient's airway. Intubation involves passing the ET tube through the glottic opening and sealing the tube with a cuff inflated against the tracheal wall, or uncuffed in the case of infants. Endotracheal intubation is indicated when there is present or impending respiratory failure or the patient is unable to protect his or her own airway as a result of coma, decreased level of consciousness, or cardiac arrest.

- **Orotracheal intubation with direct laryngoscopy (Figure 7-4):** The glottic opening is visualized with a laryngoscope while the ET tube is being inserted. *This is the most common ET intubation method in the emergency setting.*
  - **Indications:** Used on any patient when there is a need for a definitive airway
  - **Contraindications:** Intact gag reflex
  - **Advantages:** Provides a definitive airway, prevents aspiration
  - **Disadvantages:** Difficult to perform correctly in patients with anatomic abnormalities, such as obesity or an anterior trachea
  - **Complications:** Unrecognized esophageal intubation resulting in death
- **Nasotracheal intubation:** The ET tube is passed into the trachea through the nasopharynx. Intubation is performed without the visualization of the glottis, hence the term "blind" nasotracheal intubation. Use on breathing patients to prevent a worsening of their condition and when direct laryngoscopy is contraindicated.

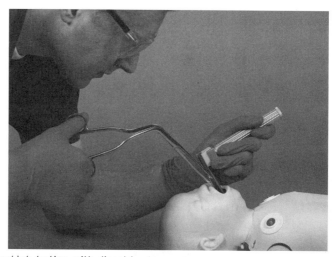

Figure 7-4 Orotracheal intubation with direct larynscopy.

- **Indications:** Patients with an intact gag reflex, in respiratory distress
  - **Contraindications:** Apneic patients; those with head trauma and possible midface fractures; basal skull fracture; blood-clotting disorders; patients taking blood-thinning medications (eg, Warfarin); in the event of anatomic abnormalities (deviated septum, nasal polyps) or frequent cocaine use
  - **Advantages:** Able to provide definitive airway placement in patients with intact gag reflex
  - **Disadvantages:** Nasal turbinate damage, uncontrollable nosebleed; may still cause gag reflex, emesis, and aspiration.
  - **Complications:** Epistaxis
- **Digital intubation (Figure 7-5):** Digital intubation is performed by placing the fingers of the intubator's hand into the patient's mouth, in an attempt to guide the ET tube into the trachea.
  - **Indications:** Patients without an intact gag reflex, who are unconscious
  - **Contraindications:** Patients who are alert and have an intact gag reflex
  - **Advantages:** Able to insert ET tube without need for direct visualization; useful in patients trapped in vehicles or in cases of equipment failure
  - **Disadvantages:** Possible esophageal intubation
  - **Complications:** Possible esophageal intubation, as well as the possibility of the patient becoming alert while an attempt is made, biting the fingers of the intubator
- **Transillumination technique (Figure 7-6):** Using a malleable fiberoptic stylet with a lighted tip, this method allows for intubation without the need for manipulating the head and neck or the need for direct visualization of the vocal cords.
  - **Indications:** Patients without an intact gag reflex, who are unconscious
  - **Contraindications:** Patients who are alert and have an intact gag reflex
  - **Advantages:** Able to insert ET tube without need for direct visualization; useful in patients trapped in vehicles or in cases of equipment failure

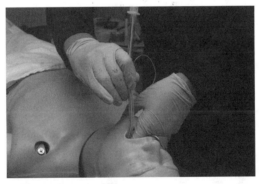

Figure 7-5 Digital intubation.

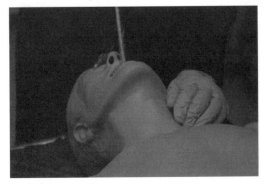

Figure 7-6 Transillumination technique.

- **Disadvantages:** Possible esophageal intubation
- **Complications:** Possible esophageal intubation

Rapid-Sequence Intubation

- Rapid-sequence intubation (RSI) refers to sedation and paralysis prior to an intubation procedure. Medications (see **Table 7-3**) are used to allow rapid placement of an ET tube between the vocal cords, while the cords are being visualized with the help of a laryngoscope. The neuromuscular blocking agents paralyze the patient's smooth muscles, especially the laryngeal muscles to prevent laryngospasm, and diaphragm.

  - **Indications:** Patients with an intact gag reflex who are in respiratory distress and need definitive airway management
  - **Contraindications:** None in the emergency setting
  - **Advantages:** Able to insert ET tube via direct visualization in a patient who had an intact gag reflex prior to paralytic administration
  - **Disadvantages:** Difficult to perform correctly in patients with anatomic abnormalities, such as obese patients and patients with an extremely anterior trachea
  - **Complications:** Unrecognized esophageal intubation resulting in potential death.

  It is important to remember that you now have a patient who is in respiratory arrest, requiring total ventilator support.

Table 7-3 Common Medications Used in Rapid-Sequence Intubation

Medication	Purpose	Initial Adult Dose	Initial Pediatric Dose
Etomidate	Short-acting nonbarbiturate hypnotic agent	IV: 0.2-0.3 mg/kg	IV: 0.2-0.3 mg/kg Not approved for patients < 10 years
Fentanyl	Short-acting opiate with short duration of action and no histamine release	IV: 25-100 µg/kg	IV: 2.0-10.0 µg/kg
Midazolam	Potent benzodiazepine, long-lasting amnesic with rapid onset	IV: 2.0-2.5 mg/kg	Not recommended for pediatric use
Lidocaine	May decrease intracranial pressure in potentially head-injured patients	IV: 1.0-1.5 mg/kg	IV: 1.0 mg/kg
Atropine	To counteract bradycardia; decreases secretions	IV: 0.5 mg	IV: 0.01 mg/kg in all patients younger than 3 years
Vecuronium	Nondepolarizing neuromascular blocker to prevent fasciculations	IV: 0.1 mg/kg; maintenance dose within 25-40 min: 0.01-0.05 mg/kg	IV: 0.1 mg/kg in all patients younger than 3 years; maintenance dose within 20-35 min: 0.01-0.05 mg/kg
Succinylcholine	Depolarizing neuromuscular blocker, with rapid onset, that causes complete short-term paralysis	IV: 1-2 mg/kg	IV: 1-1.5 mg/kg
Pancuronium	Long-lasting, nondepolarizing neuromuscular blocker	IV: 0.1 mg/kg	IV: 0.1 mg/kg
Rocuronium	Nondepolarizing neuromuscular blocker	IV: 0.5 mg/kg	IV: 0.5 mg/kg

Confirmation Techniques for Endotracheal Tube Placement

- Assess correct placement of the ET tube by three or more of the following methods:
  - Visualization of the tube passing through the vocal cords
  - Condensation in the ET tube with each breath
  - Positive waveform and CO_2 value, when using waveform capnography
  - Change in the CO_2 capnometry color
  - Negative aspiration via esophageal intubation detector or esophageal detector device
- Assess epigastric region for negative sounds, and bilateral lung fields for clear and equal breath sounds.

Alternative Airway Procedures

Needle Thoracostomy (Chest Needle Decompression)

Needle thoracostomy is an emergency procedure used to both diagnose and initially treat a tension pneumothorax.

- Indications
  - Tension pneumothorax
- Contraindications
  - None in the emergency setting

Procedure

Place a large-bore IV catheter needle between the second and third intercostal space. Insert the needle just above the third rib to avoid puncturing the intercostal vascular structures located underneath each rib.

Capnography

Continuous end-tidal CO_2 monitoring can confirm a tracheal intubation. A good waveform indicating the presence of CO_2 ensures that the ET tube is in the trachea.

In colorimetric capnography, a filter attached to an ET tube changes color from purple to yellow when it detects CO_2. This device has several drawbacks when compared with waveform capnography. It is not continuous; has no waveform, number, or alarms; is easily contaminated; is hard to read in the dark; and can give false readings.

Surgical Cricothyrotomy

A surgical cricothyrotomy is an incision made through the cricothyroid membrane to secure a patient's airway for emergency relief from an upper airway obstruction (**Figure 7-7**). It is a procedure that is usually performed as a last resort in cases where a definitive airway is needed and all other attempts at securing an airway have failed. Creating a surgical incision bypasses the upper airway, giving a direct path to the lower airway.

- Indications
  - Clenched teeth (making oral insertion of an ET tube impossible)
  - Severe cases of choking, such as a foreign body airway obstruction in the upper airway
  - Patient who needs airway management but cannot be intubated by the oral or nasal route
  - When the need for airway management exists, and basic airway techniques are ineffective
  - Significant facial trauma

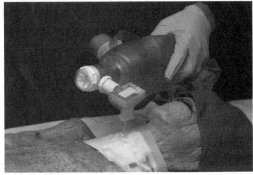

Figure 7-7 Surgical cricothyrotomy.

- Contraindications
  - Inability to identify landmarks (**cricothyroid membrane**)
  - Underlying anatomic abnormality (**tumor**)
  - Tracheal transection
  - Acute laryngeal disease caused by infection or trauma

Procedure

A surgical cricothyrotomy is generally performed by making an incision on the skin of the neck just below the thyroid cartilage, followed by another incision in the cricothyroid membrane, which lies deep to this point. An ET tube is then inserted to allow for ventilations.

Rescue Airways

Combitube

The Combitube is a dual-lumen device designed for use in emergency situations and difficult airways (**Figure 7-8**). It can be inserted without the need for visualization of the oropharynx and is designed to be inserted into the esophagus.

If the tube is inserted into the trachea, ventilation is achieved through the distal lumen as with a standard ET tube. More commonly, the device enters the esophagus and ventilation is via the proximal lumen, with oxygen entering the trachea through multiple openings situated above the distal cuff. The Combitube has a low-volume inflatable distal cuff and a much larger proximal cuff designed to occlude the oropharynx and nasopharynx.

- Indications
  - Ventilation in normal and abnormal airways
  - Failed intubation
  - Airway management in trapped patients
- Contraindications
  - Patients with intact gag reflexes
  - Patients with known esophageal pathology
  - Patients shorter than 4 feet (in such cases, use the Combitube SA [small adult])

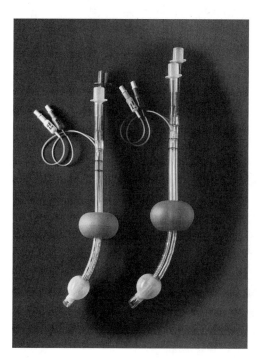

Figure 7-8 Combitube.

- Advantages
  - Requires minimal training
  - May be more useful in nonfasted patients
  - Successful passage and ventilation in many patients via the esophageal route
  - Portable, useful in remote settings
  - Functions in either the trachea or esophagus
- Disadvantages
  - Mostly adult sizes
  - Potential for esophageal trauma
  - Problems maintaining seal in some patients

KING LT-D Airway

The King airway is a single-lumen supraglottic device designed for use in emergency situations and difficult airways (**Figure 7-9**). It can be inserted without the need for visualization of the oropharynx, and is designed to be inserted into the esophagus.

Once the device is inserted into the esophagus, ventilation is accomplished via the single lumen, with oxygen entering the trachea through multiple openings situated above the distal cuff.

- Indications
  - Ventilation in normal and abnormal airways
  - Failed intubation
  - Airway management in trapped patients
- Contraindications
  - Patients with intact gag reflexes
  - Patients with known esophageal pathology
  - Patients shorter than 35"
- Advantages
  - Requires minimal training
  - May be more useful in nonfasted patients
  - Successful passage and ventilation in many patients via the esophageal route

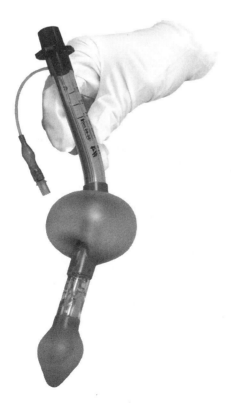

Figure 7-9 King airway.

– Available in a variety of sizes
– Portable, useful in remote settings
- Disadvantages
  – Potential for esophageal trauma
  – Problems maintaining seal in some patients

Types of Respiratory Problems
- Pulmonary edema (cardiogenic pulmonary edema, noncardiogenic pulmonary edema)
- Obstructive airway diseases (COPD, chronic bronchitis, emphysema, asthma)
- Acute respiratory distress syndrome
- Hyperventilation
- Hypoventilation

Pulmonary Edema

Pulmonary edema is caused by increased pulmonary capillary hydrostatic pressure and/or increased capillary permeability. Increased hydrostatic pressure leading to pulmonary edema may result from many causes, including excessive intravascular volume administration, pulmonary venous outflow obstruction, or left ventricular failure. There are two types of pulmonary edema: cardiogenic and noncardiogenic.

Cardiogenic Pulmonary Edema

In pulmonary circulation, a normal exchange of fluid occurs between the **interstitium** and the **vascular bed**. When there is an increase in pulmonary venous hydrostatic pressure, fluid is forced from the pulmonary capillaries into the interstitial spaces of the lungs and its tissues. This accumulation of fluid occurs when the venous return exceeds the left ventricular output; the interstitial spaces and/or the alveoli fill with low-protein fluids.

Cardiogenic pulmonary edema leads to progressive deterioration of alveolar gas exchange and acute respiratory failure. Without prompt recognition and treatment, patients deteriorate rapidly. The steps leading to cardiogenic pulmonary edema are as follows:

1. Ischemia causes left ventricular failure.
2. Increased ventricular pressure causes blood to back up into the left atrium. This action increases residual volume in the pulmonary vessels, which results in increased venous pressure in the pulmonary vessels.
3. The elevated venous pressure causes an increase in capillary hydrostatic pressure.
4. The pulmonary vessels become engorged and the fluid leaks into the interstitial space as a result of the elevated hydrostatic pressure.
5. This fluid accumulates and causes the interstitial space to expand.
6. Expansion impairs gas exchange, causing hypoxia.
7. Hypoxia worsens ischemia.

Noncardiogenic Pulmonary Edema

Noncardiogenic pulmonary edema results from changes in the permeability of the pulmonary capillary membrane as a result of either a direct or an indirect pathologic insult. The two major components that contribute to noncardiogenic pulmonary edema are elevated intravascular pressure and increased pulmonary capillary permeability.

- Causes of noncardiogenic pulmonary edema
  – Drowning
  – Fluid overload
  – Aspiration
  – Inhalation injury

- Allergic reaction
- Acute respiratory distress syndrome

Signs and Symptoms
- Tachypnea (rapid breathing)
- Tachycardia (rapid heart rate, > 100 beats/min)
- Jugular venous distention
- **Tripoding** (sitting in the tripod position with hands on knees to increase air intake)
  - Peripheral edema
  - Chest pain
  - Anxiety
- **Diaphoresis** (extreme sweating)
  - **Ascites**
  - Use of chest accessory muscles

Assessment
- Scene size-up
  - Ensure BSI.
- Initial/primary assessment
  - Assess LOC.
  - Manage ABCs.
  - Treat life-threatening illnesses/injuries.
  - Transport considerations: Transport patient in a position of comfort—usually upright with legs in a dependent position.
- Focused history and physical exam/secondary assessment
  - Obtain SAMPLE history and chief complaint (OPQRST).

Management
- Administer oxygen at 15 L/min via nonrebreathing mask.
- Reassure patient.
- Position semisitting, legs in dependent position
- Monitor vital signs.
- Encourage coughing.
- Establish cardiac monitoring.
- Establish IV access.

Table 7-4 summarizes the medications used to treat pulmonary edema.

Table 7-4 Initial Medications Used to Treat Pulmonary Edema

Treatment	Used for	Initial Adult Dose
Nitroglycerin	Vasodilation to reduce preload and afterload, improving cardiac output	SL: 0.4 mg
Furosemide	Vasodilation; increases lymphatic flow (drainage) from the lungs back into the circulatory system; eliminates excess fluid through renal system	IV: 0.5-1.0 mg/kg
Morphine sulfate	Vasodilation; decreases patient's anxiety, which increases the release of epinephrine, making the heart work harder	IV: 2-4 mg/kg
Dopamine infusion	In hypotensive patients, stimulates alpha-adrenergic receptors to contract vessel muscles and increases peripheral vascular resistance	IV: 2-20 µg/kg/min
Continuous positive airway pressure (CPAP)	Creates artificial positive end-expiratory pressure in an effort to maintain alveolar patency	5-10 cm H_2O

Chronic Obstructive Pulmonary Disease

Chronic obstructive pulmonary disease (COPD) is a general term for conditions that result in pulmonary obstruction that increases airway resistance. Two of the main conditions associated with COPD are chronic bronchitis and emphysema.

Pathophysiology of Chronic Bronchitis

Patients with **chronic bronchitis** are also known as "blue bloaters" because of their skin's blue appearance, resulting from an increase in arterial CO_2. Chronic bronchitis is characterized by excessive production of tracheobronchial mucus, chronic cough, and airflow obstruction. Chronic inflammation (or irritation) of the tracheobronchial tree leads to increased mucus production and a narrowed or blocked airway. As inflammation continues, goblet and epithelial cells hypertrophy. Because the body's natural defense mechanisms are blocked, debris accumulates in the respiratory tract.

Signs and Symptoms of Chronic Bronchitis
- Productive cough (due to hypersecretion of goblet cells)
- Dyspnea (due to obstruction of airflow to lower bronchus as the result of narrowed airways)
- Tachypnea, cyanosis
- Wheezing and rhonchi (due to narrow passageways)
- Prolonged expiration (a compensatory mechanism attempting to keep the alveoli patent)

Assessment of Chronic Bronchitis
- Scene size-up
  - Ensure BSI.
- Initial/primary assessment
  - Assess LOC.
  - Manage ABCs.
  - Treat life-threatening illness/injuries.
  - Transport considerations: Transport patient in a position of comfort.
- Focused history and physical exam/secondary assessment
  - Obtain SAMPLE history and chief complaint (OPQRST).

Management of Chronic Bronchitis
- Apply supplemental oxygen for respiratory distress.
- Reassure patient.
- Loosen restrictive clothing.
- Monitor vital signs.
- Encourage coughing.
- Apply cardiac monitor.
- Establish IV access.

Table 7-5 summarizes the initial medications used to treat COPD.

Table 7-5 Initial Medications Used to Treat COPD

Treatment	Used for	Initial Adult Dose
Albuterol	Bronchodilation; adrenergic effects	Nebulizer: 1.25-2.5 mg
Methylprednisolone	Anti-inflammatory	IV/IM: 1-2 mg/kg
Epinephrine	Vasoconstriction of the peripheral and bronchial vessels; increases contractility, rate, and overall cardiac output; smooth muscle relaxant	SQ: 0.3 mg

Table 7-5 Initial Medications Used to Treat COPD (Continued)

Treatment	Used for	Initial Adult Dose
Magnesium sulfate	Important for muscle contraction and nerve transmission	IV: 2 g
Levalbuterol	Asthma, emphysema, chronic bronchitis	Nebulizer: 1.25 mg
Terbutaline	Asthma, emphysema, chronic bronchitis	SQ: 0.25 mg

Pathophysiology of Emphysema

Patients with emphysema are commonly known as "pink puffers" because of their pink, frail appearance, attributed to an increase in red blood cell production. Emphysema is characterized by destruction of alveolar walls and a loss of elastic recoil in the lungs. Damage to the connective tissue structure in the terminal airways results in groups of alveoli merging into large blebs, or bullae, that are far less efficient and collapse more easily than normal lung tissue, causing obstruction. In these patients, breathing is stimulated by increased levels of CO_2.

Signs and Symptoms of Emphysema

- Anxiety, tachypnea, dyspnea (due to decreased oxygen levels)
- Use of accessory muscles (due to prolonged expiration)
- Barrel chest (due to hyperinflation of the lungs)
- Clubbed fingers and toes (due to chronic hypoxia) (Figure 7-3)
- Wheezing (due to bronchiolar collapse)
- Decreased or absent breath sounds
- *Note:* Although wheezing represents a problem, lack of wheezing, or a silent chest, can represent an even more dangerous patient situation, where air movement is so poor that wheezing is not possible.

Assessment of Emphysema

- Scene size-up
  - Ensure BSI.
- Initial/primary assessment
  - Assess LOC.
  - Manage ABCs.
  - Treat life-threatening illness/injuries.
  - Transport considerations: Transport patient in a position of comfort.
- Focused history and physical exam/secondary assessment
  - Obtain SAMPLE history and chief complaint (OPQRST).

Management of Emphysema

- Administer oxygen at 15 L/min via nonrebreathing mask for patients presenting at the point of death.
- Establish IV.
- Establish cardiac monitoring.
- Reassure patient.
- Encourage coughing in an attempt to ensure patent alveoli.

Table 7-6 summarizes the initial medications used to treat emphysema.

Table 7-6 Initial Medications Used to Treat Emphysema

Treatment	Used for	Initial Adult Dose
Albuterol	Bronchodilation; adrenergic effects	Nebulizer: 1.25-2.5 mg
Methylprednisolone	Anti-inflammatory	IV/IM: 1-2 mg/kg

Continues

Table 7-6 Initial Medications Used to Treat Emphysema (Continued)

Treatment	Used for	Initial Adult Dose
Epinephrine	Vasoconstriction of the peripheral and bronchial vessels; increases contractility, rate, and overall cardiac output; smooth muscle relaxant	SQ: 0.3 mg
Magnesium sulfate	Important for muscle contraction and nerve transmission	IV: 2 g
Levalbuterol	Asthma, emphysema, chronic bronchitis; relaxes bronchiole smooth muscles, helping to dilate them	Nebulizer: 1.25 mg
Terbutaline	Asthma, emphysema, chronic bronchitis; relaxes bronchiole smooth muscles, helping to dilate them	SQ: 0.25 mg
IV, intravenous; IM, intramuscular; SQ, subcutaneous		

Asthma

Pathophysiology

Bronchial asthma is characterized by increased reactivity of the trachea, bronchi, and bronchioles to a variety of stimuli. This hyperreactivity results in widespread, reversible narrowing of the airways, or bronchospasm.

The extrasensitive bronchial airway is easily irritated by **allergens**, dust, cold, smoke, or other triggers, which lead to bronchospasm, edema (swelling or inflammation) of the airways, as well as increased mucus production that can cause significant airway obstruction. Asthma most often occurs in children and young adults.

- Histamines attach to receptor sites in larger bronchi, causing contraction of the smooth muscles.
- Leukotrienes attach to the receptor sites in the smaller bronchi, also causing swelling and the release of prostaglandins into the bloodstream.
- Increased histamine levels in the blood stimulate the mucous membranes in the lungs to secrete excessive mucus, which causes a narrowing of the bronchial lumen.
- During inhalation the bronchi expand slightly, but during exhalation, they close completely. Mucus fills lung bases.
- Types of asthma
  - **Intrinsic asthma:** Can be triggered by irritants, emotional stress, fatigue, endocrine changes, temperature variations, humidity, fumes, or anxiety
  - **Extrinsic asthma:** Can be triggered by pollen, pet dander, dust, mold, feather pillows, or food additives containing sulfites, among other allergens
  - **Status asthmaticus:** An acute form of asthma that is defined as two or more acute attacks in rapid succession or a sustained attack; status asthmaticus is not responsive to initial treatment with inhaled bronchodilators because air movement is insufficient to carry the medication to the bronchioles.

Signs and Symptoms

- Bronchial constriction
  - Dyspnea
  - Wheezing
  - Tightness in chest
  - Diminished breath sounds
- Anxiety
- Excessive mucus production
- Diaphoresis (extreme sweating) and pallor
- Tripod position (sitting with hands on knees in order to breathe better)

- Hypertension
- Tachycardia (rapid heart rate, > 100 beats/min)
- Altered LOC
- Silent chest (late sign; lack of wheezing due to complete lack of air movement)
- Cyanosis (very late sign; bluish skin due to decreased blood oxygen levels)
- Extreme exhaustion
- Pulsus paradoxus

Assessment
- Scene size-up
  - Ensure BSI.
- Initial/primary assessment
  - Assess LOC.
  - Manage ABCs.
  - Treat life-threatening illnesses/injuries.
  - Transport considerations: Transport patient in a position of comfort.
- Focused history and physical exam/secondary assessment
  - Obtain SAMPLE history and chief complaint (OPQRST).

Management
- Administer oxygen at 15 L/min via nonrebreathing mask.
- Try to calm and reassure the patient.
- Monitor vital signs.
- Establish IV access.
- Attach cardiac monitor.

Table 7-7 summarizes the initial medications used to treat asthma.

Table 7-7 Initial Medications Used to Treat Asthma

Treatment	Used for	Initial Adult Dose	Initial Pediatric Dose
Albuterol	Bronchodilation; adrenergic effects	Nebulizer: 1.25-2.5 mg	Nebulizer: 2.5 mg (0.5 mL of the 0.083% solution) added to 2 mL of normal saline
Methylprednisolone	Anti-inflammatory	IV/IM: 1-2 mg/kg	IV: 1-2 mg/kg/dose
Epinephrine	Increases contractility, rate, and overall cardiac output; smooth muscle relaxant; dilates bronchioles; helps reverse allergic reactions	SQ: 0.3 mg	SQ: 0.01 mg/kg
Magnesium sulfate	Important for muscle contraction and nerve transmission	IV: 2 g	IV/10: 25-50 mg/kg
Levalbuterol	Asthma, emphysema, chronic bronchitis	Nebulizer: 1.25 mg	Nebulizer: 0.625 mg > 6 years, 1.25 mg
Terbutaline	Asthma, emphysema, chronic bronchitis	SQ: 0.25 mg	Not indicated for pediatric use
Ipratropium bromide	Asthma, emphysema, chronic bronchitis	Nebulizer: 500 µg	Safety and efficacy in children < 12 years not established for aerosol and solution

Acute Respiratory Distress Syndrome

Pathophysiology

- Acute respiratory distress syndrome (ARDS) is caused by diffuse damage to the alveoli that reduces normal gas exchange.

  ARDS may be caused by:
  - Indirect or direct lung trauma
  - Anaphylaxis
  - Aspiration of gastric contents
  - Diffuse pneumonia
  - Drug overdose
  - Inhalation of noxious gases
  - Near drowning
  - Oxygen toxicity
  - Sepsis
  - Spinal cord injury
  - Multiple trauma (usually does not present in the prehospital setting)

  - Platelets aggregate, releasing histamine, serotonin, and bradykinin, causing inflammation and damage to the alveolar-capillary membrane, resulting in an increase in capillary permeability.
  - Fluids shift into the interstitial space and proteins and fluids leak out, increasing interstitial osmotic pressure and causing pulmonary edema.
  - Decreased blood flow and oxygenation in the alveoli impairs the cells' ability to produce **surfactant**. As a result, the alveoli collapse, impairing gas exchange and oxygenation.
  - Inflammation and pulmonary edema worsen, leading to decreased gas exchange.
  - If not rapidly identified and treated, the patient's risk of mortality increases.

Signs and Symptoms

- Tachycardia, rapid and shallow breathing, dyspnea (due to decreased oxygen levels in blood)
- Tachypnea (due to hypoxemia and its effects on the pneumotaxic center)
- Intercostal and suprasternal retractions (due to increased effort to expand stiff lungs)
- Crackles and rhonchi (due to fluid accumulation in lungs)
- Altered LOC (due to hypoxia)

Assessment

- Scene size-up
  - Ensure BSI.
- Initial/primary assessment
  - Assess LOC.
  - Manage ABCs.
  - Treat life-threatening illness/injuries.
  - Transport considerations: Transport patient in a position of comfort.
- Focused history and physical exam/secondary assessment
  - Monitor vital signs.
  - Obtain SAMPLE history and chief complaint (OPQRST).

Management

- Administer oxygen at 15 L/min via nonrebreathing mask.
- Try to calm and reassure the patient.
- Establish IV access.
- Attach a cardiac monitor.
- Prepare for intubation if respiratory distress increases.

Table 7-8 summarizes the medications used to treat ARDS.

Table 7-8 Medications Used to Treat Acute Respiratory Distress Syndrome

Treatment	Used for	Initial Adult Dose	Initial Pediatric Dose
Albuterol	Bronchodilation; adrenergic effects	Nebulizer: 1.25-2.5 mg	Nebulizer: 2.5 mg (0.5 mL of the 0.083% solution added to 2 mL of normal saline)
Methylprednisolone	Anti-inflammatory	IV/IM: 1-2 mg/kg	IV: 1-2 mg/kg
Ipratropium bromide	Asthma, emphysema, chronic bronchitis	Nebulizer: 500 µg	Safety and efficacy in children < 12 years not established for aerosol and solution
Levalbuterol	Asthma, emphysema, chronic bronchitis	Nebulizer: 1.25 mg	Nebulizer: 0.625 mg > 6 years, 1.25 mg
Epinephrine	Vasoconstriction of the peripheral and bronchial vessels; increases contractility, rate, and overall cardiac output; smooth muscle relaxant	SQ: 0.3 mg	SQ: 0.01 mg/kg

Pulmonary Embolism

Pathophysiology

A pulmonary embolism is the blockage of a pulmonary artery, most commonly as a result of a thrombus or clot that has formed in the pelvis or leg vein, become dislodged, and traveled into the pulmonary arteries, blocking the blood flow distal to the obstruction. Causes include fat; tumor tissue; catheter shear; air or amniotic fluid; deep vein thrombosis; pelvic, renal, and hepatic vein thrombosis; right heart thrombosis; atrial fibrillation; heart failure; and/or valvular heart disease.

Risk factors include a sedentary lifestyle, sitting in the same position for extended periods of time (such as during travel), pregnancy, thrombophlebitis, oral contraceptive usage, pelvic and lower extremity fracture, recent surgery, or cancer.

Signs and Symptoms
- Sudden-onset pleuritic chest pain
- Pain may be localized or diffuse
- Anxiety
- Respiratory distress
- Tachypnea
- Hypoxemia
- Hemoptysis
- Cyanosis
- Loss of consciousness
- Distended neck veins
- Shock
- Cardiac arrest may result

Assessment
- Scene size-up
  - Ensure BSI.

- Initial/primary assessment
  - Assess LOC.
  - Manage ABCs.
  - Treat life-threatening illnesses/injuries.
  - Transport considerations: Transport patient in a position of comfort.
- Focused history and physical exam/secondary assessment
  - Obtain SAMPLE/OPQRST.

Management
- Administer supplemental oxygen via nonrebreathing mask at 12 to 15 L/min.
- Establish IV access.
- Monitor vital signs.
- Apply cardiac monitor.

Table 7-9 summarizes the medications used to treat pulmonary embolism.

Table 7-9 Medications Used to Treat Pulmonary Embolism

Treatment	Used for	Initial Adult Dose	Initial Pediatric Dose
Oxygen	Increase oxygenation	15 L/min	15 L/min

Hyperventilation

Pathophysiology

Hyperventilation leads to excessive blowing off of CO_2 during exhalation, which reduces blood levels of CO_2, increases blood pH, and leads to respiratory alkalosis.

Respiratory alkalosis is characterized by low hydrogen ion levels, low arterial partial pressure of CO_2 ($Paco_2$) (less than 35 mm Hg), high pH (greater than 7.45), high bicarbonate levels, and low carbonic acid levels. The excessive exhalation of CO_2 results in a carbonic acid deficit. The drop in $Paco_2$ (**hypocapnia**) also causes a reduction in carbonic acid production and a loss of hydrogen ions and bicarbonate ions, which in turn causes the increase in blood pH.

When blood pH is high, hydrogen ions are pulled from the cells into the blood in exchange for potassium ions. The hydrogen ions entering the blood combine with bicarbonate ions to form carbonic acid, which causes the pH to drop. Hypocapnia stimulates the aortic and carotid bodies and the medulla, which causes an increase in heart rate without increasing the blood pressure.

In first-degree hyperventilation, decreased $Paco_2$ causes vasoconstriction, which results in a reduction of cerebral blood flow. Over time, the kidneys increase secretion of bicarbonate and reduce the excretion of hydrogen, creating a compensatory metobolic acidosis. Severe alkalosis can result. Lack of calcium ionization causes increased nerve excitability and muscle contractions.

Hyperventilation can be caused by anxiety, but it is important to consider serious conditions as well. Hyperventilation often occurs to create respiratory alkalosis as compensation for metabolic acidosis. Causes of metabolic acidosis include myocardial infarction, pulmonary embolism, certain drugs and toxins, infection, and diabetic ketoacidosis.

Signs and Symptoms
- Chest pain/palpitation
- Dizziness
- Paresthesia of fingers and toes
- Tightness or a lump in throat
- Tachycardia
- Carpopedal spasm
- Altered mental status
- Tachypnea

> **Tip**
>
> Medications associated with a high risk of hyperventilation include:
> - Cocaine
> - Amphetamines
> - Aspirin overdose
> - Epinephrine

Assessment

- Scene size-up
  - Ensure BSI.
- Initial/primary assessment
  - Assess LOC.
  - Manage ABCs.
  - Treat life-threatening illnesses/injuries.
  - Transport considerations: Transport patient in a position of comfort.
- Focused history and physical exam/secondary assessment
  - Obtain SAMPLE history and chief complaint (OPQRST).
  - Look for treatable causes of hyperventilation, such as diabetic ketoacidosis.

Management

- Use careful psychological support and coaching to slow the patient's breathing.
- The goal of treatment is to maximize and optimize oxygen intake. Encourage the patient to take deep, slow breaths.
- Apply oxygen at 15 L/min via nonrebreathing mask in an attempt to balance oxygen and CO_2 levels.

Hypoventilation

Pathophysiology

<u>Respiratory acidosis</u> occurs when exhalation of CO_2 is inhibited as a result of hypoventilation, such as in CNS depression or obstructive lung disease. Retention of CO_2 leads to an increase in hydrogen ion levels and in Pa_{CO_2} (> 45 mm Hg). The result is a lowered pH and an increase in carbonic acid. As pH levels drop, hemoglobin releases O_2. The CO_2 reacts with water to form carbonic acid. CO_2, along with the free hydrogen ions, stimulates the respiratory center to increase the respiratory rate to expel more CO_2 and helps reduce the CO_2 level in the blood and tissue.

Carbon dioxide and hydrogen ions dilate cerebral blood vessels, increasing blood flow to the brain. This increased blood flow can worsen cerebral edema. But as the respiratory mechanism fails, the increasing Pa_{CO_2} triggers the kidneys to conserve bicarbonate and sodium ions and to excrete hydrogen ions. Two major causes of hypoventilation are CNS depression and obstructive lung diseases. Other causes include respiratory depression, respiratory or cardiac arrest, neuromuscular impairment, medications (sedatives, hypnotics), chest wall injury, COPD, foreign body airway obstruction, and pulmonary edema.

Signs and Symptoms

- Shallow, inefficient respirations
- Altered LOC
- Cyanosis
- Tachycardia
- Hypoxemia
- Hypercapnia

Assessment

- Scene size-up
  - Ensure BSI.
- Initial/primary assessment
  - Assess LOC.
  - Manage ABCs.
  - Treat life-threatening illnesses/injuries.
  - Transport considerations: Transport patient in a position of comfort.

- Focused history and physical exam/secondary assessment
  - Obtain SAMPLE history and chief complaint (OPQRST).
  - Look for correctible causes of hypoventilation, such as diabetes, overdose, and head injury.

Management
- Assess the patient's Glasgow Coma Scale score. If an adult has a score of 8 or less, consider intubation; in pediatric patients, a score of less than 10 also warrants aggressive measures.
- Administer oxygen at 15 L/min via bag-mask ventilation at 12 to 20 breaths/min.
- Establish IV access.
- Correct reversible causes of hypoventilation.

Adult Respiratory Pharmacology

Table 7-10 through **Table 7-15** list various medications used for respiratory emergencies.

Table 7-10 Gases

Drug	Trade Name	Used for	Initial Adult Dosage
Oxygen (O_2)	N/A	Correction of hypoxia, hypoxemia, or any O_2-deficient conditions	Nasal cannula: 1 to 6 L/min Nonrebreathing mask: 12-15 L/min Bag-mask ventilation: 12-15 L/min

Table 7-11 Adrenergics

Drug	Trade Name	Used for	Initial Adult Dosage	Initial Pediatric Dosage
Epinephrine	Adrenaline	Asthma, emphysema, chronic bronchitis	SQ: 0.3 mg	SQ: 0.01 mg/kg
Racemic epinephrine	Micronefrin, Vaponefrin	Croup	Inhalation: 2-3 inhalations, repeated every 5 min PRN	Inhalation: 0.25-0.75 mL of a 2.5% solution in 2.5 mL normal saline
SQ, subcutaneous; PRN, as needed				

Table 7-12 Bronchodilators

Drug	Trade Name	Used for	Initial Adult Dosage	Initial Pediatric Dosage
Albuterol	Ventolin	Asthma, emphysema, chronic bronchitis	Nebulizer: 2.5 mg in 2.5 mL normal saline (NS) every 4-6 hr	Nebulizer: 2.5mg (0.5 mL of the 0.083% solution added to 2 mL of normal saline)
Terbutaline (beta-2 agonist)	Brethine	Asthma, emphysema, chronic bronchitis	SQ: 0.25 mg	Not indicated for pediatric use
Metaproterenol (adrenergic)	Alupent	Asthma, emphysema, chronic bronchitis	Nebulizer: 0.2-0.3 mL in 2.5 mL NS	Not indicated for pediatric use
Levalbuterol	Xopenex	Asthma, emphysema, chronic bronchitis	Nebulizer: 1.25 mg	Nebulizer: 0.63 mg

Table 7-13 Anticholinergics

Drug	Trade Name	Used for	Initial Adult Dosage	Initial Pediatric Dosage
Ipratropium bromide	Atrovent	Asthma, emphysema, chronic bronchitis	Nebulizer: 500 µg	Safety and efficacy in children < 12 years not established for aerosol and solution

Table 7-14 Anti-inflammatories

Drug	Trade Name	Used for	Initial Adult Dose	Initial Pediatric Dose
Methylprednisolone	Solu-Medrol	Asthma, emphysema, chronic bronchitis; to decrease inflammation	IV: 1-2 mg/kg	IV: 1-2 mg/kg
Dexamethasone	Decadron	Allergic reactions	SIVP: 1 mg/kg	IV: 0.25-1.0 mg/kg
Hydrocortisone	Solu-Cortef	Asthma, emphysema, chronic bronchitis	IV: 4 mg/kg	IV: 0.16-1.0 mg/kg

Table 7-15 Electrolytes

Drug	Trade Name	Treatment of	Initial Adult Dosage	Initial Pediatric Dosage
Magnesium sulfate	Magnesium sulfate	Asthma, emphysema, chronic bronchitis	IV: 2 g	IV: 25-50 mg/kg

Vital Vocabulary

adenoids Lymphatic tissues located on the posterior nasopharyngeal wall that filter bactreia.

allergens Substances that cause a hypersensitivity reaction.

apneustic center Portion of the brainstem that influences the respiratory rate by increasing the number of inspirations per minute.

ascites Abnormal accumulation of fluid in the peritoneal cavity.

carina Point at which the trachea divides into the left and right mainstem bronchi.

chronic bronchitis Chronic inflammatory condition affecting the bronchi that is associated with excess mucus production that results from overgrowth of the mucous glands in the airways.

cricothyroid membrane A thin, superficial membrane located between the thyroid and cricoid cartilages that is relatively avascular and contains few nerves; the site for emergency surgical and nonsurgical access to the airway.

diaphoresis Extreme sweating.

glottis The space in between the vocal chords that is the narrowest portion of the adult's airway; also called the glottic opening.

hilum Point of entry of all of the blood vessels and the bronchi into each lung.

hypocapnia Decreased carbon dioxide content in arterial blood.

interstitium An area of tissue between the alveoli and capillaries that allows for exchange of oxygen, nutrients, and waste to occur. During inspiration, the alveoli expand with air, and the interstitium stretches into a very thin layer, allowing for diffusion.

larynx A complex structure formed by many independent cartilaginous structures that all work together; where the upper airway ends and the lower airway begins.

medulla Continuous inferiorly with the spinal cord; serves as a conduction pathway for ascending and descending nerve tracts; coordinates heart rate, blood vessel diameter, breathing, swallowing, vomiting, coughing, and sneezing. Also refers to part of the internal anatomy of the kidney, namely, the middle layer.

pneumotaxic center Area of the brainstem that has an inhibitory influence on inspiration.

pons The portion of the brainstem that lies below the midbrain and contains nerve fibers that affect sleep and respiration.

pulmonary edema Congestion of the pulmonary air spaces with exudate and foam, often secondary to left-sided heart failure.

pulsus paradoxus A drop in the systolic blood pressure of 10 mm Hg or more; commonly seen in patients with pericardial tamponade or severe asthma.

respiratory acidosis A condition that occurs when exhalation of carbon dioxide is inhibited as a result of hypoventilation due to central nervous system depression or obstructive lung disease. Carbon dioxide retention leads to an increase in hydrogen ion levels and Pa_{CO_2} (> 45 mm Hg). The results are lowered pH and an increase in carbonic acid.

respiratory alkalosis A condition in which the amount of carbon dioxide found in the blood drops to a level below normal range. This condition produces a shift in the body's pH balance and causes the body's system to become more alkaline (basic). This condition is brought on by rapid, deep breathing called hyperventilation.

rhythmicity area Portion of the medulla oblongata that controls inspiratory and expiratory phases.

surfactant A liquid protein substance that coats the alveoli in the lungs, decreases alveolar surface tension, and keeps the alveoli expanded.

tripoding An abnormal position to keep the airway open; involves leaning forward with the hands on the knees with elbows facing outward.

tumor An abnormal anatomic mass or growth, resulting from uncontrolled cell division.

turbinates Three bony shelves that protrude from the lateral walls of the nasal cavity and extend into the nasal passageway, parallel to the nasal floor; serve to increase the surface area of the nasal mucosa, thereby improving the processes of warming, filtering, and humidifying inhaled air.

uvula A soft-tissue structure located in the posterior aspect of the oral cavity.

vallecula An anatomic space or "pocket" located between the base of the tongue and the epiglottis; an important anatomic landmark for endotracheal intubation.

vascular bed Describes the blood vessels of a particular organ.

CHAPTER 8

Cardiovascular Emergencies

The cardiovascular system consists of the heart and blood vessels. It transports blood to all parts of the body in two circulations: pulmonary (lungs) and systemic (the rest of the body). It also delivers oxygenated blood and nutrients to the cells, moves chemicals around, and transports the waste products of cell metabolism back to the lungs for excretion. Understanding the cardiovascular system is essential to understanding its link to airway management.

The Cardiovascular System

The Heart

The heart is a hollow, muscular organ surrounded by a tough, fibrous, fluid-containing sac called the **pericardium**. Located in the left chest above the diaphragm, the heart consists of three distinct layers:

- **Epicardium**: Thin, external membrane
- **Endocardium**: Innermost layer of smooth connective tissue
- **Myocardium**: Muscular layer between the epicardium and endocardium, consisting of the cardiac muscle

The heart consists of four chambers (**Figure 8-1**). The upper chambers are the right **atrium** (RA) and left atrium (LA). The lower chambers are the right **ventricle** (RV) and left ventricle (LV). The right side of the heart consists of the right atrium and right ventricle; the left side of the heart consists of the left atrium and left ventricle. The atria are reservoirs that act as a forward pump for blood being sent to the ventricles. The ventricles are the main pumping chambers of the heart.

The heart has four valves that open and close passively in response to pressure changes in the heart. The atria are separated from the ventricles by two atrioventricular (AV) valves:

- **Tricuspid valve** between the RA and RV
- **Bicuspid (or mitral) valve** between the LA and LV

The other two valves are the semilunar valves (named because of their half-moon shape):

- **Pulmonic valve** between the RV and the pulmonary artery
- **Aortic valve** between the LV and the aorta

Each of these two valves acts as a one-way door preventing the backflow of blood into the pumping chamber.

Circulation

It is important to be familiar with how blood flows through the heart to understand the overall function of the heart and how changes in electrical activity affect peripheral blood flow.

Deoxygenated blood from the body returns to the heart via the superior and inferior vena cava and empties into the RA. Deoxygenated blood is pumped from the RA through the tricuspid valve into the RV, which then pumps it through the pulmonic valve into the pulmonary artery. This deoxygenated blood passes into the lungs from the pulmonary artery and is distributed through the pulmonary circulation system, contacting alveoli and

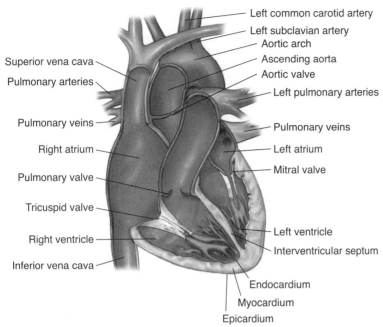

Figure 8-1 Anatomy of the heart.

exchanging gases. The pulmonary vein carries newly oxygenated blood from the lungs back to the heart, into the LA, which pumps it through the mitral (bicuspid) valve into the LV. The LV pumps this oxygenated blood through the aortic valve into the aorta and then to the capillary beds throughout the whole body for gas exchange.

Blood supply to the heart is provided by the right and left coronary arteries, which arise from the aorta, just above and behind the aortic valve.

Blood Vessels

The blood vessels constitute the vascular component of the cardiovascular system (**Figure 8-2**).

Arteries

<u>Arteries</u> are the vessels responsible for carrying blood from the heart to body tissues.

- Arteries serve as pressure reservoirs when the elastic walls contract inward during ventricular diastole (less blood in the arteries).
- Blood pressure averages 120 mm Hg during systole (systolic pressure) and 80 mm Hg during diastole (diastolic pressure).
- Pulse pressure is the difference between systolic and diastolic pressures.

Arterioles

<u>Arterioles</u> are small arteries that distribute cardiac output among systemic organs. Vasodilation and vasoconstriction in these vessels regulate blood flow. Factors that influence the diameter of arterioles are as follows:

- **Intrinsic (or local) control:** Changes *within* a tissue that alter the radius of blood vessels and adjust blood flow. Increased blood flow in an active tissue results from active hyperemia, the increase in organ blood flow that is associated with increased metabolic activity of an organ or tissue.
- **Extrinsic control:** The sympathetic division of the nervous system innervates blood vessels throughout the body. The parasympathetic division innervates blood vessels of the external genitals. Varying degrees of stimulation of these two divisions, therefore, can influence arterioles (and blood flow) throughout the body.

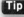

Tip

Remember, pulmonary arteries are the only arteries that carry *de*oxygenated blood, and pulmonary veins are the only veins that carry oxygenated blood.

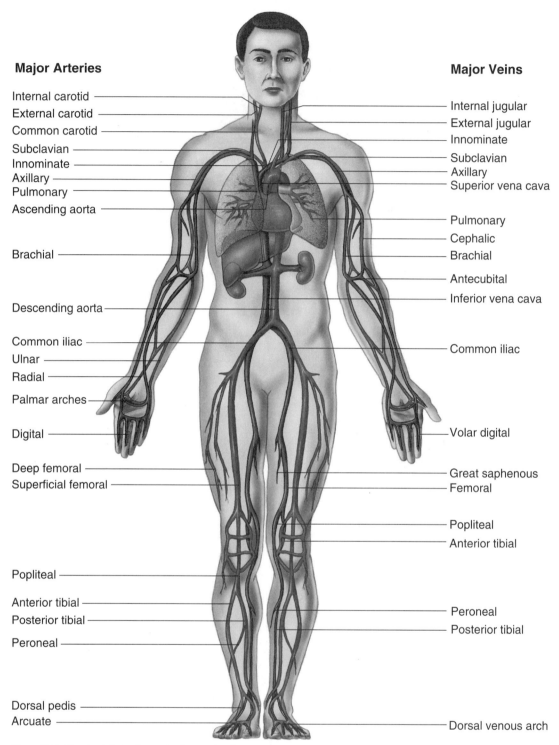

Major Arteries

- Internal carotid
- External carotid
- Common carotid
- Subclavian
- Innominate
- Axillary
- Pulmonary
- Ascending aorta
- Brachial
- Descending aorta
- Common iliac
- Ulnar
- Radial
- Palmar arches
- Digital
- Deep femoral
- Superficial femoral
- Popliteal
- Anterior tibial
- Posterior tibial
- Peroneal
- Dorsal pedis
- Arcuate

Major Veins

- Internal jugular
- External jugular
- Innominate
- Subclavian
- Axillary
- Superior vena cava
- Pulmonary
- Cephalic
- Brachial
- Antecubital
- Inferior vena cava
- Common iliac
- Volar digital
- Great saphenous
- Femoral
- Popliteal
- Anterior tibial
- Peroneal
- Posterior tibial
- Dorsal venous arch

Figure 8-2 The body's major arteries and veins.

Veins

The **veins** are responsible for returning deoxygenated blood and waste products from the tissues (and oxygenated blood from the lungs) to the heart. In resting conditions, nearly two thirds of all blood is in the veins. Veins play an important role in regulating stroke volume, or the volume of the blood pumped from a ventricle of the heart with each beat.

Venules

A *venule* is a small blood vessel that allows deoxygenated blood to return from the capillary beds to the larger veins.

Capillaries

The exchange of gases and nutrients between blood and tissues takes place in minute blood vessels called **capillaries**. The walls of capillaries are extremely thin (only one cell thick), and the diameter of a capillary is so small that red blood cells must pass through it single file.

Exchange of gases and nutrients occurs through:

- Pores between the cells that form the capillary walls.
- Vesicular transport: Mechanism for transcellular transport in which the cell encloses extracellular material in an invagination (opening) of the cell membrane to form a vesicle (cavity). The vesicle then moves through the cell to eject the material through the opposite cell membrane by reversing the process of vesicle formation.
- Bulk flow: The tendency of fluid to move through the pores. The rate of fluid moving through the pores is affected by a variety of factors, such as pore size, contraction of epithelial cells, and the number of pores.

Blood Flow

The *flow rate through blood vessels* is determined by pressure and resistance.

- **Pressure gradient:** Difference in pressure between beginning and end of vessel. (Pressure is the force exerted by blood against the vessel wall and is measured in millimeters of mercury.)
- **Resistance:** Impedance to blood flow in a vascular network. Resistance depends on the size of the vessel or vascular network and the viscosity of the blood.

Pressure gradient and resistance are directly proportional. If resistance goes up, the pressure gradient goes up.

The Heart at Work

- **Cardiac output (CO):** The amount of blood that is pumped out by either ventricle. The left and right ventricles are approximately equal in interior size, so the two ventricles have relatively equivalent outputs. Normal CO for an average adult is 5 to 6 L/min.
- **Stroke volume (SV):** The amount of blood pumped out by either ventricle in a single contraction (heartbeat). Normally, the SV is 60 to 100 mL, but the healthy heart has considerable spare capacity and can easily increase SV by at least 50%.
- **Heart rate (HR):** The number of cardiac contractions (heartbeats) per minute—in other words, the pulse rate. The normal HR for adults is 60 to 100 beats/min.

To meet changing demands, the heart must be able to increase its output several times over in response to the body's increased demand for oxygen.

The heart has several ways of increasing SV. When cardiac muscle is stretched, it contracts with greater force to a limit—a property called the **Frank-Starling mechanism**. If an increased volume of blood is returned from the systemic veins to the right side of the heart or from the pulmonary veins to the left side of the heart, the muscle surrounding the cardiac chambers must stretch to accommodate the larger volume. The more the cardiac muscle stretches, the greater the force of its contraction, the more completely it empties, and, therefore, the greater the SV.

The pressure under which a ventricle fills is called the **preload**. Preload is influenced by the volume of blood returned by the veins to the heart. In situations of increased oxygen demand, the body returns more blood to the heart (preload increases), and CO consequently increases through the Frank-Starling mechanism.

The heart can also vary the degree of contraction of its muscle *without* changing the stretch on the muscle—a property called **contractility**. Changes in contractility may be induced by medications that have a positive or negative inotropic effect. The ventricles are never completely emptied of blood with any single beat. However, if the heart squeezes into a tighter ball when it contracts, a larger percentage of the ventricular blood will be ejected, thereby increasing SV and overall CO. Nervous controls regulate the contractility of the heart from beat to beat. When the body requires increased CO, nervous signals increase myocardial contractility, thereby augmenting SV.

The heart can also increase its CO, given a constant SV, by increasing the number of contractions per minute—that is, by increasing the HR (positive chronotropic effect).

The Frank-Starling mechanism is an intrinsic property of heart muscle—that is, it is not under nervous system control. By contrast, contractility and changes in HR are regulated by the nervous system.

Autonomic Nervous System

The heart is supplied by two branches of the **autonomic nervous system**:

- Sympathetic (or adrenergic) nervous system
  - Accelerates the heart
  - Influenced by the chemicals epinephrine and norepinephrine, which increase heart rate, contractibility, automaticity, and AV conduction
- Parasympathetic (or cholinergic) nervous system
  - Slows heart rate and AV conduction through stimulation of the vagus nerve

The Heart's Electrical Conduction System

There are two types of cardiac cells: contractile and autorhythmic. **Autorhythmic cells** are distributed in an orderly fashion through the heart. They make up the heart's normal conduction system and are concentrated in the sinoatrial (SA) node, AV node, AV bundle (bundle of His), and Purkinje fibers (**Figure 8-3**). The properties of autorhythmic cells include:

- **Automaticity:** The ability to spontaneously generate and discharge an electrical impulse; if cell automaticity is increased or decreased, an arrhythmia can occur
- **Excitability:** The ability to respond to an electrical impulse
- **Conductivity:** The ability to transmit an electrical impulse from one cell to the next

Contractile cells make up the muscle walls of the atria and ventricles. They give the heart its ability to pump blood through the body. Contractile cell properties include:

- **Contractility:** The ability to contract, or shorten and lengthen their fibers, when stimulated
- **Extensibility:** The ability to stretch
- Depolarization and repolarization (discussed in the upcoming section)

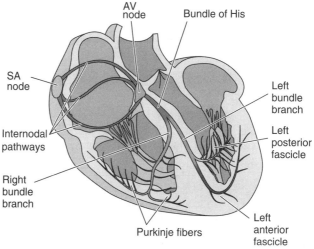

Figure 8-3 The heart's electrical conduction system.

Sinoatrial Node

The **sinoatrial (SA) node**, or **sinus node**, is a group of cells in the wall of the right atrium, near the inlet of the superior vena cava, that serves as the primary pacemaker of the heart. It has the fastest rate of the autorhythmic cells associated with the normal conduction pathway, and sets the pace of contraction for the entire heart. For that reason, the term "pacemaker" generally refers to the SA node.

The *inherent firing rate* is the rate at which the SA node or another pacemaker site normally generates electrical impulses, about 60 to 100 beats per minute. As the electrical impulse leaves the SA node, it is conducted through the left atrium by way of the Bachmann bundle, through the right atrium via the atrial tracts.

Atrioventricular Junction

Electric impulses generated in the SA node spread across the two atria through the internodal pathways (including the Bachmann bundle) in the atrial wall, causing the atrial tissue to depolarize as they pass. From there, they move to the **atrioventricular (AV) node** in the region of the AV junction. The AV junction consists of the AV node and **bundle of His**.

Impulses pass through the AV junction into the bundle of His and then move rapidly into the right and left bundle branches located on either side of the interventricular septum. Next, they spread into the **Purkinje fibers**, thousands of fibrils distributed through the ventricular muscle.

Depolarization and Repolarization

Cardiac cells at rest are considered *polarized*, meaning there is a charge differential between the inside and the outside of the cell (*resting potential*). The cell membrane of the cardiac muscle cell separates different concentrations of ions, such as sodium, potassium, and calcium. Electrical impulses are generated by the automaticity of specialized cardiac cells. This electrical impulse causes the ions to cross the cell membrane, resulting in an *action potential*. The movement of ions across the cell membrane through sodium, potassium, and calcium channels is the drive that causes contraction of the cardiac cells or muscle. **Depolarization** is the process by which the muscle fibers are stimulated to contract. It is very rapid, is caused by the inward diffusion of sodium, and moves as a wave through the heart (**Figure 8-4**).

Repolarization is the return of the ions to their previous resting state, which corresponds with the relaxation of the myocardial muscle. It results from the outward diffusion of potassium.

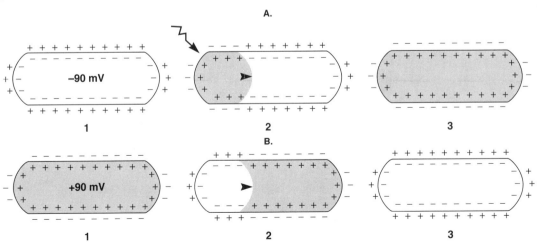

Figure 8-4 Depolarization and repolarization. **A.** Depolarization. (1) At rest, the cellular interior has a net charge of –90 mV. (2) The wave of depolarization begins as sodium ions pour into the cell. (3) Depolarized cell. **B.** Repolarization. (1) Depolarized cell. (2) The wave of repolarization begins as potassium ions leave the cell. (3) Repolarized cell.

Depolarization and repolarization are electrical activities that cause muscular activity. The action potential curve shows the electrical changes in the myocardial cell during the depolarization-repolarization cycle. This electrical activity is what is detected on an electrocardiogram (ECG), not the muscular activity.

The Cardiac Cycle

The **cardiac cycle** is the period from the end of one cardiac contraction to the end of the next. It consists of two phases: **systole** (contraction) and **diastole** (relaxation) (**Figure 8-5**).

- Atrial systole
  - Increase in ventricular volume because blood from the atria is pumped into the ventricles (to preload ventricles).
- Atrial diastole
  - Blood passively fills the atria and ventricles (after ventricular systole).
- Ventricular systole
  - The first heart sound (lub), S_1, is generated by the closing of the AV valves due to increasing pressure in the ventricles.
- Ventricular diastole
  - The second heart sound (dub), S_2, is generated by the closing of the semilunar valves, which occurs when pressure in the pulmonary trunk and aorta is greater than in the ventricles; the blood in those vessels moves toward the area of lower pressure, which closes the valves.

Electrical events are correlated with mechanical events:

- P wave = atrial depolarization = atrial systole
- QRS complex = ventricular depolarization = ventricular systole (atrial diastole occurs at the same time)
- T wave = ventricular repolarization = ventricular diastole

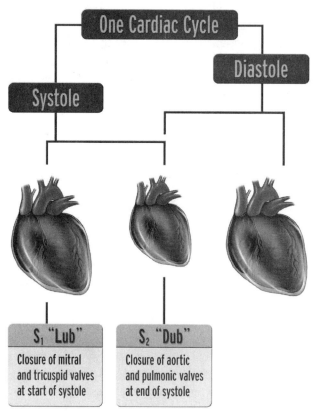

Figure 8-5 One cardiac cycle.

Action Potential

The action potential curve consists of five phases, 0 to 4:

- Phase 0, upstroke, is characterized by a sharp, tall upstroke of the action potential. The cell receives an impulse from a neighboring cell and depolarizes. During this phase the cell depolarizes and begins to contract.
- In phase 1, spike, contraction is in process. The cell begins an early, rapid, partial repolarization.
- In phase 2, plateau, contraction completes and the cell begins to relax. This is a prolonged phase of slow repolarization.
- Phase 3, downslope, is the final phase of rapid repolarization. Repolarization is complete by the end of this phase.
- Phase 4, rest, is a return to the rest period. It is the period between action potentials.

Refractory and Supernormal Periods

After the atria and ventricles have contracted, the muscles normally enter refractory periods, referred to as the absolute refractory, relative refractory, and supernormal periods.

- The refractory period begins with an absolute period characterized by a brief (1–2 msec) period in which no stimulus, no matter how strong, can result in another contraction.
- The absolute refractory period is marked by the onset of a Q wave and ends at the peak of the T wave. The absolute refractory period is followed by a relative refractory period.
- During the relative refractory period, the cell has been partially repolarized and can respond to a very strong stimulus (also referred to as the vulnerable period of repolarization). The relative refractory period corresponds with the downslope of the T wave.
- During the supernormal period, the myocardial cells will respond to a weaker than normal stimulus (despite being in a refractory period). The period is seen at the end of the T wave, just before the cell returns from its resting period.
- The supernormal period extends the relative refractory period and is generally not seen in healthy hearts.

Ectopic Beats and Arrhythmias

Any cardiac impulse originating outside the SA node is considered abnormal and is referred to as an **ectopic beat**. Ectopic beats can originate in the atria, the AV junction, or the ventricles and are named according to their point of origin. Rate suppression can occur following an ectopic beat, but after several cycles the heart rate returns to normal. A series of three or more consecutive ectopic beats is considered to be an ectopic rhythm.

The three causes of ectopic beats are as follows:

- Failure or excessive slowing of the SA node
  - Ectopic beats resulting from SA node failure serve a protective function by initiating a cardiac impulse before prolonged cardiac standstill can occur. These beats are called *escape beats*.
  - If the SA node fails to resume normal function, the ectopic site will assume the role of pacemaker and sustain a cardiac rhythm, referred to as an *escape rhythm*.
  - After the SA node resumes normal function, the escape foci are suppressed.
- Premature activation of another cardiac site
  - Impulses occur prematurely before the SA node recovers enough to initiate another beat. These beats are called *premature beats*.
- Abnormal conduction system
  - Wolff-Parkinson-White syndrome.
  - Ischemia.

Diseases of the Heart

Congestive Heart Failure

Congestive heart failure (CHF), left sided or right sided, occurs when the heart is unable, for any reason, to pump forcefully enough or fast enough to empty its chambers. Circulatory or pulmonary congestion results as blood backs up into the systemic circuit, the pulmonary circuit, or both. CHF ranges from mild to severe and may be chronic or acute. It can be caused by hypertension, drug use, thyroid disease, and coronary artery disease (CAD), independent or dependent of acute myocardial infarction (AMI).

Left-Sided Congestive Heart Failure

Pathophysiology

In left-sided congestive heart failure, the left side of the heart fails to pump, causing congestion in the lungs. The congestion in the pulmonary veins, pulmonary capillaries, and alveoli causes pulmonary edema, resulting in crackles, hypoxia, and hypotension.

Signs and Symptoms

- Altered level of consciousness (LOC)
- Dyspnea, orthopnea, paroxysmal nocturnal dyspnea
- Wheezing
- Chest pain
- Headache
- Pink, frothy sputum
- Rales (crackles)
- Weakness, anxiety
- Tachycardia
- Cyanosis
- Diaphoresis
- Jugular venous distention (JVD), positive hepatojugular reflex, hepatomegaly (due to venous congestion)
- Right upper quadrant pain (due to liver engorgement)
- Anorexia, fullness, and nausea (due to congestion of liver and intestines)
- Nocturia (nocturnal fluid redistribution and reabsorption)
- Weight gain, edema (due to fluid-volume excess)
- Ascites or anasarca (from fluid retention)

Assessment

- Scene size-up
  - Ensure body substance isolation (BSI).
  - Leave patient in a position of comfort (usually upright).
- Initial/primary assessment
  - Manage ABCs.
  - Monitor LOC.
  - Treat life-threatening illness/injuries.
  - Transport considerations: Transport patient in a position of comfort.
- Focused history and physical exam/secondary assessment
  - Obtain SAMPLE history and chief complaint (OPQRST).

Management

- Monitor vital signs.
- Apply pulse oximeter and supplemental oxygen.
- Attach cardiac monitor.
- Establish IV access.
- Administer oxygen at 15 L/min via nonrebreathing mask.
- Consider administration of a loop diuretic, such as furosemide or bumetanide.

Right-Sided Congestive Heart Failure

Pathophysiology

In right-sided CHF, ineffective right ventricular contractility leads to reduced right ventricular pumping ability and decreased cardiac output to the lungs. As a result, blood backs up in the right atrium and peripheral circulation, disrupting the excretion of sodium and water by the kidneys and causing weight gain, peripheral edema, and engorgement of the kidneys and other organs. In right-sided CHF, fluid does not back up into the lungs, so pulmonary edema and crackles do not occur.

Signs and Symptoms

- Weakness
- Anxiety
- Tachycardia
- Edema of lower extremities
- Swelling of the liver
- Chest pain
- JVD
- Fatigue (due to reduced oxygenation and inability to increase cardiac output in response to physical activity)
- Left ventricular hypertrophy (point of maximal impulse displaced toward left anterior axillary line)
- Tachycardia (due to sympathetic stimulation)
- S_3 heart tones (rapid ventricular filling)
- S_4 heart tones (atrial contraction against noncompliant ventricle)
- Cool, pale skin (due to peripheral vasoconstriction)

Assessment

- Scene size-up
  - Ensure BSI.
- Initial/primary assessment
  - Monitor LOC.
  - Manage ABCs.
  - Treat life-threatening illness/injuries.
  - Transport considerations: Transport patient with legs lower than the heart.
- Focused history and physical exam/secondary assessment
  - Obtain SAMPLE history and chief complaint (OPQRST).

Management

- Apply pulse oximeter and supplemental oxygen.
- Establish IV access.
- Monitor vital signs.
- Apply cardiac monitor.
- Obtain 12-lead ECG.

Table 8-1 summarizes treatment of congestive heart failure.

Table 8-1 Treatment of Congestive Heart Failure

Treatment	Purpose	Initial Adult Dose
Oxygen	Increases cellular perfusion.	15 L/min via nonrebreathing mask
Furosemide	Vasodilation; increases lymphatic flow (drainage) from lungs back into circulatory system; elimination of excess fluid through renal system.	IV: 0.5 mg/kg over 1-2 min

Continues

Table 8-1 Treatment of Congestive Heart Failure (Continued)

Treatment	Purpose	Initial Adult Dose
Nitroglycerin	Vasodilation to reduce preload and afterload, improving cardiac output.	SL: 0.3-0.4 mg
Nitroglycerin infusion	Vasodilation to reduce preload and afterload, improving cardiac output.	10-20 µg/min
Morphine sulfate	Vasodilation; decreases patient anxiety.	SIVP: 2-10 mg in 2-mg increments
Epinephrine infusion	Stimulates both alpha- and beta-adrenergic receptors. Alpha-1 receptors cause vasoconstriction of peripheral vessels (to improve blood pressure) and bronchial vessels (to reduce edema). Beta-1 receptors cause an increase in contractility and rate and overall cardiac output. Beta-2 receptors cause smooth bronchial muscles to relax.	2-10 µg/kg/min
Dopamine infusion	Hypotension; stimulates alpha-adrenergic receptors to increase peripheral vascular resistance by contracting vessel muscles.	2-20 µg/kg/min

Hypertensive Emergencies

Pathophysiology

Hypertension (high blood pressure) is present when the blood pressure at rest is consistently greater than about 140/90 mm Hg. Most hypertension is the result of advanced atherosclerosis or arteriosclerosis, which decreases the lumen of the arteries and reduces their elasticity. The resulting high afterload on the heart leads to an increase in filling volume and stimulates the Frank-Starling reflex, which raises the pressure behind the blood leaving the heart.

Persistent elevation of the diastolic pressure is indicative of hypertensive disease. If left untreated, hypertension significantly shortens the life span and predisposes the patient to a variety of other medical problems. The most common complications of hypertension include renal damage, stroke, and heart failure—the last a result of the left ventricle having to pump for years against a markedly increased afterload.

Signs and Symptoms

In the majority of cases, hypertension is entirely asymptomatic and is detected by chance during routine examination. By the time symptoms start to occur, hypertension is already in a more advanced stage and has probably produced at least some damage to organs such as the heart, kidneys, and brain.

The symptoms that occur in advanced hypertensive disease may be related to the elevated blood pressure or to secondary complications:

- Headache (most common symptom directly related to blood pressure elevation)
- Dizziness
- Weakness
- Epistaxis
- Blurring of vision

Hypertensive emergencies occur in about 1% of all hypertensive patients. A hypertensive emergency is defined as an acute elevation of blood pressure with evidence of end-organ damage; the evidence of end-organ dysfunction determines the urgency of the situation, not the reading on the sphygmomanometer. Two end-organ emergencies that may result from uncontrolled hypertension are left-sided heart failure and dissecting aortic aneurysm.

Assessment

- Scene size-up
  - Ensure BSI.
- Initial/primary assessment
  - Manage ABCs.
  - Monitor LOC.
  - Treat life-threatening illness/injuries.
  - Transport considerations: Transport patient in a position of comfort. If patient is unresponsive or unable to speak, rapid transport is indicated.
- Focused history and physical exam/secondary assessment
  - Obtain SAMPLE history and chief complaint (OPQRST).

Management

- Apply pulse oximeter and supplemental oxygen.
- Attach cardiac monitor.
- Monitor vital signs.
- Establish IV access.
- Obtain 12-lead ECG.
- Hypertensive crisis (sudden, marked rise in BP to levels greater than 200/130 mm Hg) may be treated with labetalol (Normodyne, Trandate), which has alpha- and beta-blocking properties. Keep the patient supine and measure his or her blood pressure at least every 3 to 5 minutes. Labetalol can be given initially by slow IV push at 20 mg, repeated in 10 minutes as necessary, or an IV drip can be started. To administer a labetalol drip, add 250 mg to 250 mL of normal saline, yielding a concentration of 1 mg/mL. Start the infusion at a rate of 2 mg/min (2 mL/min) and watch the infusion until the BP has fallen to the target level specified by your medical director.

Angina Pectoris

Pathophysiology

Angina pectoris, also called myocardial **ischemia**, is chest pain that either is self-resolving or is responsive to nitroglycerin. It is caused by a lack of oxygen to the myocardium. A narrowing or blockage of one or more arteries in the heart decreases the blood supply, and therefore the oxygen supply, causing the ischemia. Angina is commonly a symptom of impending MI but differs from MI in that it can be relieved by nitroglycerin. Angina pectoris may result from increased workload on the heart, exercise, or emotional stress. *Nitroglycerin usually relieves the pain immediately.*

Signs and Symptoms

- Tightness of the chest
- Chest pain, most often substernal and radiating to the left arm, neck, and jaw, usually lasting 3 to 5 minutes and disappearing with rest
- Dyspnea
- Vague discomfort or epigastric pain, especially in diabetes

Assessment

- Scene size-up
  - Ensure BSI.
- Initial/primary assessment
  - Monitor LOC.
  - Manage ABCs.
  - Treat life-threatening illness/injuries.
  - Transport considerations: Transport patient in a position of comfort. If patient is unresponsive or unable to speak, rapid transport is indicated.
- Focused history and physical exam/secondary assessment
  - Obtain SAMPLE history and chief complaint (OPQRST).

Management
- Apply pulse oximeter and supplemental oxygen.
- Attach cardiac monitor.
- Monitor vital signs.
- Establish IV access.
- Obtain 12-lead ECG.
- Administer nitroglycerin, if pain is not resolved with rest.

Table 8-2 summarizes the treatment of angina pectoris.

Table 8-2 Treatment of Angina Pectoris

Treatment	Purpose	Adult Dose
Oxygen	Increases cellular oxygenation	15 L/min via nonrebreathing mask
Nitroglycerin	Vasodilation to reduce preload and afterload, improving cardiac output	SL: 0.4 mg
Aspirin	Decreases platelet aggregation	PO: 160-325 mg

Pericardial Tamponade

Pathophysiology

Pericardial tamponade occurs when blood or fluid (or rarely, air) accumulates in the space between the myocardium (heart muscle) and the pericardium (outer sac covering of the heart), compressing the heart and restricting the diastolic flow, leading to reduced cardiac output. This prevents the ventricles from expanding fully, so they cannot adequately fill or pump blood effectively. Pericardial tamponade can occur from trauma or various medical conditions. It is treated in the hospital with **pericardiocentesis**. Administration of an IV fluid bolus, which increases preload, is an often-successful temporary therapy for pericardial tamponade.

Signs and Symptoms
- Muffled heart tones
- Narrowing pulse pressure
- JVD
- Pulseless electrical activity
- Hypotension
- Signs of shock

Assessment
- Scene size-up
  - Ensure BSI.
- Initial/primary assessment
  - Manage ABCs.
  - Monitor LOC.
  - Treat life-threatening illness/injuries.
  - Transport considerations: Transport patient in a position of comfort. If patient is unresponsive or unable to speak, rapid transport is indicated.
  - Assess pulse for narrowing pulse pressure.
  - Listen for muffled heart tones.
  - Inspect for JVD.
  - Assess for pulsus paradoxus with a blood pressure cuff by inflating the cuff, then deflating until the Korotkoff sound is heard, and then deflating slowly during the

respiratory cycle. If the Korotkoff sound is heard again during exhalation (with a difference of 10 mm Hg), the patient has pulsus paradoxus.

- Focused history and physical exam/secondary assessment
  - Obtain SAMPLE history and chief complaint (OPQRST).

Management
- If allowed by local protocols, pericardiocentesis is indicated.

Myocardial Infarction

Pathophysiology

Myocardial infarction (MI) occurs when the heart muscle does not get adequate oxygen because of decreased blood supply, has an increased need for oxygen, or both. MIs occur in three stages:

1. Ischemia due to lack of blood supply
2. Injury due to continued lack of blood supply
3. Infarction due to death of the myocardial cells

Signs and Symptoms
- Severe chest pain with or without diaphoresis
- Nausea
- Pain radiating to left arm, neck, and jaw
- Severe indigestion
- Epigastric pain (women)

> **How to Detect MI on an ECG**
>
> Acute MI is noted by an elevated ST segment. Chronic (previous) MIs are noted by ST-segment depression and/or pathologic Q waves. Because of the diagnostic versus monitoring capabilities of various cardiac monitors, ST-segment elevation or depression can only be accurately identified by obtaining a 12-lead ECG.
>
> *It is important to note that you cannot distinguish ST-segment elevation or depression by using a 3- or 4-lead ECG.*

Assessment
- Scene size-up
  - Ensure BSI.
- Initial/primary assessment
  - Monitor LOC.
  - Manage ABCs.
  - Treat life-threatening illness/injuries.
  - Transport considerations: Transport patient in a position of comfort. If patient is unresponsive or unable to speak, rapid transport is indicated.
- Focused history and physical exam/secondary assessment
  - Obtain SAMPLE history and chief complaint (OPQRST).

Management
- Apply pulse oximeter and supplemental oxygen.
- Establish IV access.
- Monitor vital signs.
- Attach cardiac monitor.
- Obtain 12-lead ECG.

Table 8-3 summarizes treatment of left ventricular MI. **Table 8-4** summarizes the treatment of right ventricular MI.

Table 8-3 Pharmacologic Treatment of Left Ventricular MI

Treatment	Purpose	Initial Adult Dose
Oxygen	Increases cellular perfusion	15 L/min via nonrebreathing mask
Aspirin	Decreases platelet aggregation	PO: 160-325 mg
Nitroglycerin	Vasodilation to reduce preload and afterload, improving cardiac output	SL: 0.4 mg
Morphine	Vasodilation; decreases patient's anxiety	SIVP: 2-10 mg in increments of 2-4 mg titrated

Table 8-4 Pharmacologic Treatment of Right Ventricular MI

Treatment	Purpose	Initial Adult Dose
Oxygen	Increases cellular perfusion	To cellular perfusion
Aspirin	Decreases platelet aggregation	PO: 160-325 mg
0.9% normal saline	Prevents hypotension; increases preload	IV: 500-750 mL bolus

Cardiac Arrhythmias

<u>Arrhythmias</u>, also called *dysrhythmias*, are defined by the American Heart Association as abnormal heart rhythms stemming from problems that affect the electrical system of the heart muscle. Arrhythmias reduce the effectiveness of the heart's pumping mechanism.

Placing the Leads

Most electrode cables come with either three or four cables with snaps on the ends. Snap the end of each wire into an electrode placed in accordance with its marked position. Place the LA, or left arm, electrode on the left shoulder or left pectoral muscle. Place the RA, or right arm, electrode on the right shoulder or pectoral muscle. Place the LL, or left leg, electrode anywhere on the left leg, thigh, or flank so long as it sits on a muscle, not bone, and the electrode is facing midline. If using a cardiac monitor with four cables, place the RL, or right leg, electrode anywhere on the right leg, thigh, or flank so long as it sits on a muscle and not a bone and the electrode is facing midline.

Types of Arrhythmias

There are different types of arrhythmias based on where the electrical malfunction occurs:

- SA node arrhythmias
    - Sick sinus syndrome
    - Sinus bradycardia
    - Sinus tachycardia
    - Sinus arrhythmias
    - Sinus arrest
- Atrial arrhythmias
    - Premature atrial complex (PAC)
    - Paroxysmal supraventricular tachycardia (PSVT)
    - Atrial tachycardia
    - Atrial flutter
    - Atrial fibrillation
- Conduction arrhythmias
    - First-degree AV block
    - Second-degree AV block, Mobitz type I (Wenckebach)
    - Second-degree AV block, Mobitz type II
    - Third-degree (complete) AV block
    - Bundle branch block
- AV node and tissues
    - Premature junctional complex (PJC)
    - Junctional (escape) rhythm
    - Junctional tachycardia
- Ventricular arrhythmias
    - Premature ventricular complex (PVC)
    - Ventricular tachycardia
    - Ventricular fibrillation

- Pulseless electrical activity (PEA)
- Asystole
- Idioventricular rhythm

Sinoatrial Node Arrhythmias

Sick Sinus Syndrome

Pathophysiology Sick sinus syndrome (SSS) occurs as the result of long-term damage to the SA node, which impairs its ability to effectively conduct electrical impulses through the heart. Its rate varies from fast to slow. The patient usually requires a pacemaker. Disorders that cause scarring, degeneration, or damage to the conduction system can cause SSS. It is more common in elderly adults, in whom the cause is often a nonspecific, scarlike degeneration of the conduction system. In children, cardiac surgery, especially to the atria, is a common cause of SSS. **Table 8-5** describes the ECG reading of SSS.

Table 8-5 Sick Sinus Syndrome

Rhythm	Can be regular or irregular
Rate	Any rate can occur with SSS
P waves	Normal, upright
PR interval	Within normal limits (0.12-0.20 sec in duration) and constant
QRS complex	Within normal limits (0.04-0.12 sec in duration) and constant

Sick sinus syndrome is relatively uncommon. It can result in many arrhythmias, including the following:

- Palpitations
- Tachycardia followed by extreme bradycardia
- PSVT
- Atrial fibrillation
- Sinus arrest
- Sinus node exit block
- Bradycardias

Signs and Symptoms
- Syncope
- Chest pain
- Weakness
- Nausea and vomiting
- Altered vital signs

Assessment
- Scene size-up
  - Ensure BSI.
- Initial/primary assessment
  - Monitor LOC.
  - Manage ABCs.
  - Treat life-threatening illness/injuries.
  - Transport considerations: Transport patient in a position of comfort. If patient is unresponsive or unable to speak, rapid transport is indicated.
- Focused history and physical exam/secondary assessment
  - Obtain SAMPLE history and chief complaint (OPQRST).

Management
- Apply pulse oximeter and supplemental oxygen.
- Establish IV access.

- Monitor vital signs.
- Attach cardiac monitor.
- Obtain 12-lead ECG to determine specific cause of complaint.
- Treat according to symptoms and presentation.

Sinus Bradycardia

<u>Sinus bradycardia</u> originates in the SA node. It is common in athletes.

Pathophysiology This arrhythmia is characterized by a regular heart rate of less than 60 beats per minute (**Figure 8-6**). Causes include hypothermia, an increase in parasympathetic symptoms (vagus nerve), drug side effects (especially beta-blockers), and sinus node disease. In some people, particularly well-trained athletes, sinus bradycardia is normal. **Table 8-6** describes the ECG reading of sinus bradycardia.

Table 8-6 Sinus Bradycardia

Rhythm	Regular (R-R intervals and P-P intervals are constant)
Rate	< 60 beats/min
P waves	Upright and uniform, precede each QRS complex
PR interval	Within normal limits (0.12-0.20 sec in duration) and constant
QRS complex	Within normal limits (0.04-0.12 sec in duration) and constant

Signs and Symptoms
- Syncope
- Nausea
- Vomiting
- Hypotension
- Slow pulse

Assessment
- Scene size-up
  - Ensure BSI.
- Initial/primary assessment
  - Monitor LOC.
  - Manage ABCs.
  - Treat life-threatening illness/injuries.
  - Transport considerations: Transport patient in a position of comfort. If patient is unresponsive or unable to speak, rapid transport is indicated.
- Focused history and physical exam/secondary assessment
  - Obtain SAMPLE history and chief complaint (OPQRST).

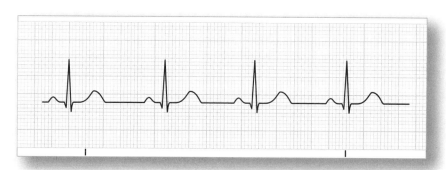

Figure 8-6 Sinus bradycardia.

Management
- Apply pulse oximeter and supplemental oxygen.
- Establish IV access.
- Monitor vital signs.
- Attach cardiac monitor.
- Obtain 12-lead ECG to determine specific cause of complaint.
- Treat according to symptoms and presentation.

Table 8-7 summarizes pharmacologic treatment of sinus bradycardia.

Table 8-7 Pharmacologic Treatment of Sinus Bradycardia

Treatment	Purpose	Initial Adult Dose
Transcutaneous pacing	To electrically increase heart rate in symptomatic patients	Set pacer at 70 beats/min and 30 mA, increasing mA until capture
Atropine	Parasympatholytic; increases heart rate	IV: 0.5 mg
Oxygen	Increases cellular perfusion	15 L/min via nonrebreathing mask
Note: Treat the underlying cause, not just the symptoms.		

Sinus Tachycardia

Pathophysiology Sinus tachycardia is characterized by a regular heart rate of more than 100 beats per minute (**Figure 8-7**). Causes include exertion, excitability, drug side effects, and sinus node disease. **Table 8-8** describes the ECG reading of sinus tachycardia.

Table 8-8 Sinus Tachycardia

Rhythm	Regular (R-R intervals and P-P intervals are constant)
Rate	Between 100 and 180 beats/min
P waves	Upright and uniform, precede each QRS complex
PR interval	Within normal limits (0.12-0.20 sec) and constant
QRS complex	Within normal limits (0.04-0.12 sec) and constant

Signs and Symptoms
- Rapid pulse
- Palpitations
- Nausea and vomiting
- Profuse sweating
- Chest pain
- Hypotension

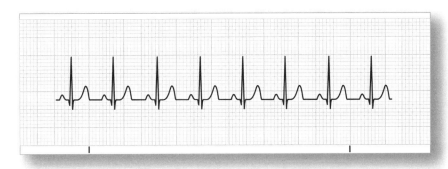

Figure 8-7 Sinus tachycardia.

Assessment
- Scene size-up
  - Ensure BSI.
- Initial/primary assessment
  - Monitor LOC.
  - Manage ABCs.
  - Treat life-threatening illness/injuries.
  - Transport considerations: Transport patient in a position of comfort. If patient is unresponsive or unable to speak, rapid transport is indicated.
- Focused history and physical exam/secondary assessment
  - Obtain SAMPLE history and chief complaint (OPQRST).

Management
- Apply pulse oximeter and supplemental oxygen.
- Establish IV access.
- Monitor vital signs.
- Attach cardiac monitor.
- Obtain 12-lead ECG to determine specific cause of complaint.
- Treat according to symptoms and presentation.

Atrial Arrhythmias

Premature Atrial Complex

Pathophysiology A **premature atrial complex (PAC)** is characterized by beats originating from the atrium and occurring premature to the beat coming from the SA node (**Figure 8-8**). **Table 8-9** describes the ECG reading of a premature atrial complex.

Table 8-9 Premature Atrial Complex

Rhythm	Irregular (underlying rhythm is disrupted by premature atrial contractions).
Rate	Dependent on the rate of the underlying rhythm.
P waves	Present with the underlying rhythm and premature beats.
PR interval	Present with the underlying rhythm and premature beats.
QRS complex	Premature beats are narrow (< 0.10 sec) and look the same as QRS complexes of the underlying rhythm. T waves of the premature beats are of the same direction as the R waves. PACs are not usually followed by a compensatory pause.

Causes
- AMI
- CHF
- Chronic obstructive pulmonary disease (COPD)
- Hypokalemia

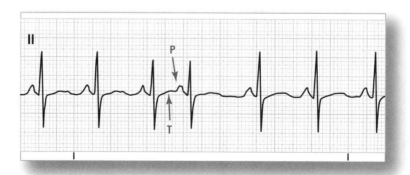

Figure 8-8 Premature atrial complex.

- Myocardial ischemia
- Use of caffeine, tobacco, or alcohol

Signs and Symptoms
- Chest pain
- Palpitations
- Dyspnea
- Syncope
- Altered LOC
- Hypotension

Assessment
- Scene size-up
  - Ensure BSI.
- Initial/primary assessment
  - Monitor LOC.
  - Manage ABCs.
  - Treat life-threatening illness/injuries.
  - Transport considerations: Transport patient in a position of comfort. If patient is unresponsive or unable to speak, rapid transport is indicated.
- Focused history and physical exam/secondary assessment
  - Obtain SAMPLE history and chief complaint (OPQRST).

Management
- Apply pulse oximeter and supplemental oxygen.
- Establish IV access.
- Monitor vital signs.
- Attach cardiac monitor.
- Obtain 12-lead ECG to determine specific cause of complaint.
- Treat according to symptoms and presentation.

Supraventricular Tachycardia

Pathophysiology In **supraventricular tachycardia (SVT)**, impulses originate above the ventricles. It is caused by a rapid firing of ectopic foci with a rate of 150 to 250 beats per minute. SVT is classified based on the patient's hemodynamic status (stable vs. unstable) and can be either **paroxysmal SVT (PVST)** or sustained (**Figure 8-9**). **Table 8-10** describes the ECG reading of supraventricular tachycardia.

Table 8-10 Supraventricular Tachycardia

Rhythm	Regular
Rate	150-250 beats/min.
P waves	One P wave precedes each QRS complex. The P wave is typically buried in the T wave of the preceding beat. If present, the P waves may be flattened or notched.
PR interval	If determinable and not buried in the T wave, the PR interval will be within normal limits.
QRS complex	Typically within normal limits (0.04-0.12 sec).

Causes
- AMI
- CHF
- COPD
- Hypokalemia
- Myocardial ischemia
- Use of caffeine, tobacco, or alcohol

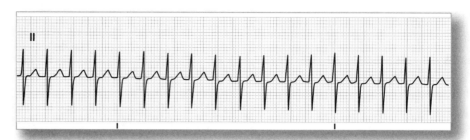

Figure 8-9 Supraventricular tachycardia.

Signs and Symptoms
- Palpitations
- Anxiety

Assessment
- Scene size-up
  - Ensure BSI.
- Initial/primary assessment
  - Monitor LOC.
  - Manage ABCs.
  - Treat life-threatening illness/injuries.
  - Transport considerations: Transport patient in a position of comfort. If patient is unresponsive or unable to speak, rapid transport is indicated.
- Focused history and physical exam/secondary assessment
  - Obtain SAMPLE history and chief complaint (OPQRST).

Management
- Apply pulse oximeter and supplemental oxygen.
- Establish IV access.
- Monitor vital signs.
- Attach cardiac monitor.
- Obtain 12-lead ECG to determine specific cause of complaint.

Table 8-11 summarizes treatment of stable SVT, and **Table 8-12** outlines treatment of unstable SVT.

Table 8-11 Treatment of Stable SVT

Treatment	Purpose	Initial Adult Dose
Vagal stimulation	Decreases heart rate	Have patient attempt to bear down like he or she is having a bowel movement, or blow through a straw
Adenosine	Interrupts reentry in AV node to restore normal sinus rhythm; slows conduction time through AV node; vasodilation of coronary artery	IV: 6 mg

Table 8-12 Treatment of Unstable SVT

Treatment	Purpose	Initial Adult Dose
Synchronized cardioversion	Restores normal heart rate	50 J
Diltiazem	Slows conduction velocity to increase AV node refractory period	SIVP: 0.25 mg/kg over 2 min
Amiodarone	Blocks sodium and myocardial potassium channels	IV: 150 mg over 10 min

Multifocal Atrial Tachycardia

Pathophysiology In multifocal **atrial tachycardia**, the pacemaker of the heart moves within various areas of the atria. Multifocal atrial tachycardia is characterized by a rate of more than 100 beats per minute and is, in effect, a tachycardic wandering atrial pacemaker (**Figure 8-10**). **Table 8-13** describes the ECG reading of multifocal atrial tachycardia.

Table 8-13 Multifocal Atrial Tachycardia

Rhythm	Irregular.
Rate	> 100 beats/min.
P waves	There is one P wave preceding each QRS complex. The P wave is typically buried in the T wave of the preceding beat. If present, the P waves may be flattened or notched.
PR interval	If determinable and not buried in the T wave, the PR interval will be within normal limits.
QRS complex	Typically within normal limits (0.04–0.12 sec).

Causes
- Use of tobacco, caffeine, or alcohol
- Hypokalemia
- COPD
- CHF
- AMI
- Myocardial ischemia

Signs and Symptoms
- Chest pain
- Dyspnea
- Syncope
- Palpitations
- Altered LOC
- Pulmonary congestion
- Hypotension

Assessment
- Scene size-up
  - Ensure BSI.
- Initial/primary assessment
  - Monitor LOC.
  - Manage ABCs.

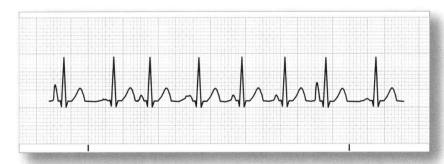

Figure 8-10 Multifocal atrial tachycardia.

- Treat life-threatening illness/injuries.
- Transport considerations: Transport patient in a position of comfort. If patient is unresponsive or unable to speak, rapid transport is indicated.
  - Focused history and physical exam/secondary assessment
    - Obtain SAMPLE history and chief complaint (OPQRST).

Management
- Apply pulse oximeter and supplemental oxygen.
- Establish IV access.
- Monitor vital signs.
- Attach cardiac monitor.
- Obtain 12-lead ECG to determine specific cause of complaint.
- Treat according to symptoms and presentation.

Atrial Flutter

Pathophysiology Atrial flutter is characterized by a sawtooth atrial baseline at a rapid rate of greater than 250 beats per minute (**Figure 8-11**). It presents in ratios of 2:1, 3:1, and 4:1. Causes include congestive heart failure, AMI, hypoxia, and pulmonary embolism. **Table 8-14** describes the ECG reading of atrial flutter.

Table 8-14 Atrial Flutter

Rhythm	Atrial rhythm is regular, depending on conduction ratio; ventricular rhythm may be regular or irregular.
Rate	Depends on ventricular response; may be normal, slow, or fast.
P waves	There are no identifiable P waves. The atrial activity is represented by flutter waves, which produce a characteristic sawtooth appearance.
PR interval	None.
QRS complex	Within normal limits (0.04–0.12 sec).

Signs and Symptoms
- Chest pain
- Dyspnea
- Syncope
- Altered LOC
- Pulmonary congestion
- CHF
- AMI
- Hypotension

Assessment
- Scene size-up
  - Ensure BSI.
- Initial/primary assessment
  - Monitor LOC.
  - Manage ABCs.
  - Treat life-threatening illness/injuries.

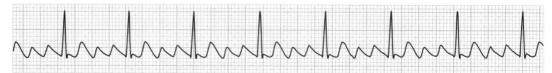

Figure 8-11 Atrial flutter.

- Transport considerations: Transport patient in a position of comfort. If patient is unresponsive or unable to speak, rapid transport is indicated.
- Attach cardiac monitor and obtain ECG.
- Focused history and physical exam/secondary assessment
  - Obtain SAMPLE history and chief complaint (OPQRST).

Management **Table 8-15** summarizes treatment of atrial flutter.

Table 8-15 Treatment of Atrial Flutter

Treatment	Purpose	Initial Adult Dose
Oxygen	Increases cellular perfusion	15 L/min via nonrebreathing mask
Synchronized cardioversion	Restores normal heart rate	50 J
Diltiazem	Slows conduction velocity to increase AV node refractory period	IV: 0.25 mg/kg

Atrial Fibrillation

Pathophysiology <u>Atrial fibrillation</u> (**Figure 8-12**) occurs as a result of the many ectopic foci (nonpacemaker heart cells that automatically depolarize) in the atria. It often occurs after heavy drinking. Causes include hypoxia, digitalis toxicity, AMI, and heart disease. **Table 8-16** describes the ECG reading of atrial fibrillation. If the ventricular response rate is rapid, hemodynamic instability may result.

Table 8-16 Atrial Fibrillation

Rhythm	Irregular.
Rate	Depends on ventricular response; may be normal, slow, or fast.
P waves	There are no discernible P waves–the baseline is chaotic because the atrial activity is represented by fibrillatory waves.
PR interval	None.
QRS complex	Within normal limits (0.04-0.12 sec).

Signs and Symptoms
- Hypotension
- Hypoxia
- Altered LOC
- Pulmonary congestion
- Confusion
- Dyspnea

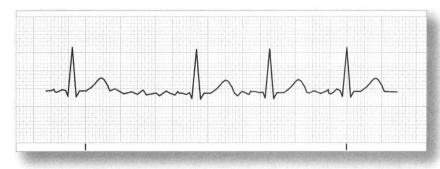

Figure 8-12 Atrial fibrillation.

- Chest pain
- Heart rate of greater than 150 beats/min

Assessment
- Scene size-up
  - Ensure BSI.
- Initial/primary assessment
  - Monitor LOC.
  - Manage ABCs.
  - Treat life-threatening illness/injuries.
  - Transport considerations: Transport patient in a position of comfort. If patient is unresponsive or unable to speak, rapid transport is indicated.
- Focused history and physical exam/secondary assessment
  - Obtain SAMPLE history and chief complaint (OPQRST).

Management
- Apply pulse oximeter and supplemental oxygen.
- Establish IV access.
- Monitor vital signs.
- Attach cardiac monitor.
- Obtain 12-lead ECG to determine specific cause of complaint.
- Treat according to symptoms and presentation.

Table 8-17 summarizes treatment of atrial fibrillation.

Table 8-17 Treatment of Atrial Fibrillation

Treatment	Purpose	Initial Adult Dose
Synchronized cardioversion	Restores normal atrial contraction	50 J
Oxygen	Increases cellular perfusion	15 L/min via nonrebreathing mask
Adenosine*	Interrupts reentry in the AV node to restore normal sinus rhythm; slows conduction time through the AV node; vasodilation of the coronary artery	RIVP: 6 mg
Diltiazem	Slows conduction velocity to increase AV node refractory period	IV: 0.25 mg/kg
Labetalol	Negative inotropic effect; negative chronotropic effect; antihypertensive	IV: 5-20 mg
Amiodarone	Prolongs action potential and refractory period; slows the sinus rate; prolongs PR and QT intervals; vasodilation	IV: 150 mg over 10 min

*Adenosine is not indicated in atrial fibrillation. However, it may be given if one is unable to determine baseline rhythm, in an attempt to slow rhythm and differentiate atrial fibrillation from SVT.

Conduction Arrhythmias ("Heart Blocks")

First-Degree AV Block

Pathophysiology **First-degree AV block**, also known as first-degree heart block, occurs when the electrical impulse moves through the AV node slower than normal (**Figure 8-13**). **Table 8-18** describes the ECG reading of first-degree AV block.

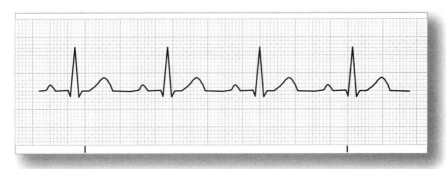

Figure 8-13 First-degree AV block.

Table 8-18 First-Degree AV Block

Rhythm	Regular
Rate	60-100 beats/min (normal)
P waves	Upright and uniform, one P wave to a QRS complex
PR interval	Constant, > 0.20 sec
QRS complex	Within normal limits (0.04-0.12 sec)

Causes
- An increase in vagal tone (parasympathetic system)
- Myocardial ischemia
- Myocardial infarction

Signs and Symptoms
- Usually asymptomatic

Assessment
- Scene size-up
  - Ensure BSI.
- Initial/primary assessment
  - Monitor LOC.
  - Manage ABCs.
  - Treat life-threatening illness/injuries.
  - Transport considerations: Transport in position of comfort. If patient is unresponsive or unable to speak, rapid transport is indicated.
- Focused history and physical exam/secondary assessment
  - Obtain SAMPLE history and chief complaint (OPQRST).

Management
- Apply pulse oximeter and supplemental oxygen.
- Establish IV access.
- Monitor vital signs.
- Attach cardiac monitor.
- Obtain 12-lead ECG to determine specific cause of complaint.

Second-Degree AV Block: Mobitz Type I (Wenckebach)
Pathophysiology In **second-degree AV block, Mobitz type I**, electrical impulses are intermittently blocked, producing a progressively longer PR interval until an impulse is blocked (**Figure 8-14**). **Table 8-19** describes the ECG reading of Mobitz type I second-degree AV block.

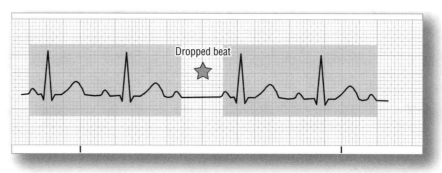

Figure 8-14 Second-degree AV block: Mobitz type I.

Table 8-19 Second-Degree AV Block: Mobitz Type I (Wenckebach)

Rhythm	Irregular; cycle recurs as a pattern.
Rate	Ventricular rate is slightly slower than normal.
P waves	Upright and uniform. There are more P waves than QRS complexes because some of the QRS complexes are blocked.
PR interval	Gets progressively longer until a QRS complex is "dropped." After the blocked beat, the cycle starts all over again.
QRS complex	Within normal limits (0.04–0.12 sec).

Signs and Symptoms
- Chest pain
- Dyspnea
- Syncope
- Altered LOC
- Pulmonary congestion
- Hypotension

Assessment
- Scene size-up
  - Ensure BSI.
- Initial/primary assessment
  - Monitor LOC.
  - Manage ABCs.
  - Treat life-threatening illness/injuries.
  - Transport considerations: Transport in position of comfort. If patient is unresponsive or unable to speak, rapid transport is indicated.
- Focused history and physical exam/secondary assessment
  - Obtain SAMPLE history and chief complaint (OPQRST).

Management
- Apply pulse oximeter and supplemental oxygen.
- Establish IV access.
- Monitor vital signs.
- Attach cardiac monitor.
- Obtain 12-lead ECG to determine specific cause of complaint.
- Treat according to symptoms and presentation.

Table 8-20 summarizes treatment of Mobitz type I second-degree AV block.

Table 8-20 Treatment of Symptomatic Second-Degree AV Block, Mobitz Type I

Treatment	Purpose	Initial Adult Dose
Atropine	Parasympatholytic: increases heart rate	IV: 0.5 mg
Transcutaneous pacing	**If atropine is ineffective:** Set pacer to 70 beats/min and 30 mA, increasing mA until capture	
Note: Treat the cause.		

Second-Degree AV Block: Mobitz Type II

Pathophysiology In **second-degree AV block, Mobitz type II**, there is an intermittent block, where P waves are not conducted to the ventricles (**Figure 8-15**). This is less common yet more severe than type I because it is more likely to progress to complete heart block (third-degree AV block). Mobitz type II second-degree AV block differs from first-degree AV block because *most* of the P waves conduct to a QRS complex, unlike in first-degree AV block, in which all of the P waves conduct to a QRS complex. **Table 8-21** describes the ECG reading of Mobitz type II second-degree AV block.

Table 8-21 Second-Degree AV Block: Mobitz Type II

Rhythm	Typically regular. Irregular if the conduction ratio (number of P waves to each QRS complex) varies.
Rate	The ventricular rate is slower than normal (< 60 beats/min), while the atrial rate is within normal limits.
P waves	Upright and uniform. There are more P waves than QRS complexes.
PR interval	Constant; can be normal or longer than normal (> 0.20 sec).
QRS complex	Within normal limits (0.04–0.12 sec).

Signs and Symptoms
- Chest pain
- Dyspnea
- Syncope
- Altered LOC
- Pulmonary congestion
- Hypotension

Assessment
- Scene size-up
  - Ensure BSI.
- Initial/primary assessment
  - Monitor LOC.
  - Manage ABCs.

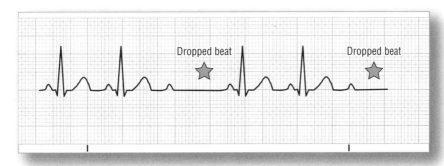

Figure 8-15 Second-degree AV block: Mobitz type II.

- Treat life-threatening illness/injuries.
- Transport considerations: Transport patient in a position of comfort. If patient is unresponsive or unable to speak, rapid transport is indicated.
- Focused history and physical exam/secondary assessment
  - Obtain SAMPLE history and chief complaint (OPQRST).

Management
- Apply pulse oximeter and supplemental oxygen.
- Establish IV access.
- Monitor vital signs.
- Attach cardiac monitor.
- Obtain 12-lead ECG to determine specific cause of complaint.

Table 8-22 summarizes treatment of Mobitz type II second-degree AV block.

Table 8-22 Treatment of Symptomatic Second-Degree AV Block: Mobitz Type II

Treatment	Purpose	Adult
Transcutaneous pacing	Electrically increase heart rate	Set pacer to 70 beats/min and 30 mA, increasing mA until capture
Note: Atropine is not effective for infranodal AV block (Mobitz type II and third-degree block with wide QRS complexes).		

Third-Degree (Complete) AV Block

Pathophysiology In **third-degree (complete) AV block** the heart's electrical signals do not pass from the upper to the lower chambers. Instead they operate independently of each other. When this occurs, the ventricular pacemaker takes over. The ventricles contract and pump blood at a slower rate than the atrial pacemaker (**Figure 8-16**). **Table 8-23** describes the ECG reading of third-degree (complete) AV block.

Table 8-23 Third-Degree (Complete) AV Block

Rhythm	Regular atrial rate and regular ventricular rate, each independent of the other.
Rate	The ventricular rate is slower than normal (< 60 beats/min), while the atrial rate is within normal limits.
P waves	Upright and regular.
PR interval	There is no relationship between P waves and QRS complexes. They beat independently and regularly.
QRS complex	May be normal or wide, depending on how low in the conduction pathway the escape beats are.

Signs and Symptoms
- Chest pain
- Dyspnea

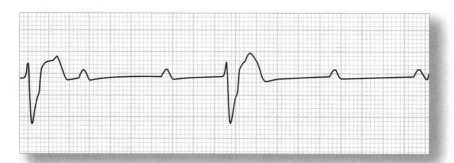

Figure 8-16 Third-degree (complete) AV block.

- Syncope
- Altered LOC
- Pulmonary congestion
- Hypotension

Assessment
- Scene size-up
  - Ensure BSI.
- Initial/primary assessment
  - Monitor LOC.
  - Manage ABCs.
  - Treat life-threatening illness/injuries.
  - Transport considerations: Transport in position of comfort. If patient is unresponsive or unable to speak, rapid transport is indicated.
- Focused history and physical exam/secondary assessment
  - Obtain SAMPLE history and chief complaint (OPQRST).

Management
- Apply pulse oximeter and supplemental oxygen.
- Establish IV access.
- Monitor vital signs.
- Attach cardiac monitor.
- Obtain 12-lead ECG to determine specific cause of complaint.

Table 8-24 summarizes treatment of third-degree (complete) AV block.

Table 8-24 Treatment of Third-Degree (Complete) AV Block

Treatment	Purpose	Initial Adult Dose
Transcutaneous pacing	Electrically increase heart rate	Set pacer to 70 beats/min and 30 mA, increasing mA until capture
Note: Atropine is not effective for infranodal AV block (Mobitz type II and third-degree block). *Caution:* Never use lidocaine for third-degree AV block with ventricular escape beats because administration of lidocaine can suppress the only electrical activity producing perfusing beats.		

Bundle Branch Block

Pathophysiology Bundle branch blocks (BBB) are arrhythmias in which the supraventricular impulses are delayed in getting to the ventricles (**Figure 8-17**). Either bundle branch, or both, can be blocked. If both bundle branches are blocked, this is called a complete heart block. An incomplete BBB will have a wide QRS complex, but not as wide as a complete BBB.

Signs and Symptoms
- Chest pain
- Dyspnea
- Syncope
- Altered LOC
- Pulmonary congestion
- Hypotension

Assessment
- Scene size-up
  - Ensure BSI.
- Initial/primary assessment
  - Monitor LOC.
  - Manage ABCs.

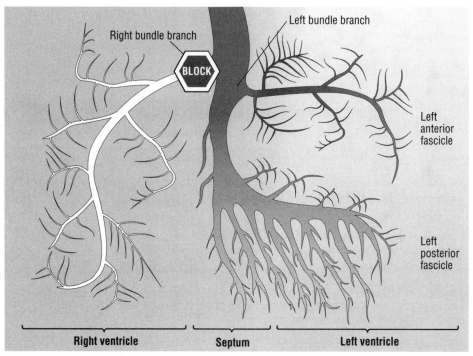

Figure 8-17 Bundle branch block.

- Treat life-threatening illness/injuries.
- Transport considerations: Transport patient in a position of comfort. If patient is unresponsive or unable to speak, rapid transport is indicated.
- Focused history and physical exam/secondary assessment
    - Obtain SAMPLE history and chief complaint (OPQRST).

Management
- Apply pulse oximeter and supplemental oxygen.
- Establish IV access.
- Monitor vital signs.
- Attach cardiac monitor.
- Obtain 12-lead ECG to determine specific cause of complaint.

Atrioventricular Node and Tissues

Premature Junctional Complex

Pathophysiology A **premature junctional complex (PJC)** is caused by premature electrical impulses that occur in the AV junction before the next expected sinus beat (**Figure 8-18**). This condition is typically benign and does not require immediate intervention. **Table 8-25** describes the ECG reading of a premature junctional complex.

Table 8-25 Premature Junctional Complex

Rhythm	Irregular (underlying rhythm is disrupted by presence of early beats).
Rate	Dependent on the rate of the underlying rhythm.
P waves	Typically present with the underlying rhythm but not the premature beats. If present, the P waves are usually inverted.
PR interval	Typically present with the underlying rhythm. If present with the premature beats, the PR interval is < 0.12 sec.
QRS complex	Premature beats are narrow (< 0.10 sec).

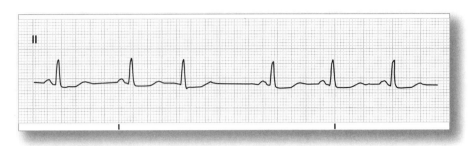

Figure 8-18 Premature junctional complex.

Causes
- CHF
- COPD
- Hypokalemia
- Myocardial ischemia
- Use of caffeine, tobacco, or alcohol
- Idiopathic
- Digitalis toxicity

Signs and Symptoms
- Usually asymptomatic

Assessment
- Scene size-up
  - Ensure BSI.
- Initial/primary assessment
  - Monitor LOC.
  - Manage ABCs.
  - Treat life-threatening illness/injuries.
- Focused history and physical exam/secondary assessment
  - Obtain SAMPLE history and chief complaint (OPQRST).

Management
- Apply pulse oximeter and supplemental oxygen.
- Establish IV access.
- Monitor vital signs.
- Attach cardiac monitor.
- Obtain 12-lead ECG to determine specific cause of complaint.
- Treat according to symptoms and presentation.

Junctional (or Escape) Rhythm

Pathophysiology **Junctional rhythms** (also called escape rhythms) are rhythms that occur when the primary pacemaker (SA node) fails and the AV node takes over as the primary pacemaker (**Figure 8-19**). **Table 8-26** describes the ECG reading of junctional rhythm.

Table 8-26 Junctional Rhythm

Rhythm	Regular.
Rate	40-60 beats/min.
P waves	May precede, be lost in (absent), or follow the QRS complex. When present, the P wave is inverted.
PR interval	If present, < 0.12 sec and constant.
QRS complex	Within normal limits (0.04-0.12 sec).

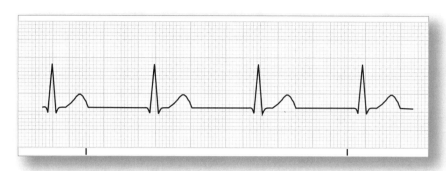

Figure 8-19 Junctional rhythm.

An *accelerated junctional rhythm* is a rhythm that occurs faster than its intrinsic rate (60–100 beats/min). A junctional rhythm normally conducts at a rate of between 40 and 60 beats/min.

Causes
- Ischemia of the AV junction

Signs and Symptoms
- Usually asymptomatic

Assessment
- Scene size-up
  - Ensure BSI.
- Initial/primary assessment
  - Monitor LOC.
  - Manage ABCs.
  - Treat life-threatening illness/injuries.
- Focused history and physical exam/secondary assessment
  - Obtain SAMPLE history and chief complaint (OPQRST).

Management
- Apply pulse oximeter and supplemental oxygen.
- Establish IV access.
- Monitor vital signs.
- Attach cardiac monitor.
- Obtain 12-lead ECG to determine specific cause of complaint.
- Treat according to symptoms and presentation.

Management for junctional rhythms is usually not indicated, because junctional and accelerated junctional rhythms are usually a compensatory mechanism and are well tolerated.

Junctional Tachycardia

Pathophysiology Junctional tachycardia occurs when impulses originate in the AV junctional pacemaker at a rate of anywhere between 100 and 220 beats/min and are conducted retrograde to the atria and antegrade to the ventricles (**Figure 8-20**). **Table 8-27** describes the ECG reading of junctional tachycardia.

Table 8-27 Junctional Tachycardia

Rhythm	Regular; R-R is constant.
Rate	100-180 beats/min; atrial and ventricular rates are equal.
P waves	May precede, be lost in (absent), or follow the QRS complex. When present, the P wave is inverted.
PR interval	If present, < 0.12 sec and constant.
QRS complex	Within normal limits (0.04-0.12 sec).

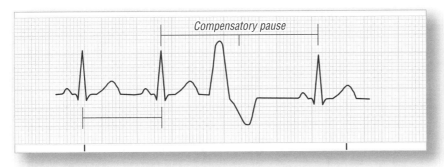

Figure 8-20 Junctional tachycardia.

Causes
- Hypokalemia
- Digitalis toxicity
- Myocardial infarction
- CHF
- COPD
- Use of caffeine, tobacco, or alcohol

Signs and Symptoms
- Altered LOC
- Pulmonary congestion
- Hypoxia
- Heart rate > 150 beats/min
- Chest pain
- Dyspnea
- Fluttering in chest
- Hypotension

Assessment
- Scene size-up
  - Ensure BSI.
- Initial/primary assessment
  - Monitor LOC.
  - Manage ABCs.
  - Treat life-threatening illness/injuries.
- Focused history and physical exam/secondary assessment
  - Obtain SAMPLE history and chief complaint (OPQRST).

Management
- Apply pulse oximeter and supplemental oxygen.
- Establish IV access.
- Monitor vital signs.
- Attach cardiac monitor.
- Obtain 12-lead ECG to determine specific cause of complaint.
- Treat according to symptoms and presentation.

Table 8-28 summarizes treatment of junctional tachycardia.

Table 8-28 Treatment of Junctional Tachycardia

Treatment	Purpose	Adult Dose
Vagal stimulation	Decreases heart rate	Have patient attempt to bear down like he or she is having a bowel movement, or blow through a straw

Continues

Table 8-28 Treatment of Junctional Tachycardia (Continued)

Treatment	Purpose	Adult Dose
Amiodarone	Prolongs action potential and refractory period; slows the sinus rate; prolongs PR and QT intervals; vasodilation	IV: 150 mg
Adenosine	Interrupts reentry in AV node to restore normal sinus rhythm; slows conduction time through AV node; vasodilation of coronary artery	IV: 6 mg
Synchronized cardioversion	Restores normal heart rate	100 J

Ventricular Arrhythmias

Premature Ventricular Complex

Pathophysiology A **premature ventricular complex (PVC)** is characterized by a premature, extra beat originating in the ventricles and a wide QRS complex without a P wave. It is usually followed by a pause, called the compensatory pause. **Table 8-29** describes the ECG reading of a premature ventricular complex.

Table 8-29 Premature Ventricular Complex

Rhythm	Irregular (underlying rhythm is disrupted by presence of the early beat or beats).
Rate	Depends on the rate of the underlying rhythm.
P waves	Typically present with the underlying rhythm but not the premature beats.
PR interval	Typically present with the underlying rhythm but not the premature beats.
QRS complex	Premature beats are wide (> 0.10 sec) and bizarre, and differ from QRS complexes of the underlying rhythm. T waves of the premature beats take an opposite direction to the R waves. PVCs are usually followed by a compensatory pause.

   Uniform PVCs originate from the same site in the ventricle and are in one or the same direction (**Figure 8-21**). *Multifocal PVCs* originate from several sites in the ventricle and appear different from each other, going in two directions (**Figure 8-22**). *Bigeminal PVCs* are

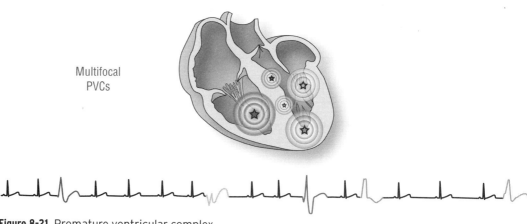

Multifocal PVCs

Figure 8-21 Premature ventricular complex.

noted by every other beat being a PVC (**Figure 8-23**). *Trigeminal PVCs* are characterized by every third beat being a PVC. *Couplets* are two PVCs together.

Causes

- Hypokalemia
- CHF
- Increased sympathetic nervous system response
- Myocardial ischemia
- Electrolyte imbalance
- Hypoxia
- Use of caffeine, tobacco, alcohol
- Heart disease
- Tricyclic antidepressants
- Acidosis
- AMI
- Stress

Signs and Symptoms

- Palpitations
- Chest pain
- Difficulty breathing
- Profuse sweating
- Nausea and vomiting

Assessment

- Scene size-up
  - Ensure BSI.

- Initial/primary assessment
  - Monitor LOC.
  - Manage ABCs.
  - Treat life-threatening illness/injuries.
- Focused history and physical exam/secondary assessment
  - Obtain SAMPLE history and chief complaint (OPQRST).

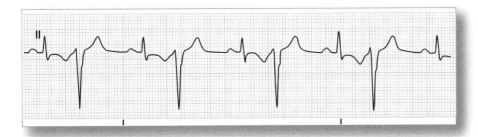

Figure 8-22 Multifocal PVCs.

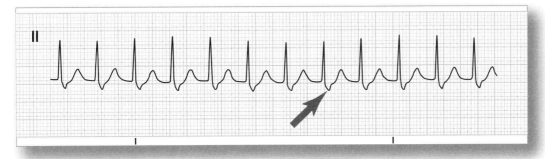

Figure 8-23 Bigeminal PVCs.

Management

- Apply pulse oximeter and supplemental oxygen.
- Establish IV access.
- Monitor vital signs.
- Attach cardiac monitor.
- Obtain 12-lead ECG to determine specific cause of complaint.
- Treat according to symptoms and presentation.

Table 8-30 summarizes treatment of premature ventricular complex.

Table 8-30 Treatment of Premature Ventricular Complex (> 6/min or Symptomatic)

Treatment	Purpose	Adult Dose
Amiodarone	Prolongs action potential and refractory period; slows the sinus rate; prolongs PR and QT intervals; vasodilation	IV: 150 mg over 10 min
Lidocaine	Suppresses automaticity and spontaneous depolarization of the ventricles	IV: 1.0-1.5 mg/kg

Ventricular Tachycardia

Pathophysiology <u>Ventricular tachycardia</u> (v-tach) is characterized by three or more PVCs in a row (typically six to ten PVC runs), without P waves, and with a wide QRS complex; the ventricular rate is 150 to 220 beats/min. T waves may not be present (**Figure 8-24**). Types of v-tach are as follows: monomorphic (all beats have the same appearance) and polymorphic (beats have different appearances). Ventricular tachycardia may present either with or without a pulse. If there is no pulse, treat as ventricular fibrillation. **Table 8-31** describes the ECG reading of ventricular tachycardia.

Table 8-31 Ventricular Tachycardia

Rhythm	Typically regular.
Rate	Ventricular rate is between 150 and 250 beats/min.
P waves	Typically absent. However, if identified, there is no association with the rhythm.
PR interval	None.
QRS complex	Wide (> 0.10 sec) and bizarre. T waves of the ventricular beats take an opposite direction to the R waves.

Ventricular Tachycardia With a Pulse

Causes

- Stress
- Hypoxia
- AMI

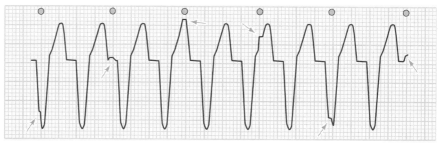

Figure 8-24 Ventricular tachycardia.

- Electrolyte imbalance
- Heart disease
- Use of caffeine, alcohol, or tobacco

Signs and Symptoms (Both Monomorphic and Polymorphic)
- Altered LOC
- Hypotension
- Pulmonary congestion
- Hypoxia
- Heart rate > 150 beats/min
- Chest pain
- Dyspnea
- Fluttering in chest (palpitations)

Assessment
- Scene size-up
  - Ensure BSI.
- Initial/primary assessment
  - Monitor LOC.
  - Manage ABCs.
  - Treat life-threatening illness/injuries.
- Focused history and physical exam/secondary assessment
  - Obtain SAMPLE history and chief complaint (OPQRST).

Management
- Apply pulse oximeter and supplemental oxygen.
- Establish IV access.
- Monitor vital signs.
- Attach cardiac monitor.
- Obtain 12-lead ECG to determine specific cause of complaint.
- Treat according to symptoms and presentation.

Table 8-32 summarizes treatment of monomorphic stable ventricular tachycardia. **Table 8-33** summarizes treatment of polymorphic ventricular tachycardia.

Table 8-32 Treatment of Monomorphic Stable Ventricular Tachycardia

Treatment	Purpose	Initial Adult Dose
Synchronized cardioversion	Cardiac reset (for unstable patients)	100 J
Lidocaine or	Suppresses automaticity and spontaneous depolarization of ventricles	IV: 1.0-1.5 mg/kg
Procainamide or	Increases threshold of ventricular fibrillation/pulseless v-tach	Up to 50 mg/min Total of 17 mg/kg
Amiodarone	Prolongs action potential and refractory period; slows the sinus rate; prolongs PR and QT intervals; vasodilation–decreases peripheral vascular resistance	IVP: 150 mg

Table 8-33 Treatment of Polymorphic Ventricular Tachycardia

Treatment	Purpose	Initial Adult Dose
Synchronized cardioversion	Cardiac reset (for unstable patients)	100 J
Magnesium sulfate	Important for muscle contraction and nerve transmission	IV: 2 g over 10 min

Ventricular Fibrillation

Pathophysiology <u>**Ventricular fibrillation**</u> (v-fib) is characterized by erratic firing from multiple sites in the ventricle (**Figure 8-25**). It is the most common cause of prehospital cardiac arrest. Treatment is the same as with pulseless v-tach. **Table 8-34** describes the ECG reading of ventricular fibrillation.

Table 8-34 Ventricular Fibrillation

Rhythm	None
Rate	None
P waves	None
PR interval	None
QRS complex	None

Signs and Symptoms
- Unconscious
- Pulseless
- Apneic

Assessment
- Scene size-up
  - Ensure BSI.
- Initial/primary assessment
  - Monitor ABCs.
  - Initiate CPR.
- Focused history and physical exam/secondary assessment
  - Obtain SAMPLE history and chief complaint (OPQRST) from bystanders or family members.

Management
- Apply pulse oximeter and supplemental oxygen.
- Establish IV or IO access.
- Attach cardiac monitor/defibrillator.

Table 8-35 summarizes treatment of ventricular fibrillation.

Table 8-35 Treatment of Ventricular Fibrillation

Treatment	Purpose	Initial Adult Dose
Defibrillation	Cardiac reset	Monophasic: 200 J Biphasic: 120 J
Epinephrine *or*	Stimulates both alpha- and beta-adrenergic receptors	IV: 1 mg
Vasopressin	Peripheral vasoconstriction (nonadrenergic) to increase blood flow to heart and brain	IV: 40 units May give one dose, in place of first or second dose of epinephrine
Lidocaine *or*	Suppresses automaticity and spontaneous depolarization of ventricles	IVP: 1 mg/kg
Amiodarone	Prolongs action potential and refractory period; slows the sinus rate; prolongs PR and QT intervals; vasodilation	IVP: 300 mg

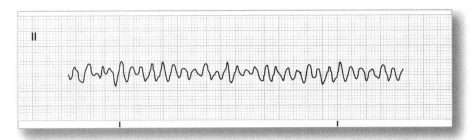

Figure 8-25 Ventricular fibrillation.

Pulseless Electrical Activity

Pathophysiology In **pulseless electrical activity (PEA)**, an electrical rhythm is present but has no ventricular response and therefore there is no pulse. It can present as any rhythm on the monitor. The goal is to treat the cause. **Table 8-36** describes the ECG reading of pulseless electrical activity.

Table 8-36 Pulseless Electrical Activity

Rhythm	May be regular or irregular
Rate	May be fast, normal, or slow
P waves	May be present or absent, depending on rhythm origin
PR interval	May be present or absent; depending on rhythm origin
QRS complex	May be normal width or wide and bizarre (> 0.10 sec), depending on rhythm origin

Table 8-37 outlines possible causes and treatment of PEA (the six Hs and Ts).

Table 8-37 Possible Causes and Treatment of PEA

Possible Causes	Corrective Action
Hypovolemia	Fluid administration
Hypoxia	Oxygenation and ventilation
Hydrogen ions	Ventilation
Hypokalemia/hyperkalemia	Managed in hospital
Hypothermia/hyperthermia	Manage body temperature
Hypoglycemia/hyperglycemia	Correct blood glucose level
Tablets	Consider naloxone and flumazenil
Tamponade, cardiac	Pericardiocentesis
Tension pneumothorax	Chest needle decompression
Thrombosis, coronary	Managed in hospital
Thrombosis, pulmonary	Managed in hospital
Trauma	Correct hypovolemia

Signs and Symptoms
- Unconscious
- Apneic
- Pulseless

Assessment

- Scene size-up
  - Ensure BSI.
- Initial/primary assessment
  - Establish ABCs.
  - Treat life-threatening illness/injuries.
  - Initiate CPR.
- Focused history and physical exam/secondary assessment
  - Obtain SAMPLE history and chief complaint (OPQRST) from bystanders or family members.

Management

- Establish IV or IO access.
- Attach defibrillator.
- Apply pulse oximeter and supplemental oxygen.

Asystole ("Cardiac Standstill")

Pathophysiology <u>Asystole</u> is the absence of cardiac activity, both electrical and mechanical. It is a terminal rhythm with almost no chance of recovery (**Figure 8-26**). *Equipment failure can mimic asystole. If this rhythm is present, be sure to confirm it in two leads.* **Table 8-38** describes the ECG reading of asystole. Fine ventricular tachycardia may be confused with asystole.

Table 8-38 Asystole

Rhythm	None
Rate	None
P waves	None
PR interval	None
QRS complex	None

Signs and Symptoms

- Unconscious
- Apneic
- Pulseless

Assessment

- Scene size-up
  - Ensure BSI.
- Initial/primary assessment
  - Establish ABCs.
  - Initiate CPR.
- Focused history and physical exam/secondary assessment
  - Obtain SAMPLE history and chief complaint (OPQRST) from bystanders or family members.

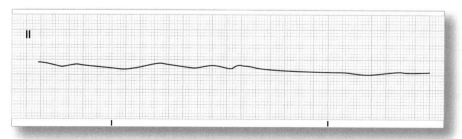

Figure 8-26 Asystole.

Management
- Apply pulse oximeter and supplemental oxygen.
- Establish IV or IO access.
- Attach cardiac monitor/defibrillator.

Table 8-39 summarizes treatment of asystole.

Table 8-39 Treatment of Asystole

Treatment	Purpose	Initial Adult Dose
Atropine	Increases heart rate; blocks parasympathetic nervous system	IV: 1 mg
Epinephrine *or*	Stimulates both alpha- and beta-adrenergic receptors	IV/IO: 1 mg
Vasopressin	Peripheral vasoconstriction (nonadrenergic) to increase blood flow to heart and brain	IV/IO: 40 units May give one dose, in place of first or second dose of epinephrine

Idioventricular Rhythm

Pathophysiology An idioventricular rhythm occurs when the SA and AV nodes have failed, forcing the ventricular muscle to act as the heart's pacemaker. Idioventricular rhythms can be either slow or fast (accelerated idioventricular rhythm).

Table 8-40 describes the ECG reading of idioventricular rhythm.

Table 8-40 Idioventricular Rhythm

Rhythm	Regular (becomes irregular as the heart dies). R-R intervals are equal.
Rate	20-40 beats/min (40-100 beats/min for accelerated).
P waves	None.
PR interval	None.
QRS complex	Wide (0.04-0.12 sec) and bizarre. T wave typically takes the opposite direction of the QRS wave.

Causes
- Myocardial infarction
- Electrolyte imbalance
- Digitalis toxicity

Signs and Symptoms
- Altered LOC
- Hypotension
- Bradycardia

Assessment
- Scene size-up
  - Ensure BSI.
- Initial/primary assessment
  - Monitor LOC.
  - Manage ABCs.
  - Treat life-threatening illness/injuries.
- Focused history and physical exam/secondary assessment
  - Obtain SAMPLE history and chief complaint (OPQRST).

Management
- Apply pulse oximeter and supplemental oxygen.
- Establish IV access.

- Monitor vital signs.
- Attach cardiac monitor.
- Obtain 12-lead ECG to determine specific cause of complaint.
- Treat according to symptoms and presentation.

Table 8-41 summarizes treatment of idioventricular rhythm.

Table 8-41 Treatment of Idioventricular Rhythm

Treatment	Purpose	Adult Dose
Transcutaneous pacing	Increases heart rate to increase cardiac output	Set pacer to 70 beats/min and 30 mA, increasing mA until capture
Atropine	Increases heart rate; blocks para-sympathetic nervous system	IV: 0.5 mg

Twelve-Lead ECGs and ECG Interpretation

ECG Leads and Lead Placement

To view difficult perspectives of the heart, electrodes must be placed in different areas. The leads I, II, III, aVR, aVL, and aVF "look" at the heart in the frontal plane (**Figure 8-27**), and the **precordial** (V$_1$–V$_6$) leads "look" at the horizontal plane (**Figure 8-28**).

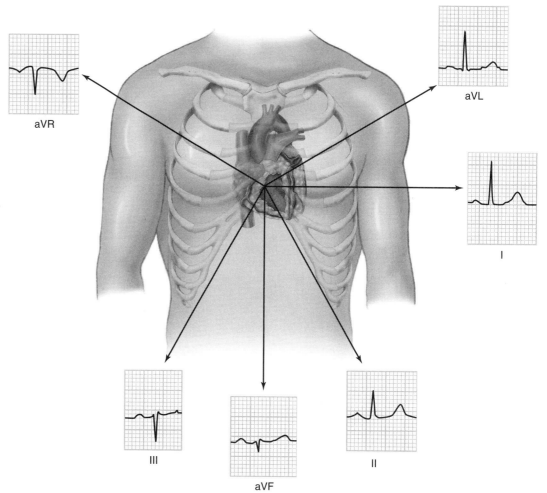

Figure 8-27 Limb leads look at the heart in the vertical plane.

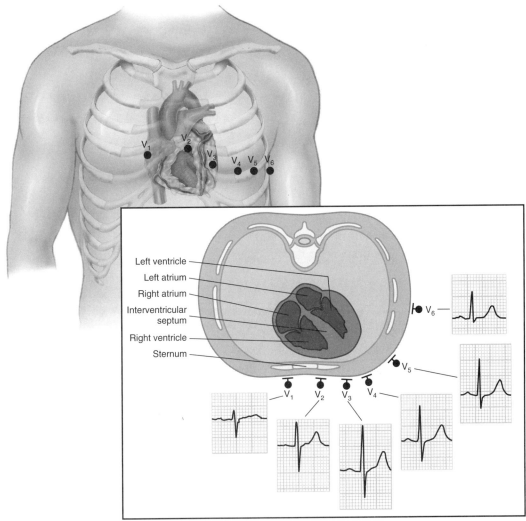

Figure 8-28 Precordial leads (chest leads) look at the heart in the horizontal plane.

Categories of Myocardial Infarction

Myocardial infarctions (MIs) are divided into two categories:

- An ST-segment-elevation MI (<u>**STEMI**</u>) is when there are visible ST-segment changes on the ECG. An elevated ST segment is defined as an ST segment rising greater than 1 mm from the isoelectric line. This elevation must be present in two or more contiguous leads, which record the effects in the same coronary artery.
- A non-ST-segment-elevation MI (<u>**NSTEMI**</u>) is when there are no visible ST-segment changes on the ECG (**Table 8-42**).

Table 8-42 Evolution of an Acute Myocardial Infarction on the ECG

Stage	ECG Changes in Overlying Leads*	Timing
Ischemia	T-wave inversion ST-segment depression	With the onset of ischemia
Injury	ST-segment elevation	Minutes to hours
Infraction	Q waves appear	Within several hours to several days
*Reciprocal changes will be seen in opposite leads.		

Tip

Location of lead placement for a 12-lead ECG:

- Lead V_1 is placed in the fourth intercostal space to the right of the sternum.
- Lead V_2 is placed in the fourth intercostal space to the left of the sternum.
- Lead V_3 is placed directly between leads V_2 and V_4.
- Lead V_4 is placed in the fifth intercostal space in the left midclavicular line.
- Lead V_5 is placed horizontally with V_4 in the anterior axillary line.
- Lead V_6 is placed horizontally with V_4 and V_5 in the midaxillary line.

The Twelve-Lead ECG in a Normal, Healthy Heart

The normal 12-lead ECG evaluates and displays the same electrical events within the heart from 12 different angles (**Figure 8-29**). Many disease processes can be detected by a 12-lead ECG. Remember, the only way to rule in or rule out ST-segment elevation or depression in the prehospital environment is via a printed 12-lead ECG.

Electrocardiograms

The keys to interpreting an ECG rhythm (**Figure 8-30**) are as follows:

- **Rhythm:** Regular vs. irregular
- **Rate:** Beats per minute
- **P-wave morphology:** Indicates the electrical impulse that travels through the atria—upright vs. inverted vs. absent
- **PR interval:** Indicates the delay in the electrical impulse traveling through the AV node
- **QRS complex:** Indicates the electrical impulse that travels along the bundle of His, right and left bundle branches, and Purkinje fibers
- **T wave:** Indicates ventricular conduction and depolarization

A normal sinus rhythm is the normal electrical activity of the healthy heart (**Figure 8-31**). **Table 8-43** describes the ECG reading of a normal sinus rhythm.

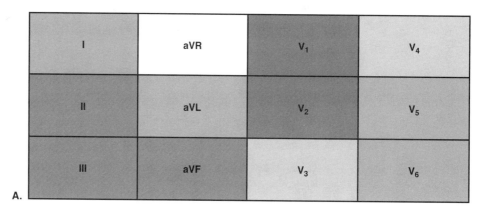

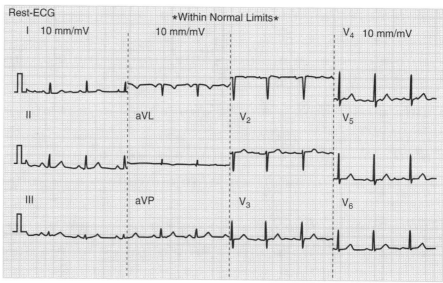

Figure 8-29 A. The areas on a 12-lead ECG correlate to views of the heart **B.** A normal ECG with standard 12-lead format.

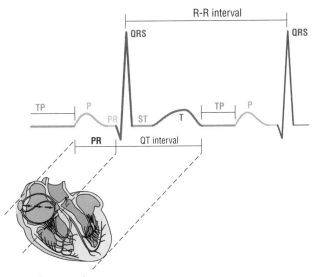

Figure 8-30 The ECG and cardiac events.

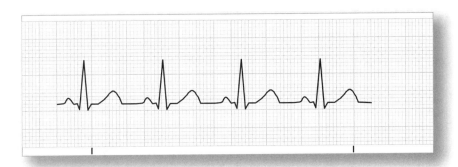

Figure 8-31 Normal sinus rhythm.

Table 8-43 Normal Sinus Rhythm

Rhythm	Regular (R-R intervals and P-P intervals are constant)
Rate	60-100 beats/min (atrial and ventricular rates are equal)
P waves	Upright and uniform, precede each QRS complex
PR interval	Within normal limits (0.12-0.20 sec in duration) and constant
QRS complex	Within normal limits (0.04-0.12 sec in duration) and constant

P Waves
- **Width:** Should be less than 0.11 seconds (lead II)
- **Height:** Should be less than 2.5 mm (lead II)
- **PR interval:** 0.12–0.20 seconds
- **Morphology:** Upright (all leads)

QRS Complex
- **Q wave:** Q waves smaller than one third the height of the R wave, less than 1 mm wide, and not in two contiguous leads are not pathologic.
- **Width:** Less than 0.12 second.
- **QT interval:** Less than 0.42 second.
- **ST segment:** Should return to isoelectric line and should not have a depression or elevation.

T Wave
- **Morphology:** Should be upright in all leads except aVR

Abnormal Twelve-Lead ECGs: Myocardial Infarctions

Table 8-44 shows the location of a myocardial ischemia and/or infarction through the use of 12-lead ECGs.

Table 8-44 Location of Myocardial Ischemia and/or Infarction

Location	ECG Changes
Anterior	V_3 and V_4
Lateral	V_5 and V_6
Anterolateral	I, aVL, V_5, and V_6
High lateral	I and aVL
Inferolateral	II, III, aVF, and V_6
Inferior	II, III, and aVF
Septal	V_1 and V_2
Right ventricle	V_4R

The Twelve-Lead ECG in an Anterior MI

Anterior infarctions are typically caused by an occlusion of the proximal left anterior descending coronary artery (LAD). Because of the placement of leads V_3 and V_4 over the anterior surface of the heart, infarction may be observed by the development of Q waves, T-wave inversion, and ST-segment elevation (**Figure 8-32**). Common complications of an anterior infarction are congestive heart failure, bundle branch blocks, and complete heart blocks.

The Twelve-Lead ECG in a Lateral MI

Lateral infarctions are typically caused by an occlusion of the circumflex. Because of the placement of leads V_5 and V_6 over the lateral surface of the heart, infarction may be observed by the development of Q waves, T-wave inversion, and ST-segment elevation (**Figure 8-33**). A complication of a lateral infarction is left ventricular dysfunction.

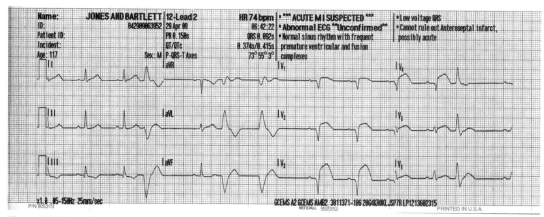

Figure 8-32 Anterior MI with septal extension.

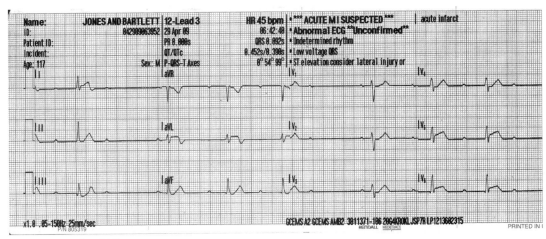

Figure 8-33 Lateral MI.

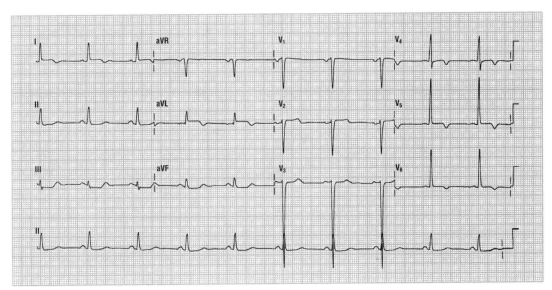

Figure 8-34 Anterolateral MI.

The Twelve-Lead ECG in an Anterolateral MI

Anterolateral infarctions are typically caused by an occlusion of the left circumflex or left anterior descending artery (LAD). Because of the placement of leads I, aVL, V_5, and V_6 over the anterior and lateral surface of the heart, infarction may be observed by the development of Q waves, T-wave inversion, and ST-segment elevation (**Figure 8-34**). Common complications of anterolateral infarctions are left ventricular dysfunction, bundle branch blocks, and congestive heart failure.

The Twelve-Lead ECG in a High Lateral MI

High lateral infarctions are typically caused by an occlusion of the circumflex. Because of the placement of leads I and aVL over the high lateral surface of the heart, infarction may be observed by the development of Q waves, T-wave inversion, and ST-segment elevation (**Figure 8-35**). A complication of a high lateral infarction is left ventricular dysfunction.

The Twelve-Lead ECG in an Inferolateral MI

Inferolateral infarctions are typically caused by an occlusion of the right coronary artery. Because of the placement of leads II, III, aVF, and V_6 over the inferior surface of the heart, infarction may be observed by the development of Q waves, T-wave inversion, and ST-segment elevation (**Figure 8-36**). Complications of an inferolateral infarction are hypotension and left ventricular dysfunction.

The Twelve-Lead ECG in an Inferior MI

Inferior infarctions are typically caused by an occlusion of the right coronary artery. Because of the placement of leads II, III, and aVF over the inferior surface of the heart, infarction may be observed by the development of Q waves, T-wave inversion, and ST-segment elevation (**Figure 8-37**). Complications of an inferior infarction are hypotension and left ventricular dysfunction.

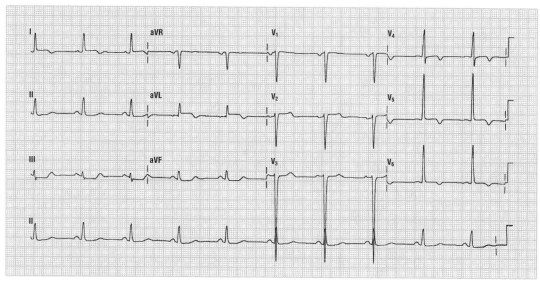

Figure 8-35 High lateral MI.

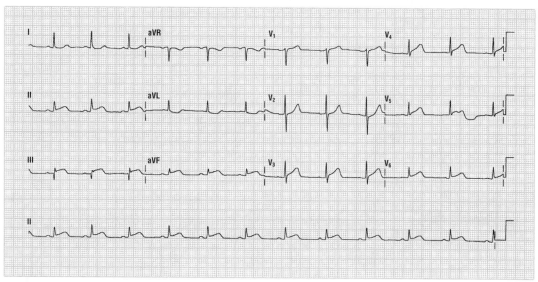

Figure 8-36 Inferolateral MI.

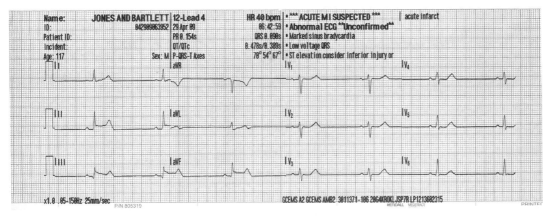

Figure 8-37 Inferior MI.

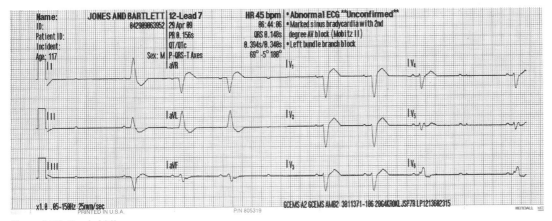

Figure 8-38 Septal MI.

The Twelve-Lead ECG in a Septal MI

Pathophysiology

Septal infarctions are typically caused by an occlusion of the left coronary artery. Because of the placement of leads V_1 and V_2 over the left ventricular septum, infarction may be observed by the development of Q waves, T-wave inversion, and ST-segment elevation (**Figure 8-38**). Complications of a septal infarction are bundle branch blocks.

The Twelve-Lead ECG in a Right Ventricular MI

Right ventricular infarctions are typically caused by an occlusion of the right coronary artery. Lead V_4 will need to be placed in the fifth intercostal space in the *right* midclavicular line to view the right ventricle. Placement of this lead on the right side of the chest now implies that this is lead V_4R. Infarction may be observed by the development of Q waves, T-wave inversion, and ST-segment elevation (**Figure 8-39**). Complications of right ventricular infarctions are profound hypotension and right ventricular dysfunction.

Bundle Branch Blocks

Pathophysiology

When a bundle branch becomes injured, it may cease to conduct electrical impulses appropriately. This results in altered pathways for ventricular depolarization. Because the electrical impulse can no longer use the preferred pathway across the bundle branch, it may move instead through muscle fibers in a way that both slows the electrical movement

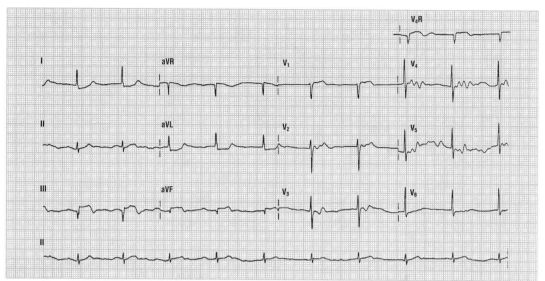

Figure 8-39 Right ventricular MI.

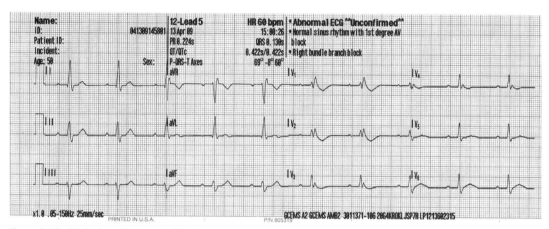

Figure 8-40 Right bundle branch block.

and changes the direction of the impulses. As a result, there is a loss of ventricular synchrony, ventricular depolarization is prolonged, and there may be a corresponding drop in cardiac output. Bundle branch blocks may result from an MI, so signs and symptoms may be similar.

A **bundle branch block** can be diagnosed when the duration of the QRS complex exceeds 120 milliseconds. A right bundle branch block (RBBB) (**Figure 8-40**) typically causes prolongation of the last part of the QRS complex, and may shift the heart's electrical axis slightly to the right. The ECG will show a terminal R wave in lead V_1 and a slurred S wave in lead I. Left bundle branch block (LBBB) (**Figure 8-41**) widens the entire QRS, and in most cases shifts the heart's electrical axis to the left. The ECG will show a QS or RS complex in lead V_1 and a monophasic R wave in lead I. In patients with a preexisting bundle branch block, the ECG may not show the usual changes if an AMI occurs.

Complications of bundle branch blocks are inability to diagnose an infarction with an LBBB, and possible complete heart blocks.

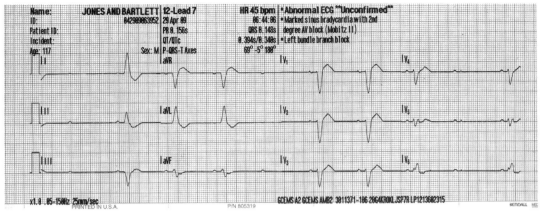

Figure 8-41 Left bundle branch block.

Cardiac Electrical Procedures and Pharmacologic Interventions

Transcutaneous Cardiac Pacing (TCP)

1. Apply pacing electrodes.
2. Turn pacer on.
3. Set rate to 70 beats/min.
4. Set current, and gradually increase until capture occurs.
   a. For symptomatic bradycardia, or high-degree heart blocks: Increase from minimal setting until capture is achieved. Capture is characterized by a wide QRS complex and a broad T wave after each pacer spike. Once capture occurs, add 10 milliamperes.

Synchronized Cardioversion

Cardioversion is performed if the patient's heart rate is over 150 beats/min and the patient is symptomatic. Cardioversion is a synchronized direct current (DC) countershock. The countershock is synchronized with the R wave (ventricular polarization) to avoid delivering the countershock during ventricular diastole (T wave). Cardioversion is indicated for unstable supraventricular tachycardia (SVT) (or paroxysmal SVT [PSVT]), atrial flutter, atrial fibrillation with rapid response, and ventricular tachycardia with a pulse.

Escalating Energy Setting for Synchronized Cardioversion
- 50 J for PSVT and atrial flutter
- 100 J
- 200 J
- 300 J
- 360 J

Defibrillation
- Defibrillation is the administration of an unsynchronized DC countershock and is indicated in ventricular fibrillation (v-fib) and pulseless ventricular tachycardia (v-tach).

Tip

It is important to remember to press the Sync button after each attempted cardioversion to ensure that the machine remains synchronized with the R wave.

- One shock is followed by immediate CPR.
  - Monophasic waveform
    - Monophasic defibrillators deliver a unidirectional countershock via a positive and negative defibrillation electrode.
    - Adults: 360 J for v-fib and pulseless v-tach
    - Infants and children: 2–4 J/kg
  - Biphasic waveform defibrillation
    - Biphasic defibrillators deliver a bidirectional countershock via a **bipolar** (both positive and negative) defibrillation electrode that is directed to another bipolar defibrillation electrode, which then redirects the impulse back to the first electrode. This process continues until the entire charge is delivered and takes approximately 10 milliseconds.
    - Adults: Initial dose 150–200 J, with the second dose being equal or higher.
    - Infants and children: 2–4 J/kg.
    - If you are unsure whether your defibrillator is monophasic or biphasic, use 200 J as a default dose.

Vasopressors

A **vasopressor** is a drug that causes the muscles of the arteries and capillaries to contract. During cardiac arrest, vasopressors are administered when an IV/IO is in place, after the first or second shock.

- 1 mg (1:10,000) of epinephrine may be given every 3 to 5 minutes *or*
- 40 units of vasopressin can be substituted for either the first or second dose of epinephrine, only to be given once.

Antiarrhythmics

Antiarrhythmics control or prevent cardiac ventricular arrhythmias. Antiarrhythmics work by relaxing electrical activity, allowing the heart to resume a normal rhythm.

- Lidocaine: 1mg/kg (to a maximum dose of 3 mg/kg)
- Amiodarone: 300 mg for first dose, 150 mg for second dose
- Magnesium sulfate: 2-gram bolus (indicated in polymorphic ventricular tachycardia)

Beta-Adrenergic Blockers

Beta-adrenergic blockers block the inhibitory effects of sympathetic nervous system agents, such as epinephrine. Their actions are as follows:

- Slow ventricular rate in atrial fibrillation or atrial flutter
- Treat class II/III heart failure
- Slow heart rate
- Increase ventricular filling by relaxing obstructing cardiac muscle to increase cardiac output
- Block sympathetic nervous system

Contraindications to using beta-adrenergic blockers include the following:

- Heart rate of less than 60 beats/min
- Systolic blood pressure (SBP) of less than 100 mm Hg
- Moderate to severe left ventricular failure (CHF)
- Signs of peripheral hypoperfusion
- PR interval of greater than 0.24 second
- Second- or third-degree blocks
- Acute asthma or reactive airways disease

Vital Vocabulary

antiarrhythmics The medications used to treat and prevent cardiac rhythm disorders.

aortic valve The valve between the left ventricle and the aorta.

arrhythmias Disturbances in cardiac rhythm. Also called *dysrhythmias*.

arteries The blood vessels that carry oxygenated blood away from the heart.

arterioles A small-diameter blood vessel that extends and branches out from an artery and leads to capillaries.

asystole A state of no cardiac electrical activity.

atrial fibrillation A rhythm in which the atria no longer contract but fibrillate or quiver without any organized contraction.

atrial tachycardia Any rapid heart rhythm originating in the atria, such as atrial fibrillation and atrial flutter.

atrioventricular (AV) node A specialized structure located in the AV junction that slows conduction through the AV junction.

atrium Upper chamber of the heart.

automaticity Spontaneous initiation of depolarizing electric impulses by pacemaker sites within the electric conduction system of the heart.

autonomic nervous system A subdivision of the nervous system that controls primarily involuntary body functions. It comprises the sympathetic and parasympathetic nervous systems.

autorhythmic cells Cells distributed in an orderly fashion through the heart. They make up the heart's conduction system and are concentrated in the sinoatrial (SA) node, atrioventricular (AV) node, atrioventricular (AV) bundle (bundle of His), and Purkinje fibers.

beta-adrenergic blockers Medical treatments that block the inhibitory effects of sympathetic nervous system agents, such as epinephrine.

bicuspid (or mitral) valve The valve located between the left atrium and the left ventricle of the heart.

bipolar Monitor leads that contain two electrodes (positive and negative). Applied to the arms and legs. Found in leads I, II, and III.

bundle branch blocks Disturbances in electric conduction through the right or left bundle branch from the bundle of His.

bundle of His The portion of the electric conduction system in the interventricular septum that conducts the depolarizing impulse from the atrioventricular junction to the right and left bundle branches.

capillaries Extremely narrow blood vessels composed of a single layer of cells through which oxygen and nutrients pass to the tissues. Capillaries form a network between arterioles and venules.

cardiac cycle The period from one cardiac contraction to the next. Each cardiac cycle consists of ventricular contraction (systole) and relaxation (diastole).

cardiac output (CO) Amount of blood pumped by the heart per minute, calculated by multiplying the stroke volume by the heart rate per minute.

conductivity The ability to transmit an electrical impulse from one cell to the next.

contractile cells Cells that make up the muscle walls of the atria and ventricles. They give the heart its ability to pump blood through the body.

contractility The strength of heart muscle contractions.

depolarization The process of discharging resting cardiac muscle fibers by an electric impulse that causes them to contract.

diastole The period of ventricular relaxation during which the ventricles passively fill with blood.

ectopic beat Any cardiac impulse originating outside the SA node; considered abnormal.

endocardium The thin membrane lining the inside of the heart.

epicardium The thin membrane lining the outside of the heart.

excitability The ability to respond to an electrical impulse.

extensibility The ability to stretch.

first-degree AV block A partial disruption of the conduction of the depolarizing impulse from the atria to the ventricles, causing prolongation of the PR interval.

Frank-Starling mechanism The increase in strength of contraction due to increased end diastolic volume (the volume of blood in the heart just before the ventricles begin to contract).

heart rate (HR) The number of cardiac contractions (heartbeats) per minute—in other words, the pulse rate.

hypertension High blood pressure, usually a diastolic pressure of greater than 90 mm Hg.

ischemia Tissue anoxia from diminished blood flow to tissue, usually caused by narrowing or occlusion of the artery.

junctional rhythms Arrhythmias arising from ectopic foci in the area of the atrioventricular junction; often show an absence of the P wave, a short PR interval, or a P wave appearing after the QRS complex.

junctional tachycardia Occurs when impulses originate in the atrioventricular junctional pacemaker at a rate of anywhere between 100 and 220 beats/min and are conducted retrograde to the atria and antegrade to the ventricles.

myocardial infarction (MI) Occurs when the heart muscle does not get adequate oxygen because of decreased blood supply, an increased need for oxygen, or both. The main site of infarct (tissue death) is the left ventricle.

myocardium The cardiac muscle.

NSTEMI Non-ST-segment-elevation myocardial infarction. Characterized as a myocardial infarction without ST-segment elevation.

paroxysmal SVT (PVST) A tachycardia that originates in tissue above the ventricles and begins and ends suddenly.

pericardial tamponade Impairment of diastolic filling of the right ventricle as the result of significant amounts of fluid in the pericardial sac surrounding the heart, leading to a decrease in the cardiac output.

pericardiocentesis A procedure in which fluid is aspirated from the pericardial sac.

pericardium The double-layered sac containing the heart and the origins of the superior vena cava, inferior vena cava, and pulmonary artery.

precordial Leads that are applied to the chest, allowing for a horizontal view of the heart. Found in leads V_1, V_2, V_3, V_4, V_5, and V_6.

preload The pressure under which a ventricle fills; it is influenced by the volume of blood returned by the veins to the heart.

premature atrial complex (PAC) Heartbeats originating from the atrium and occurring before the beat coming from the sinoatrial node.

premature junctional complex (PJC) Caused by premature electrical impulses that occur in the atrioventricular junction.

premature ventricular complex (PVC) An extra heartbeat originating in the ventricles and a wide QRS complex without a P wave. It is usually followed by a pause called the compensatory pause.

pulmonic valve The valve between the right ventricle and the pulmonary artery.

pulseless electrical activity (PEA) An electrical rhythm is present but there is no ventricular response and therefore no pulse.

Purkinje fibers A system of fibers in the ventricles that conducts the excitation impulse from the bundle branches to the myocardium.

repolarization The return of ions to their previous resting state, which corresponds with the relaxation of the myocardial muscle. It results from the outward diffusion of potassium.

second-degree AV block, Mobitz type I A progressive prolongation of the PR interval on consecutive beats, followed by a "dropped" QRS complex.

second-degree AV block, Mobitz type II Electrical impulses are delayed in an irregular fashion in the heart, such that beats are occasionally skipped. Less common yet more severe than type I, because it is more likely to progress to complete heart block (third-degree AV block).

sick sinus syndrome (SSS) The result of long-term damage to the sinoatrial node, which impairs its ability to effectively conduct electrical impulses through the heart.

sinoatrial (SA) node or **sinus node** The dominant pacemaker of the heart, located at the junction of the superior vena cava and the right atrium.

sinus bradycardia A sinus rhythm with a heart rate of less than 60 beats/min.

sinus tachycardia A sinus rhythm with a heart rate of greater than 100 beats/min.

STEMI ST-segment-elevation myocardial infarction. Characterized as a myocardial infarction with ST-segment elevation.

stroke volume The amount of blood pumped out by either ventricle in a single contraction (heartbeat).

supraventricular tachycardia (SVT) An abnormal heart rhythm with a rapid, narrow QRS complex.

systole The period during which the ventricles contract.

third-degree (complete) AV block When the heart's electrical signals do not pass from the upper to the lower chambers, and instead operate independently of each other. When this occurs, the ventricular pacemaker takes over. The ventricles contract and pump blood at a slower rate than the atrial pacemaker.

tricuspid valve The valve between the right atrium and right ventricle of the heart.

vasopressor A drug that causes the muscles of the arteries and capillaries to contract. Administered during cardiac arrest when an IV/IO is in place, after the first or second shock.

veins The blood vessels that carry deoxygenated blood to the heart.

ventricle Lower chamber of the heart.

ventricular fibrillation Heart condition characterized by erratic firing from multiple sites in the ventricle; the most common cause of prehospital cardiac arrest.

ventricular tachycardia Heart condition characterized by three or more PVCs in a row (typically six to ten PVC runs), without P waves, and with a wide QRS complex; ventricular rate is 150–220 beats/min. T wave may not be present.

Neurologic Emergencies

Neurology Overview

The nervous system (**Figure 9-1**) is composed of the central nervous system (CNS) and the peripheral nervous system. The CNS is responsible for thought, perception, feelings, and autonomic body functions. The peripheral nervous system transmits commands from the brain to the body and transmits messages from the body to the brain. The nervous system in turn is made up of two systems:

- **The somatic nervous system:** Responsible for voluntary movement of the skeletal muscles.
- **The autonomic nervous system:** Responsible for involuntary actions of the body and maintaining homeostasis. The autonomic system is broken further into the sympathetic and parasympathetic nervous systems.

Table 9-1 shows the structures and general functions of the nervous system.

- The sympathetic nervous system secretes the neurotransmitter norepinephrine, which causes the fight-or-flight response, meaning this neurotransmitter causes *increases* in certain functions of major organs, such as blood pressure, heart rate, and respirations.
- The parasympathetic nervous system secretes the neurotransmitter acetylcholine (ACh). This stimulates the feed-and-breed response, which causes *decreases* in certain functions of major organs, such as blood pressure, heart rate, and respirations.

The CNS processes the staggering amount of information it receives from the peripheral nervous system, using the **diencephalon** and the **brainstem**. Within the brainstem, the **midbrain** regulates level of consciousness (LOC), whereas the **pons** controls respiratory rate and breathing patterns, and the **medulla oblongata** controls the blood pressure and heart rate. **Figure 9-2** and **Figure 9-3** show the key structures of the brain and the activities they control.

Anatomy and Physiology

- Definitions
  - The **ganglion** is a tissue structure that contains the synapses between CNS neurons and peripheral neurons.
  - **Synapse:** Nerve cells (neurons) do not directly touch each other; instead, there are slight gaps between nerve cells called synapses.
  - **Neurotransmitters:** Chemicals that carry an electrically conducted signal across the synapse from one neuron to the next neuron, thus connecting the nerve cells and relaying messages throughout the nervous system. Dopamine, ACh, epinephrine, and serotonin are examples of neurotransmitters. The main neurotransmitters of the autonomic nervous system are:
    - **Acetylcholine (ACh):** A cholinergic neurotransmitter used in the preganglionic nerves of the sympathetic nervous system and in both the **preganglia** and the **postganglia** of the parasympathetic nervous system.

Tip
To remember the difference between the sympathetic and parasympathetic nervous systems, use the acronym SNAP: 1. **S**ympathetic–**N**orepinephrine 2. **A**cetylcholine–**P**arasympathetic

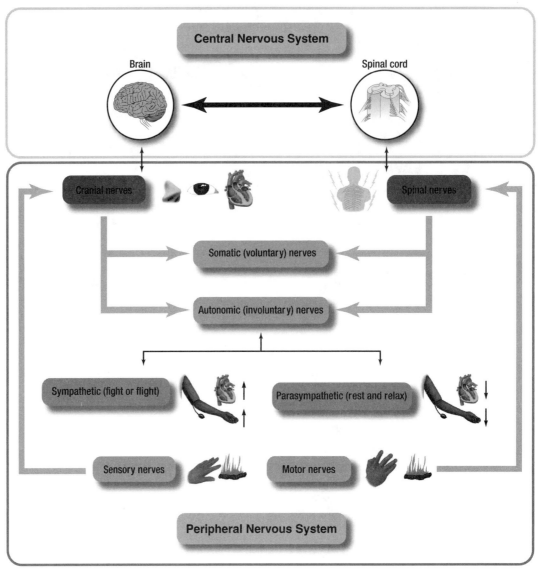

Figure 9-1 Organization of the nervous system.

- **Norepinephrine:** An adrenergic neurotransmitter located in the postganglia of the sympathetic nervous system.
- Drugs that affect the sympathetic nervous system (sympathomimetics) act by directly stimulating the adrenal medulla and are known as **adrenergic drugs**. See **Table 9-2**.

Table 9-1 Structures of the Nervous System and General Functions

Major Structure	Subdivision	General Function
Central nervous system		
Brain	Occipital	Vision and storage of visual memories
	Parietal	Sense of touch and texture; storage of those memories
	Temporal	Hearing and smell; language; storage of sound and odor memories
	Frontal	Voluntary muscle control; storage of those memories
	Prefrontal	Judgment and predicting consequences of actions; abstract intellectual functions

Table 9-1 Structures of the Nervous System and General Functions (Continued)

Major Structure	Subdivision	General Function
	Limbic system	Basic emotions; basic reflexes (eg, chewing, swallowing)
	Diencephalon (thalamus)	Relay center; filters important signals from routine signals
	Diencephalon (hypothalamus)	Emotions; temperature control; interaction with endocrine system
Brainstem	Midbrain Pons Medulla oblongata	LOC; RAS; muscle tone and posture Respiratory patterning and depth Heart rate; blood pressure; respiratory rate
Spinal cord		Reflexes; relays information to and from body
Peripheral nervous system		
Cranial nerves		Brain to body part communication; special peripheral nerves that connect directly to body parts
Peripheral nerves		Brain to spinal cord to body part communication; receive stimuli from body; send commands to body
LOC, level of consciousness; RAS, reticular activating system.		

- Drugs that affect the parasympathetic nervous system are known as *parasympathomimetics*.
- Cholinergic drugs act either directly or indirectly to stimulate the parasympathetic nervous system; excessive cholinergics can cause defecation, urination, meiosis, bronchospasms, emesis, lacrimation, and salivation. Cholinergics include the following:
  - Cholinesterase inhibitors: Organophosphates (eg, insecticides, herbicides, nerve gases)
  - Anticholinergics: Substances that block the neurotransmitter acetylcholine in the central and peripheral nervous system (eg, dicyclomine)
  - Muscarinic cholinergic antagonists: Atropine
  - Ganglionic blocking agents: Benzohexonium
  - Ganglionic stimulating agents: Nicotine

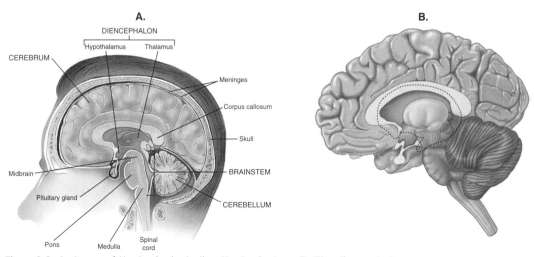

Figure 9-2 A. Areas of the brain, including the brainstem. **B.** The diencephalon.

Cerebral cortex
- Receives sensory information from skin, muscles, glands, and organs
- Sends messages to move skeletal muscles
- Integrates incoming and outgoing nerve impulses
- Performs associative activities such as thinking, learning, and remembering

Basal nuclei
- Play a role in the coordination of slow, sustained movements
- Suppress useless patterns of movement

Thalamus
- Relays most sensory information from the spinal cord and certain parts of the brain to the cerebral cortex
- Interprets certain sensory messages such as those of pain, temperature, and pressure

Hypothalamus
- Controls various homeostatic functions such as body temperature, respiration, and heartbeat
- Directs hormone secretions of the pituitary

Cerebellum
- Coordinates subconscious movements of skeletal muscles
- Contributes to muscle tone, posture, balance, and equilibrium

Brainstem
- Origin of many cranial nerves
- Reflex center for movements of eyeballs, head, and trunk
- Regulates heartbeat and breathing
- Plays a role in consciousness
- Transmits impulses between brain and spinal cord

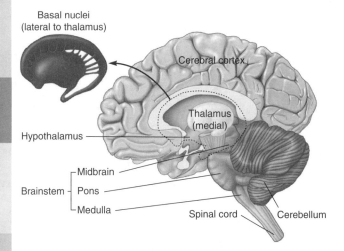

Figure 9-3 Activities controlled by each brain structure.

- There are two types of ACh receptors in the parasympathetic nervous system:
  - **Nicotinic:** Nicotinic N is found in all autonomic ganglia; nicotinic M initiates muscular contraction.
  - **Muscarinic:** Found in many organs throughout the body, and are primarily responsible for the parasympathetic response.
  - Results of stimulation to the parasympathetic nervous system:
    - Secretion from digestive glands
    - Reduction of heart rate and cardiac contractile force
    - Bronchoconstriction
    - Pupillary constriction
    - Increased smooth muscle activity along the digestive tract

Spinal Nerves

Thirty-one pairs of spinal nerves emerge from each side of the spinal cord and are named for the vertebral region and level from which they arise (cervical, thoracic, lumbar); each

Table 9-2 Actions of the Sympathetic and Parasympathetic Nervous Systems

System Affected	Sympathetic Stimulation	Parasympathetic Stimulation
Cardiovascular	Increases heart rate Increases contractility	Decreases heart rate Decreases contractility
Coronary arteries	Initially coronary artery dilation, but eventually stimulation of alpha-receptors will cause vasoconstriction	Coronary artery dilation
Respiratory	Bronchodilation	Bronchoconstriction

Table 9-2 Actions of the Sympathetic and Parasympathetic Nervous Systems (Continued)

System Affected	Sympathetic Stimulation	Parasympathetic Stimulation
Renal	Decreases output	No change
Abdominal blood vessels	Constricts	None
Muscle blood vessels	Dilates	None
Skin blood vessels	Constricts	None
Liver	Increases blood glucose levels	Slight glycogen synthesis
Ciliary muscle (eye)	Relaxes, for far vision	Contracts, for near vision
Pupil	Dilates	Constricts
Sweat glands	Copious sweating	None
Basal metabolism	Increases up to 100% of normal metabolic rates	None
Skeletal muscle	Breaks down glycogen into glucose	None
Adrenal glands	Release epinephrine and norepinephrine	None
Salivary glands	Constrict blood vessels; slight production of thick, viscous secretion	Dilates blood vessels; thin, copious secretions
Gastric glands	Inhibition	Stimulation
Pancreas	Inhibition	Stimulation
Lacrimal glands	None	Increase secretion of tears
Gastrointestinal (GI) tract lining	Decreases peristalsis/motility	Increases peristalsis/motility
Sphincter tone (GI tract)	Increases	Decreases
Erector pili muscles (skin)	Contracts	None
Urinary bladder lining	Relaxes	Contracts
Sphincter (urinary bladder)	Contracts	Relaxes

influences a different body function. For example, the upper thoracic nerves help with coughing and breathing; the lower thoracic nerves help maintain abdominal control. Nerve roots occasionally converge in a cluster called a **plexus**, where they rejoin and function as a group (**Figure 9-4**). The functions of the nerves in each plexus are as follows:

- **Cervical plexus (C1 through C5):** The phrenic nerve arises from this plexus and provides motor innervations to the diaphragm.
- **Brachial plexus (C5 through T1):** Controlling the upper extremities, the main nerves arising from this plexus are the axillary, median, musculocutaneous, radial, and ulnar nerves.
- **Lumbar plexus (L1 through L4):** The femoral nerve supplies the skin and muscles of the abdominal wall, external genitalia, and part of the lower limbs.
- **Sacral plexus (L4 through S4):** The pudendal nerve and the sciatic nerve (the largest nerve in the body, which forms the tibial and common peroneal nerves), supply the buttocks and perineum as well as most of the lower limbs.

Table 9-3 describes the three types of spinal nerves in the body.

Cranial Nerves

Cranial nerves are composed of 12 pairs of nerves that originate in the medulla. To reach their targets, they must enter and exit the cranium through openings in the skull. Cranial nerves function much like spinal nerves. They innervate the face, head, and parts of the neck, except

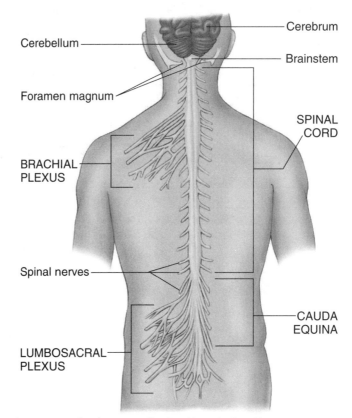

Figure 9-4 Nerve roots converge in plexuses, allowing them to function as a group.

the vagus nerve, which runs down the neck and into the chest and abdomen. They play roles in a wide variety of motor and sensory functions that involve both the voluntary and autonomic nervous systems (**Table 9-4**).

Pathophysiology of Neurologic Conditions

There are many potential sources of neurologic impairment:

- **Cancer:** Neoplasms may take over blood supplies and grow to surround or compress other tissues, including nerves.
- **Degenerative causes:** Naturally occurring alterations in tissue due to the aging process; autoimmune disorders that cause the body to attack its own cells.
- **Developmental causes:** Genetic differences and other problems with fetal development that may become apparent or might not emerge for years.
- **Vascular causes:** Blockages or tears in the veins or arteries (as a result of hypertension, aneurysm, emboli, plaque, and blood clots) that cut off blood supplies to the brain arteries (**Figure 9-5**).

Table 9-3 Types of Spinal Nerves

Sensory nerves: Receive sensory stimuli (such as pain). Electrical impulses are transmitted from the sensory organ through the ganglia via the sensory branch and into the brain.
Motor nerves: Cells inside the brain transmit nerve impulses from the brain directly to the target tissue. The motor components of the cranial nerves are derived from cells that are located inside the brain. Each cell has an axon that extends out of the cranium to the muscle or body part it will control.
Mixed fibers (sensory and motor): Mixed fiber nerves contain both motor and sensory tracts, allowing two-way communication.

Table 9-4 Cranial Nerve Types and Function

Cranial Nerve Number	Name	Type	Function
I	Olfactory	Sensory	Transmits sense of smell
II	Optic	Sensory	Transmits visual information
III	Occulomotor	Motor	Controls most eye movements
IV	Trochlear	Motor	Controls lateral eye movement
V	Trigeminal	Sensory and motor	Receives sensation from the face and innervates the muscles of mastication
VI	Abducens	Sensory and motor	Controls eye abduction
VII	Facial	Sensory	Receives sense and taste from anterior two thirds of tongue; innervates facial muscles
VIII	Vestibulocochlear	Sensory	Senses sound, rotation, and gravity
IX	Glossopharyngeal	Sensory and motor	Receives sense and taste from posterior one third of tongue
X	Vagus	Sensory and motor	Innervates most laryngeal and pharyngeal muscles; controls muscles for voice
XI	Accessory	Motor	Controls muscles in the neck
XII	Hypoglossal	Motor	Innervates muscles for swallowing and speech

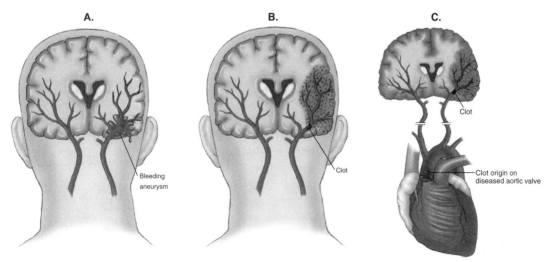

Figure 9-5 Vascular causes of neurologic conditions. **A.** Aneurysms are areas of weakness in the walls of arteries that can dilate (bulge out) and eventually rupture or leak. **B.** Atherosclerosis can damage the wall of a cerebral artery, producing narrowing and/or a clot. When the vessel is completely blocked, blood flow may be blocked and cells begin to die. **C.** An embolus, a blood clot usually formed on a diseased heart valve, can travel through the body's vascular system, lodge in a cerebral artery, and cause a stroke.

- **Intracranial pressure (ICP):** Increased ICP can lead to brain ischemia or herniation of the brain (the brain is pushed down and through the foramen magnum, increasing pressure on the medulla oblongata).
- **Infectious processes:** Certain infections can cause diffuse brain injury, such as infectious meningitis. Abcesses can form, causing focal problems. Patients usually have other signs of infection, such as fever.

Specific Injuries and Illness

Cerebrovascular Accident

Pathophysiology

A cerebrovascular accident (CVA), also known as a stroke, is caused by an interruption of circulation in a portion of the brain, which results in ischemia and braintissue damage. Patients often experience paralysis or hemiparesis. Stroke in one hemisphere of the brain can cause paralysis on the contralateral side of the body. If the stroke damages cranial nerves, it will affect structures on the same side of the body. Patients may regain function over a period of weeks or months or may not regain function at all, depending on the severity of the damage.

There are two types of stroke:

- **Occlusive/thrombotic stroke** (most common) is caused by a blockage in a blood vessel caused by an embolus. It develops slowly, and patients often have a past history of vessel disease.
  - Usually results from atherosclerosis or tumor within the brain
  - May be associated with valvular heart disease and atrial fibrillation, history of angina, and/or previous stroke
- **Hemorrhagic stroke** (less common) is caused by intracranial bleeding caused by the rupture of blood vessels; it develops suddenly. Although rare, a seizure may be followed by a stroke, producing a similar set of symptoms. The underlying problem should be treated promptly.
  - Usually results from cerebral aneurysms, atrioventricular malformation, hypertension
  - May be associated with use of cocaine and other sympathomimetics
  - May be asymptomatic, preceding vessel rupture

Risk Factors for Stroke
- Advanced age
- Chronic alcohol consumption
- Elevated cholesterol level
- Race
- History of transient ischemic attack (TIA)
- Cardiac disease, hypertension
- Cocaine use
- Smoking
- Cardiac arrhythmias
- Oral contraceptive use
- Diabetes

Signs and Symptoms
- Dizziness
- Severe headache
- Nausea and vomiting
- Gradual- or rapid-onset neurologic deficits
- Inability to maintain a patient's airway
- Inability to manage secretions

Tip

The three types of aphasia are as follows:
- **Receptive:** Patient cannot understand speech but can speak clearly; indicates damage to the temporal lobe of the brain.
- **Expressive:** Patient cannot speak but can understand speech; indicates damage to the frontal lobe.
- **Global:** Patient cannot speak or understand what you say, but can think clearly.

- Hemiplegia
- Hypoventilation
- Facial droop
- Cardiac arrhythmias
- Dysphagia
- Aphasia
- Seizure
- Unequal pupils
- Altered LOC
- Elevated blood pressure

Stroke Screening Tools

The most common stroke screening tool used by prehospital providers is the Cincinnati Prehospital Stroke Screen (CPSS). The CPSS evaluates three areas: facial droop (**Figure 9-6**), arm drift (**Figure 9-7**), and speech. If any of these items is abnormal, there is a high likelihood of stroke.

Assessment

- Scene size-up
  - Ensure body substance isolation (BSI).
- Initial/primary assessment
  - Assess LOC.
  - Manage ABCs (airway, breathing, circulation).
  - Treat life-threatening illness/injuries.
  - Transport considerations: Rapidly transport patient, in a position of comfort, to a facility with computed tomography (CT) capabilities.
- Focused history and physical exam/secondary assessment
  - Determine the last time patient was seen to be "normal," without signs and symptoms.
  - Obtain SAMPLE history and chief complaint (OPQRST).

Management

- Apply supplemental oxygen.
- Establish an intravenous line (IV) access.
- Reassure patient.
- Monitor vital signs.
- Apply cardiac monitor.
- Monitor blood glucose level.

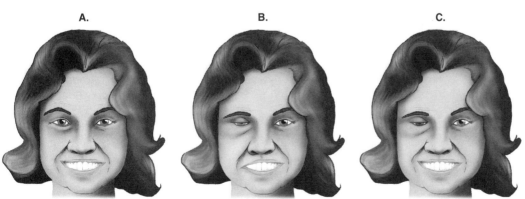

Figure 9-6 Facial Droop: Have your patient smile and show his or her teeth. **A.** A normal smile. **B.** Facial droop, including a drooping eyelid (ptosis), which may or may not be present. **C.** A normal smile with ptosis present.

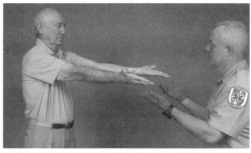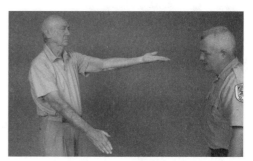

Figure 9-7 Arm drift: Have the patient close his or her eyes and hold both arms out in front of him or her.

- Provide supportive, symptomatic care.
- Suction if unable to manage secretions.

Transient Ischemic Attack

Pathophysiology

A TIA, often called a mini-stroke, is a temporary interruption in blood flow to an area of the brain. The decreased blood flow leads to a lack of cellular perfusion in the brain, resulting in ischemia. To be classified as a TIA, the neurologic deficit(s) must self-resolve within 24 hours. Risk factors for a TIA are the same as for a CVA.

Signs and Symptoms

- Dizziness
- Severe headache
- Nausea and vomiting
- Gradual- or rapid-onset neurologic deficits
- Inability to maintain a patient's airway
- Inability to manage secretions
- Hemiplegia
- Hypoventilation
- Facial droop
- Cardiac arrhythmias
- Dysphagia
- Aphasia
- Seizure
- Unequal pupils
- Altered LOC
- Elevated blood pressure

> **Tip**
>
> A TIA is a precursor to a CVA, occurring within 1 year in approximately 50% of the population.

Assessment

- Scene size-up
  - Ensure BSI.
- Initial/primary assessment
  - Assess LOC.
  - Manage ABCs.
  - Treat life-threatening illness/injuries.
  - Transport considerations: Rapidly transport patient, in a position of comfort, to a facility with CT capabilities.
- Focused history and physical exam/secondary assessment
  - Determine the last time patient was seen to be "normal," without signs and symptoms.
  - Obtain SAMPLE history and chief complaint (OPQRST).

Management

- Apply supplemental oxygen.
- Establish IV access.
- Reassure patient.
- Monitor vital signs.
- Apply cardiac monitor.
- Monitor blood glucose level.
- Provide supportive, symptomatic care.
- Suction if unable to manage secretions.

Tip

Hypertension in stroke patients is a compensatory mechanism and should not be treated prehospitally.

Seizures

Pathophysiology

Seizures involve sudden, erratic firing of neurons. Patients who have epilepsy commonly have seizures. Knowing the cause of the patient's seizures will help direct management. Some of the causes of seizures include the following:

- Abscess
- AIDS
- Alcohol
- Birth defect
- Brain infections (meningitis, encephalitis)
- Brain trauma
- Diabetes mellitus
- Fever
- Inappropriate medication dosage
- Organic brain syndromes
- Recreational drugs
- Stroke or TIA
- Systemic infection
- Tumor
- Uremia (buildup of toxins due to kidney failure)

Classification of Seizures

Seizures can be classified as generalized (affecting large portions of the brain) or partial (affecting a limited area of the brain).

Within the category of generalized seizures are the grand mal and petit mal types. Grand mal seizures, also called tonic–clonic seizures, usually follow a pattern, traveling through each of the following steps in order, although sometimes skipping a step:

1. **Aura**: A sensation the patient experiences before the seizure occurs (eg, muscle twitch, funny taste, seeing lights, hearing a high-pitched noise).
2. Loss of consciousness.
3. Tonic phase: Body-wide rigidity.
4. Hypertonic phase: Arched back and rigidity.
5. Clonic phase: Rhythmic contraction of major muscle groups. Arm, leg, head movement; lip smacking; biting; teeth clenching.
6. Postseizure: Major muscles relax; nystagmus may still be occurring. Eyes may be rolled back.
7. **Postictal**: Reset period of the brain. It can take several minutes to hours before the patient gradually returns to the preseizure LOC. During this time patients are often initially aphasic (unable to speak), confused or unable to follow commands, combative, very emotional, and tired or sleeping. They may present with a headache.

During the seizing process, respirations may become very erratic, loud, and obviously abnormal; the patient may also stop breathing and become cyanotic. These periods of apnea are usually very short-lived and do not require assistance. If the patient is apneic for more than 30 seconds, immediately begin positive pressure ventilatory assistance. The patient may also become incontinent.

Petit mal or absence seizures present with little to no movement. The typical patient with petit mal seizures is a child. Classically the child will simply stop moving. The child will rarely fall. These seizures usually last no more than several seconds. There is no postictal period and no confusion.

Partial seizures are classified as either simple partial or complex partial. Such seizures involve only a limited portion of the brain. They may be localized to just one spot within the brain or may begin in one spot and move in wavelike fashion to other locations.

Signs and Symptoms

Patients may experience a wide array of signs and symptoms when having seizures, ranging from one hand shaking or having a taste of pennies in the mouth to movement of every limb or the complete loss of consciousness. They may be aware of the seizure, or they may wake up afterward not knowing what happened.

Assessment

- Scene size-up
  - Ensure BSI.
- Initial/primary assessment
  - Assess LOC.
  - Manage ABCs.
  - Treat life-threatening illness/injuries.
  - Transport considerations: Unless a clear and easily reversible cause for the seizure is found, all patients should be transported because seizures can be a warning sign of more serious nervous system problems.
- Focused history and physical exam/secondary assessment
  - Attempt to determine cause of seizure.
  - Obtain SAMPLE history and chief complaint (OPQRST).

Management

Monitor and protect patients from injuring themselves. Prehospital management of patients with seizure begins with standard care. Quickly determine whether trauma is a concern.

- Where was the patient before the seizure?
- What was the patient doing before the seizure?
- How did the patient get to the current position?
- If the situation is unclear or there is confirmed trauma, perform manual in-line immobilization.

Never restrain the patient or attempt to stop the seizing movement. Prevent the patient from striking objects and becoming injured. Place nothing within the patient's mouth while the seizure is ongoing. If bystanders have placed objects (eg, spoons, butter knives) in the mouth, remove them.

Provide ventilatory assistance only if the seizure or apnea is prolonged. Ventilation of the actively seizing patient will be very difficult. Oral or nasotracheal intubation will be next to impossible during a seizure.

In the postictal phase, emotional support is very important. Provide privacy. Speak calmly and slowly. Be prepared to repeat yourself. Reorient the patient to place and time. If a child is febrile, remove the patient's clothing in an attempt to lower the core body temperature.

Any patient who you suspect could experience a seizure should have the following care.

- Establish IV access. Diazepam, lorazepam, and midazolam are the drugs of choice to stop seizures. In patients who are seizing and in whom IV access cannot be established, diazepam can be administered rectally at 0.2 mg/kg, or 5 mg of intranasal midazolam can be given.
- Place blankets over the rails of the ambulance cot.
- Place blankets over hard surfaces near the patient.
- Ensure that the patient's cot straps are not too tight.
- In-hospital management will seek to identify the cause of the seizure. Blood studies, including drug and blood glucose level determinations, will be done. CT or MRI scans may be performed.

Status Epilepticus

Pathophysiology

<u>Status epilepticus</u> is a seizure that lasts for longer than 4 to 5 minutes or two or more consecutive seizures that occur without consciousness returning between seizure episodes. This time frame is arbitrary, however; you should refer to your local protocols for guidelines on how long a seizure can continue before you should intervene.

During a seizure, neurons are in a hypermetabolic state (using huge amounts of glucose and producing lactic acid). For a short period, this state does not produce long-term damage. If the seizure continues, however, the body cannot remove the waste products effectively or ensure adequate glucose supplies. Such a hypermetabolic state can result in neurons being damaged or killed.

Signs and Symptoms

Status epilepticus may be convulsive (dramatic involuntary muscle contraction, spasms, and loss of consciousness) or nonconvulsive (patient appears dazed). Convulsive status epilepticus is more serious and is associated with a worse prognosis if treatment is delayed.

Assessment

- Scene size-up
  - Ensure BSI.
- Initial/primary assessment
  - Assess LOC.
  - Manage ABCs.
  - Treat life-threatening illness/injuries.
- Focused history and physical exam/secondary assessment
  - Attempt to determine cause of seizure.
  - Obtain SAMPLE history and chief complaint (OPQRST).

Management

Management of status epilepticus begins with standard care. Administer benzodiazepines (diazepam, 5.0 mg IV/IM; lorazepam, 0.05 mg/kg [maximum 4 mg]; or midazolam, 2.5–5.0 mg IV or 5.0 mg intranasally). You may repeat diazepam every 10 to 15 minutes to a total dose of 30 mg. If you are unable to obtain IV access, you may give diazepam rectally. You may repeat the lorazepam dose in 10 to 15 minutes, with a maximum dose of 8 mg in 12 hours.

Be prepared to completely control airway and ventilation, because benzodiazepines can cause respiratory depression and respiratory arrest. Continue to use airway positioning and bag-mask ventilations until the seizure stops. If benzodiazepines do not quickly control the seizure and the patient cannot be ventilated, paralytics may be needed to allow for adequate airway management.

Syncope

Pathophysiology

<u>Syncope</u> (fainting) is sudden and temporary loss of consciousness with accompanying loss of postural tone. It affects mainly adults and accounts for nearly 3% of all emergency department visits. The brain uses glucose at a high rate and has no ability to store glucose, so even a 3- to 5-second interruption in blood flow can cause loss of consciousness. The role of the EMS provider is to determine what caused the sudden decrease in cerebral perfusion.

Signs and Symptoms

Classically, the patient with syncope is in a standing position when the event occurs. With young adults, the pattern is usually one of vasovagal syncope. The person will experience fear, emotional stress, or pain, the room will seem to spin, and the individual will pass out. In older adults, cardiac arrhythmia is a more typical cause of syncope. The patient experiences a sudden run of ventricular tachycardia, the blood pressure drops, and the person falls to the floor. The rhythm terminates, the blood pressure rises, and the individual regains consciousness. In either case, the whole process takes less than 60 seconds.

Patients with syncope usually experience **prodrome**, signs or symptoms that precede a disease or condition. For syncope, prodromal complaints include feelings of dizziness, weakness, shortness of breath, chest pain, headache, or visual disturbances.

Assessment

- Scene size-up
  - Ensure BSI.
- Initial/primary assessment
  - Assess LOC.
  - Manage ABCs.
  - Treat life-threatening illness/injuries.
- Focused history and physical exam/secondary assessment
  - Attempt to determine cause of syncope.
  - Obtain SAMPLE history and chief complaint (OPQRST).

Management

Begin with standard care. Determine whether the patient may have experienced trauma during the fall, and take cervical spine precautions as needed. Focus on blood glucose level and likely cardiac causes. Obtain orthostatic vital signs if possible.

Provide emotional support, because syncope can be very embarrassing. Transport the patient to the hospital. Syncope can be a sign of life-threatening cardiac arrhythmias, stroke, or another serious medical condition.

Alzheimer's Disease

Pathophysiology

Alzheimer's disease is a progressive, irreversible brain disorder and the most common form of dementia. Dementia is a chronic deterioration of a person's personality, memory, and ability to think. Alzheimer's disease is a progressive organic condition in which neurons die; there is no definitive treatment for the destroyed neurons.

Signs and Symptoms

Symptoms are subtle at onset. Over time, patients lose their ability to think, reason clearly, solve problems, and concentrate; they may present with altered behavior that includes paranoia, delusions, and social inappropriateness. In the later stages of Alzheimer's disease, patients cannot take care of themselves and may lose the ability to speak.

Assessment

- Scene size-up
  - Ensure BSI.

- Initial/primary assessment
  - Assess LOC.
  - Manage ABCs.
  - Treat life-threatening illness/injuries.
- Focused history and physical exam/secondary assessment
  - Attempt to determine cause of syncope.
  - Obtain SAMPLE history and chief complaint (OPQRST).

Management

Prehospital management is standard care.

Myasthenia Gravis

Pathophysiology

Acetylcholine is an important neurotransmitter needed to allow for muscular contraction. In **myasthenia gravis**, the body creates antibodies against the acetylcholine receptors. The thymus gland (where T cells mature) is believed to play a role in the production of these antibodies. As acetylcholine levels fall, muscle weakness begins.

Myasthenic crisis is a sudden increase in the destruction of acetylcholine, resulting in weakness in the respiratory muscles. As a result, patients can become hypoxic. Infections, emotional stress, or reactions to medications can trigger this crisis.

Signs and Symptoms

This weakness most commonly affects the eyes, eyelids, and facial muscles. Some patients will have difficulty swallowing or speaking, or leg or arm weakness. Patients suffer no sensory impairment. Myasthenia gravis usually affects women younger than 40 years and men older than 60 years.

Assessment

- Scene size-up
  - Ensure BSI.
- Initial/primary assessment
  - Assess LOC.
  - Manage ABCs.
  - Treat life-threatening illness/injuries.
- Focused history and physical exam/secondary assessment
  - Attempt to determine cause of syncope.
  - Obtain SAMPLE history and chief complaint (OPQRST).

Management

Standard care will effectively manage these patients in the field. Be prepared to assist with ventilations in patients with crisis. In-hospital management includes removal of the thymus gland, medications to boost neurotransmitter levels, and immunosuppressants.

Peripheral Neuropathy

Peripheral neuropathy comprises a group of conditions in which the nerves leaving the spinal cord become damaged. As a consequence, the signals moving to or from the brain become distorted. Causes of peripheral neuropathy include trauma, toxins, tumors, autoimmune attacks, and metabolic disorders. Trigeminal neuralgia and Guillain-Barré syndrome are examples. The remainder of this discussion focuses on the most common form, diabetic neuropathy. Diabetic neuropathy is frequently seen in diabetic patients older than 50 years; more males than females are affected. Its onset is gradual, occurring over months and years.

Signs and Symptoms

As blood glucose levels rise, the peripheral nerves may become damaged, resulting in mis-firing and shorting of signals. Affected individuals may then experience sensory or motor impairment. Loss of sensation, numbness, burning sensations, pain, paresthesia, and muscle weakness are common. Patients may eventually lose the ability to feel their feet or other areas.

Assessment
- Scene size-up
  - Ensure BSI.
- Initial/primary assessment
  - Assess LOC.
  - Manage ABCs.
  - Treat life-threatening illness/injuries.
- Focused history and physical exam/secondary assessment
  - Attempt to determine cause of syncope.
  - Obtain SAMPLE history and chief complaint (OPQRST).

Management
Management in the prehospital setting is supportive. Provide standard care. In-hospital management will include pain medication. The use of antidepressants and anticonvulsants seems to have a positive effect on calming the peripheral nerves.

Parkinson's Disease
Pathophysiology
Parkinson's disease is a degenerative disease of the brain that often impairs motor skills, speech, and other functions and can present as chronic or progressive. Parkinson's disease results from a decreased stimulation of the motor cortex by the basal ganglia, normally caused by the insufficient formation and action of dopamine. In patients with Parkinson's disease, 80% or more of these dopamine-producing cells are damaged or dead. This causes the nerve cells to fire wildly, leaving patients unable to control their movements.

Signs and Symptoms
- Muscle rigidity
- Tremors
- Bradykinesia/akinesia
- Cognitive dysfunction
- Postural instability

Guillain-Barré Syndrome
Pathophysiology
Guillain-Barré syndrome is an autoimmune disease affecting the peripheral nervous system, usually triggered by an acute infectious process. The end result of such an autoimmune attack on the peripheral nerves is inflammation of myelin and conduction block, leading to a muscle paralysis that may be accompanied by sensory or autonomic disturbances. It is frequently severe and usually exhibits as an ascending paralysis noted by weakness in the legs that spreads to the upper limbs and the face along with complete loss of deep tendon reflexes.

As the weakness progresses upward, usually over periods of hours to days, the arms and facial muscles also become affected. Frequently, the lower cranial nerves may be affected, leading to difficulty swallowing, drooling, and/or maintaining an open airway, as well as respiratory distress. Most patients require hospitalization, and about 30% require ventilatory assistance. Sensory loss, if present, usually takes the form of loss of **proprioception**.

Signs and Symptoms
- Ascending paralysis
- Weakness
- Difficulty swallowing
- Respiratory distress/failure

Spinal Cord Injuries

Although a majority of spinal injuries are a direct result of trauma, they can be caused by medical problems as well. Understanding neural innervations allows you to understand the presenting signs and symptoms.

Anterior Cord Syndrome

<u>Anterior cord syndrome</u> occurs when the blood supply to the anterior portion of the spinal cord is interrupted as a result of an incomplete spinal cord injury, a lesion encroaching on the spinal cord itself, or a blockage in a spinal artery (known as spinal stroke). It is characterized by the loss of motor function below the level of injury, loss of sensations carried by the anterior columns of the spinal cord (pain and temperature), and preservation of sensations carried by the posterior columns (fine touch and proprioception). Patients can typically feel some sensations through the intact path of the posterior spinal cord, but movements are absent.

Signs and Symptoms
- Complete motor paralysis below the level of the lesion because of interruption of the corticospinal tract
- Loss of pain and temperature sensation at and below the level of the lesion because of interruption of the spinothalamic tract
- Retained proprioception and vibratory sensation because of intact dorsal columns

Central Cord Syndrome

Central cord syndrome is a form of incomplete spinal cord injury characterized by impairment in the arms and hands and to a lesser extent in the legs. The brain's ability to send and receive signals to and from parts of the body below the site of injury is reduced but not entirely blocked. This syndrome is associated with damage to the central area of the spinal cord. These nerves are particularly important for hand and arm function.

Signs and Symptoms
- Loss of fine motor control in the upper extremities
- Sensory loss below the site of the injury
- Loss of bladder control

Brown-Séquard Syndrome
Pathophysiology
Brown-Séquard syndrome is an incomplete spinal cord lesion characterized by hemisection of the spinal cord. Most commonly caused by penetrating trauma to the spinal cord, it can also be caused by tumors, tuberculosis, and multiple sclerosis. Brown-Séquard syndrome causes a loss of pain and temperature sensation on the opposite side of the injury, with motor paralysis on the side of the injury.

The presentation can be progressive and incomplete. It can advance from a typical Brown-Séquard syndrome to complete paralysis. It is not always permanent, and progression or resolution depends on the severity of the original spinal cord injury and the underlying pathology that originally caused the syndrome.

Signs and Symptoms
- Ipsilateral hemiplegia
- Contralateral pain and temperature deficits

Vital Vocabulary

adrenergic drugs Drugs that affect the sympathetic nervous system (sympathomimetics), which act by directly stimulating the adrenal medulla.

anterior cord syndrome A condition that occurs with flexion injuries or fractures resulting in the displacement of bony fragments into the anterior portion of the spinal cord; findings include paralysis below the level of the insult and loss of pain, temperature, and touch sensation.

aura Sensations experienced by a patient before an attack occurs. Common in seizures and migraine headaches.

brainstem The area of the brain between the spinal cord and cerebrum, surrounded by the cerebellum; controls functions that are necessary for life, such as respiration.

diencephalon The part of the brain between the brainstem and the cerebrum that includes the thalamus, the subthalamus, hypothalamus, and epithalamus.

ganglion Groupings of nerve cell bodies located in the peripheral nervous system.

medulla oblongata The inferior portion of the midbrain, which serves as a conduction pathway for both ascending and descending nerve tracts.

midbrain The part of the brain that is responsible for helping to regulate level of consciousness.

myasthenia gravis An abnormal condition characterized by the chronic fatigability and weakness of muscles, especially in the face and throat. It is the result of a defect in the conduction of nerve impulses at the nerve junction. This deficit is caused by a lack of acetylcholine.

peripheral neuropathy A group of conditions in which the nerves leaving the spinal cord become damaged.

plexus A cluster of nerve roots that permits peripheral nerve roots to rejoin and functions as a group.

pons The portion of the brainstem that lies below the midbrain and contains nerve fibers that affect sleep and respiration.

postganglia Occurring after the ganglia.

postictal The period of time after a seizure during which the brain is reorganizing activity.

preganglia Occurring before the ganglia.

prodrome Signs or symptoms that precede a disease or condition.

proprioception The ability to perceive the position and movement of one's body or limbs.

status epilepticus A seizure that lasts for longer than 4 to 5 minutes or two or more consecutive seizures that occur without a return to consciousness between seizure episodes.

syncope Fainting; brief loss of consciousness caused by transient and inadequate blood flow to the brain.

Endocrine Emergencies

Anatomy and Physiology

The endocrine system is a network of glands that produce and secrete chemical messengers called hormones. The main function of the endocrine system and its hormone messengers is to promote permanent structural changes and maintain homeostasis. Maintaining homeostasis means responding to any change in the body, such as low glucose or calcium levels in the blood. There are two major types of glands:

- **Exocrine glands:** Excrete chemicals for elimination (*exo* = outside). Exocrine glands (eg, sweat glands, salivary glands, and the liver) have ducts that carry their secretions to the surface of the skin or inside the body cavity.
- **Endocrine glands:** Secrete or release hormones that are used inside the body (*endo* = inside). Endocrine glands have no ducts; they release hormones directly into tissue or the bloodstream, transferring information from one cell to another to coordinate body functions (eg, mood regulation, metabolism, tissue function, growth and development, and sexual development and function).

Components of the endocrine system include the following:

- **Hypothalamus:** A small region of the brain (not a gland) that controls several body functions and is the primary link between the endocrine system and the nervous system.
- **Pituitary gland:** Regulates the function of other endocrine glands, and is thus known as the "master gland" (**Table 10-1**).
- **Thyroid:** Secretes **thyroxine**, which stimulates energy production in the cells when the body's metabolic rate decreases, and **calcitonin**, which helps maintain normal calcium levels in the blood. When excessive calcium is detected in the bloodstream, calcitonin is secreted, thus decreasing the excessive calcium.
- **Parathyroid:** Assists in the regulation of calcium. When calcium levels in the blood are low, it secretes **parathyroid hormone (PTH)**, which stimulates the bone-dissolving cells to break down bone and release calcium into the blood. This hormone is a calcitonin antagonist.
- **Adrenal glands:** Located on top of each kidney, the adrenal glands consist of an outer **adrenal cortex**, which produces hormones called **corticosteroids**, and an inner **adrenal medulla**, which produces the hormones called **catecholamines** (epinephrine and norepinephrine). Corticosteroids regulate the body's metabolism, its salt/water balance, the immune system, and sexual function. Catecholamines increase heart and respiratory rates, as well as the blood pressure when the body is under physical or emotional stress.
- **Pancreas:** Considered both an endocrine and an exocrine gland, the pancreas is a digestive gland that regulates blood glucose levels through secretion of **insulin** and **glucagon** into the blood. It secretes digestive enzymes into the intestine.
- **Gonads:** The main source of sex hormones. In men, the gonads are the **testes**, which produce hormones called **androgens** (eg, **testosterone**). In women, the gonads are the **ovaries**, which release eggs and secrete **estrogen** and **progesterone**.

The endocrine system regulates hormone levels using negative or positive feedback to maintain the optimal internal operating environment in the body (**Figure 10-1**).

Table 10-1 Hormones Secreted by the Pituitary Gland

Growth hormone (GH)	Regulates metabolic processes related to growth and adaptation to physical and emotional stressors
Thyroid-stimulating hormone (TSH)	Increases production and secretion of thyroid hormone
Adrenocorticotropic hormone (ACTH)	Stimulates the adrenal gland to secrete cortisol and adrenal proteins that contribute to the maintenance of the adrenal gland
Luteinizing hormone (LH)	In women: ovulation, progesterone production In men: regulates spermatogenesis, testosterone production
Follicle-stimulating hormone (FSH)	In women: ovarian follicle maturation, estrogen production In men: spermatogenesis
Prolactin	Milk production
Antidiuretic hormone (ADH)	Controls plasma osmolality; increases the permeability of the distal renal tubules and collecting ducts, which leads to an increase in water reabsorption
Oxytocin	Contracts the uterus during childbirth and stimulates milk production

Endocrine disorders can be caused by either oversecretion or undersecretion of a gland, which leads to overactivity or underactivity in the organ regulated by that gland. Despite their intricate pathophysiology, most clinically significant endocrine emergencies result in alterations of fluid balance, mental status, vital signs, and blood glucose levels.

Types of Endocrine Disorders

- Diabetes mellitus
- Hypoglycemia
- Hyperglycemia and diabetic ketoacidosis (DKA)
- Hyperosmolar hyperglycemic nonketotic syndrome (HHNS)
- **Hypokalemia** and **hyperkalemia**
- Metabolic alkalosis
- Metabolic acidosis
- Grave's disease (hyperthyroidism)
- Myxedema (hypothyroidism)

Diabetes Mellitus

Pathophysiology

Diabetes is a disease that results from either inadequate insulin secretion from the pancreas (type 1) or insensitivity of target tissues to insulin (type 2). Diabetes results in increased levels of blood glucose. The pancreas is the primary regulator of blood glucose. The endocrine portion of the pancreas, the islets of Langerhans, secretes the hormones insulin, glucagons, somatostatin, and amylin. These hormones work synergistically to maintain blood glucose levels within the normal range.

The pancreas also has exocrine glands that secrete digestive enzymes and bicarbonate (to neutralize acid coming from the stomach) into the duodenum.

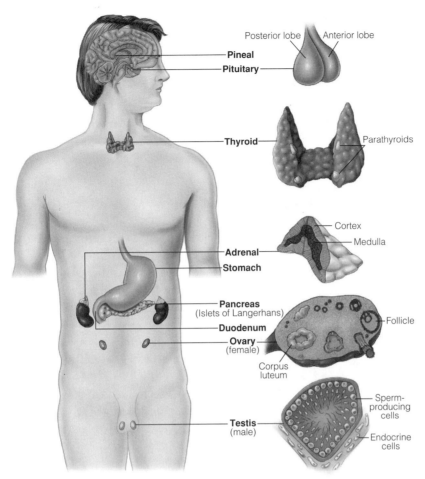

Figure 10-1 The endocrine system uses the various glands within the system to deliver chemical messages to organ systems throughout the body.

Glucose that is not used immediately for energy is stored in the liver and muscles as glycogen or converted by adipose tissue into fat. The liver releases glucose back into the bloodstream when glucose levels drop and removes it when glucose levels are too high. Only the glycogen in the liver can be converted back to glucose; the glycogen stored in muscle can be used only by the muscle for energy.

Insulin is secreted by the beta cells of the pancreas in response to blood glucose levels. After a meal, blood glucose levels rise, stimulating the pancreas to release insulin. The more glucose in the blood, the more insulin the pancreas releases. Insulin transports glucose into the cells via facilitated diffusion, where it is converted into energy. It also has an effect on many cells that play a part in absorbing the glucose, causing the blood glucose levels to return to normal.

Glucagon has the opposite effect. When blood glucose levels are low, the pancreas releases more glucagon. The presence of glucagon stimulates the release of the glucose that is stored in liver cells, making energy available to the tissues between meals.

Diabetes mellitus results from an impairment of the body's ability to produce or use insulin. There are two major types of diabetes mellitus.

Type 1 Diabetes

- **Type 1 diabetes** is predominantly an autoimmune disorder, in which the immune system produces antibodies that mistakenly attack the patient's pancreatic islet beta cells.
- It was formerly known as juvenile-onset diabetes because it is known to strike children more often than adults, although adults can also develop type 1 diabetes.

- The beta cells of the pancreas no longer produce insulin or produce too little insulin.
  - Without insulin, glucose cannot enter the cells, depriving them of nourishment and energy.
  - Glucose builds up in the bloodstream instead.
  - Patients with type 1 diabetes require insulin replacement therapy to help regulate blood glucose levels.
  - For this reason, type 1 diabetes was also once known as insulin-dependent diabetes mellitus, although this term is no longer officially used.

Type 2 Diabetes

- **Type 2 diabetes** was formerly referred to as adult-onset diabetes because it traditionally develops in middle age (> age 40 years).
- It is becoming more common in younger people.
- It is more common than type 1 diabetes, afflicting an estimated 90% of all diabetic people in the United States.
- Type 2 diabetes can also be the result of a deficiency in insulin production, but more often is characterized by insulin resistance, a condition in which insulin production is generally or nearly adequate; however, for reasons that are not completely understood, the body cannot effectively utilize the insulin.
  - There is a strong genetic component in type 2 diabetes that is not yet fully defined; environmental factors such as aging, sedentary lifestyle, or obesity are also thought to play a role.
  - Treatment involves reducing blood glucose levels to normal.

Although the pathophysiology of each type of diabetes is different, the complications are the same. Both forms result in high blood glucose levels and glucose deprivation in the cells. Diabetes carries wide-ranging complications: it increases the risk of cardiovascular disease and stroke, neurologic problems, kidney problems, and vision problems (blurred vision).

Tip
The normal range for blood glucose level is 70 to 130 mg/dL.

Signs and Symptoms

- Hyperglycemia
- Excessive thirst
- Frequent urination
- Exceptional hunger
- Fatigue
- Unexplained, rapid weight loss
- Visual disturbances
- Irritability
- Ketoacidosis causes sweet acetone smell on breath
- Tremors or shakiness
- Dizziness
- HHNS

Hypoglycemia

Pathophysiology

Hypoglycemia means low blood glucose levels (< 70 mg/dL), which deprive the central nervous system (CNS), especially the brain, of energy, in effect "starving" the brain. Hypoglycemia develops rapidly and, if untreated, can result in cerebral dysfunction and, ultimately, permanent brain damage and death. In diabetics, hypoglycemic reactions may be caused by taking too much insulin or too little food. Hypoglycemia is also seen in alcoholics and in patients who have ingested certain poisons or overdosed with certain drugs (notably, aspirin). Hypoglycemia must be treated immediately.

Signs and Symptoms
- Weakness and dizziness
- Impaired coordination
- Slurred speech
- Diaphoresis (excessive sweating)
- Altered level of consciousness (LOC)
- Neurologic deficit
- Seizures

Assessment
- Scene size-up
  - Ensure body substance isolation (BSI).
- Initial/primary assessment
  - Assess LOC.
  - Manage ABCs.
  - Treat life-threatening illness/injuries.
  - Transport considerations: Transport in a position of comfort.
- Focused history and physical exam/secondary assessment
  - Obtain SAMPLE history and chief complaint (OPQRST).

Management
- Administer oxygen at 15 L/min via nonrebreathing mask.
- Assess blood glucose level.
- Establish intravenous line (IV) of 5% dextrose, or IV of 0.9% normal saline.
- Monitor vital signs.
- Apply cardiac monitor.
- Administer IV bolus of D_{50} if blood glucose level is low.
- Administer glucagon per local protocol.

Table 10-2 summarizes treatment of hypoglycemia.

Table 10-2 Treatment of Hypoglycemia

Treatment	Used For	Adult Dose	Pediatric Dose
0.9% normal saline	Perfusion; increase or maintain radial pulses	IV: 250-500 mL	IV: 20 mL/kg
Dextrose 50%	Increase blood glucose levels in patients without an intact gag reflex	IV: 25 g	Not indicated for pediatric use
Dextrose 25%	Increase blood glucose levels in patients without an intact gag reflex	Not indicated for adult use	IV: 2 mL/kg
Oral glucose	Increase blood glucose levels in patients with an intact gag reflex	PO: 15-30 g	PO: 15 g
Glucagon	Increase blood glucose levels in patients without an intact gag reflex, when unable to establish an IV	IM or intranasal: 1 mg	IM or intranasal: 0.5 mg
IV, intravenous; PO, by mouth; IM, intramuscular.			

Hyperglycemia and Diabetic Ketoacidosis

Pathophysiology

Hyperglycemia, or abnormally high levels of blood glucose (> 120 mg/dL), is a classic symptom of diabetes mellitus. It is also an independent medical condition with other causes, ranging from excessive food intake, infection or illness, injury, recent surgery, or emotional stress. In diabetics, hyperglycemia may be caused by undermedication with their daily insulin. Depending on the cause, onset may be rapid or gradual (hours to days). The signs and symptoms of hypoglycemia and hyperglycemia can be quite similar and are described in **Table 10-3**.

Table 10-3 Characteristics of Hyperglycemia and Hypoglycemia

	Hyperglycemia	Hypoglycemia
History		
Food intake	Excessive	Insufficient
Insulin dosage	Insufficient	Excessive
Onset	Gradual (hours to days)	Rapid, within minutes
Skin	Warm and dry	Pale and moist
Infection	Common	Uncommon
Gastrointestinal tract		
Thirst	Intense	Absent
Hunger	Absent	Intense
Vomiting	Common	Uncommon
Respiratory system		
Breathing	Rapid, deep (Kussmaul respirations)	Normal or rapid
Odor of breath	Sweet, fruity	Normal
Cardiovascular system		
Blood pressure	Normal to low	Low
Pulse	Normal or rapid and full	Rapid, weak
Nervous system		
Consciousness	Restless merging to coma	Irritability, confusion, seizure, or coma
Urine		
Sugar	Present	Absent
Acetone	Present	Absent
Treatment		
Response	Gradual, within 6 to 12 hours following medical treatment	Immediately after administration of glucose

Untreated hyperglycemia can lead to serious conditions known as DKA and HHNS. The absence of or resistance to insulin prevents the cells from taking up glucose, thereby starving them and triggering the release of stress hormones. At the same time, because the body must compensate for the lack of glucose in the cells, it turns to other energy sources, principally fat. The metabolization of fat leaves behind acids and ketones as waste products. The unabsorbed blood glucose is excreted in the urine, which leads to excessive loss of water and electrolytes (sodium and potassium). This causes continued excessive urine output, resulting in dehydration and, potentially, shock.

Signs and Symptoms

- Hyperglycemia
  - Frequent and excessive thirst
  - Frequent urination
  - Exceptional hunger
  - Fatigue
  - Unexplained, rapid weight loss

- Visual disturbances
- Irritability
- DKA
  - Diuresis
  - Warm, dry skin
  - Dry mucous membranes
  - Tachycardia, thready pulse
  - Postural hypotension
  - Excessive, rapid weight loss
  - Polyuria
  - Polydipsia
  - Polyphagia
- Acidosis
  - Abdominal pain
  - Anorexia
  - Nausea/vomiting
  - Acetone (fruity-smelling) breath odor
  - Kussmaul respirations
  - Altered LOC

Assessment
- Scene size-up
  - Ensure BSI.
- Initial/primary assessment
  - Assess LOC.
  - Manage ABCs.
  - Treat life-threatening illness/injuries.
  - Transport considerations: Transport in a position of comfort.
- Focused history and physical exam/secondary assessment
  - Obtain SAMPLE history and chief complaint (OPQRST).

Management
- Administer oxygen at 15 L/min via nonrebreathing mask.
- Assess blood glucose level.
- Establish IV of 0.9% normal saline, with judicious fluid boluses.
  - Decrease blood glucose by 50 to 75 mg/dL per hour if appropriate. A decrease that is too rapid can lead to encephalopathy.
- Monitor vital signs.
- Apply cardiac monitor.

  Table 10-4 summarizes treatment of hypoglycemia and DKA.

Table 10-4 Treatment of Hypoglycemia and Diabetic Ketoacidosis

Treatment	Used For	Initial Adult Dose	Initial Pediatric Dose
0.9% normal saline	Perfusion; increase or maintain radial pulses; attempt to "dilute" circulating glucose	IV: 500–1,000 mL	IV: 20 mL/kg

Hyperosmolar Hyperglycemic Nonketotic Syndrome

Pathophysiology

This syndrome is a serious hyperglycemic condition that is most often seen in older patients with type 2 diabetes and may occur in those previously undiagnosed, or in diabetics who have improperly managed their medications and diet. The condition may be precipitated by an infection (especially pneumonia or a urinary tract infection) or by certain medications that impair glucose tolerance or increase fluid loss.

The added stress of the illness may lead to increased insulin resistance and further reductions of insulin levels in the bloodstream. Although ketogenesis and ketoacidosis do not develop, insulin levels are not sufficient to permit glucose use by peripheral tissues or to decrease glucogenesis by the liver.

Hyperosmolarity is a condition in which the blood has high concentrations of sodium, glucose, and other molecules that normally attract water into the bloodstream. Normally the kidneys compensate for high glucose levels in the blood by excreting excess glucose in the urine. However, when the patient is in a dehydrated state, the kidneys conserve fluid, driving glucose levels to become higher. This creates a vicious cycle of increasing blood glucose levels and increasing dehydration. The resulting hyperglycemia produces CNS dysfunction. Pathophysiologic changes may develop over a period of days or weeks. Typically, HHNS presents with blood glucose levels of more than 600 mg/dL.

Signs and Symptoms

- Weakness
- Polyuria
- Polydipsia
- Polyphagia
- Lethargy
- Loss of feeling or function in muscles
- Seizures
- Nausea
- Altered LOC, occurring gradually over 4 to 5 days
- Neurologic deficits
- Dehydration
- Absence of ketones (no fruity breath odor)

Assessment

- Scene size-up
  - Ensure BSI.
- Initial/primary assessment
  - Assess LOC.
  - Manage ABCs.
  - Treat life-threatening illness/injuries.
  - Transport considerations: Transport in a position of comfort.
- Focused history and physical exam/secondary assessment
  - Obtain SAMPLE history and chief complaint (OPQRST).

Management

- Administer oxygen at 15 L/min via nonrebreathing mask.
- Assess blood glucose level.
- Establish IV of 0.9% normal saline, with judicious fluid boluses.
  - Decrease blood glucose by 50 to 75 mg/dL per hour if appropriate. Too rapid a decrease can lead to encephalopathy.
- Monitor vital signs.
- Apply cardiac monitor.

The goal of treatment is to correct the dehydration and thus improve the blood pressure, urine output, and circulation. **Table 10-5** summarizes treatment of HHNS.

Table 10-5 Treatment of Hyperosmolar Hyperglycemic Nonketotic Syndrome

Treatment	Used For	Initial Adult Dose	Initial Pediatric Dose
0.9% normal saline	Perfusion; increase or maintain radial pulses; attempt to "dilute" circulating glucose	IV: 500–1,000 mL	IV: 20 mL/kg

Metabolic Alkalosis

Pathophysiology

In metabolic alkalosis, the level of available bicarbonates is high in relation to the level of carbonic acid in the bloodstream, thereby increasing blood pH. This rise in pH depresses the chemoreceptors in the medulla, causing the respiratory rate to decrease, thus increasing the low arterial pressure of carbon dioxide ($Paco_2$). The additional carbon dioxide combines with water to form carbonic acid. Thus, a compensatory respiratory acidosis develops.

When the bicarbonate level exceeds the norm, the renal glomeruli can no longer reabsorb excess bicarbonate. This excess is excreted in the urine, but the hydrogen ions are retained. To maintain homeostasis, the kidneys excrete excess sodium, water, and bicarbonate.

Causes
- Chronic vomiting or nasogastric suctioning
- Use of corticosteroids
- Massive blood transfusions
- Cushing syndrome
- Excessive bicarbonate retention, usually caused by renal perfusion
- Excessive intake of antacids
- Hypokalemia
- Drugs such as diuretics and glucocorticoids

Signs and Symptoms
- Mental dullness
- Muscular tension
- Slow, shallow breaths
- Tetany

Assessment
- Scene size-up
  - Ensure BSI.
- Initial/primary assessment
  - Assess LOC.
  - Manage ABCs.
  - Treat life-threatening illness/injuries.
  - Transport considerations: Transport in a position of comfort.
- Focused history and physical exam/secondary assessment
  - Obtain SAMPLE history and chief complaint (OPQRST).

Management
- Administer oxygen at 15 L/min via nonrebreathing mask.
- Assess blood glucose level.
- Monitor vital signs.
- Apply cardiac monitor.

Metabolic Acidosis

Pathophysiology

In metabolic acidosis, the level of available bicarbonates is low in relation to the level of carbonic acid in the bloodstream, thereby decreasing blood pH. As hydrogen ions start to accumulate in the body, chemical buffers in the cells and extracellular fluid bind with them. The excess hydrogen ions that the buffers cannot bind with decrease the pH and stimulate chemoreceptors in the medulla to increase the respiratory rate. The increased respiratory rate lowers the $Paco_2$, which creates a compensatory respiratory alkalosis.

Healthy kidneys try to compensate for acidosis by secreting excess hydrogen ions into the renal tubules. Each time a hydrogen ion is secreted into the renal tubules, a sodium ion and a bicarbonate ion are absorbed from the tubules and returned to the blood.

Causes

- Excessive acid load
  - Ingestion, such as salicylates or ethylene glycol
  - DKA
  - Lactic acidosis
  - Malnutrition
  - Poor nutritional intake
  - Chronic alcoholism
- Excessive loss of bicarbonate
  - Diarrhea
  - Renal loss
  - Salicylate ingestion
  - Decreased tissue oxygenation or perfusion

Signs and Symptoms

- Rapid, deep breaths
- Altered LOC
- Nausea, vomiting
- Headache, malaise, and lethargy
- CNS depression
- Hypotension
- Gastrointestinal distress
- Warm, flushed skin

Assessment

- Scene size-up
  - Ensure BSI.
- Initial/primary assessment
  - Assess LOC.
  - Manage ABCs.
  - Treat life-threatening illness/injuries.
  - Transport considerations: Transport in a position of comfort.
- Focused history and physical exam/secondary assessment
  - Obtain SAMPLE history and chief complaint (OPQRST).

Management

- Administer oxygen at 15 L/min via nonrebreathing mask.
- Assess blood glucose level.
- Monitor vital signs.
- Apply cardiac monitor.

Table 10-6 summarizes treatment of metabolic acidosis.

Table 10-6 Treatment of Metabolic Acidosis

Treatment	Used For	Adult	Pediatric
Normal saline or lactated Ringer's solution	Increase perfusion; increase hydration status	IV: 250–500 mL	IV: 20 mL/kg
Sodium bicarbonate	Neutralize blood acidity	IV: 1 mEq/kg	IV: 1 mEq/kg

Hyperthyroidism

Pathophysiology

Grave's disease is an autoimmune disorder that causes hyperthyroidism (overproduction of the thyroid hormone). It is the most common cause of hyperthyroidism and is more common in women than in men. Untreated, it may lead to a condition known as **thyrotoxicosis** or thyroid storm, a life-threatening disorder. Family history of the disease is a risk factor; otherwise, the cause is unknown.

Signs and Symptoms

- Goiter (an enlarged thyroid)
- Bulging eyes (exophthalmos)
- Non-pitting edema
- Nervousness
- Irritability
- Excessive perspiration
- Fine, brittle hair
- Muscle weakness, especially in the upper arms and thighs
- Shaky hands (tremors)
- Tachycardia
- Hypertension
- Increased bowel activity
- Weight loss, despite normal or increased appetite
- Sleep disturbances
- Sensitivity to light
- Confusion
- Irregular menstrual cycles

Assessment

- Scene size-up
  - Ensure BSI.
- Initial/primary assessment
  - Assess LOC.
  - Manage ABCs.
  - Treat life-threatening illness/injuries.
  - Transport considerations: Transport in a position of comfort.
- Focused history and physical exam/secondary assessment
  - Obtain SAMPLE history and chief complaint (OPQRST).

Management

- Administer oxygen at 15 L/min via nonrebreathing mask.
- Assess blood glucose level.
- Monitor vital signs.
- Apply cardiac monitor.

Hypothyroidism
Pathophysiology

Myxedema is a term sometimes used to describe hypothyroidism, a deficiency in the production of the thyroid hormone. The disorder also sometimes results from the treatment of hyperthyroidism. In hypothyroidism, there is a general slowing of the metabolic processes as a result of the reduction or absence of the thyroid hormone. All organ systems may be affected to a degree of seriousness proportionate to the amount of hormone loss. Hypothyroidism is often characterized by localized accumulations of mucinous material in the skin, hence its name (*myx* = mucin; *edema* = swelling). Myxedema often occurs in women older than 40 years.

Untreated, longstanding hypothyroidism can lead to a potentially life-threatening condition known as **myxedema coma**.

Risk Factors
- Family history
- Treatment for hyperthyroidism
- Radiation to the neck
- Previous thyroid surgery

Signs and Symptoms
- Myxedema
  - Facial swelling
  - Bradycardia
  - Fatigue/sleepiness
  - Feeling cold
  - Dry skin
  - Altered LOC
  - Weakness
  - Weight gain
- Myxedema coma
  - Deterioration of mental status (hallmark sign)
  - Hyperthermia
  - Absence of fever in the presence of infection

Assessment
- Scene size-up
  - Ensure BSI.
- Initial/primary assessment
  - Assess LOC.
  - Manage ABCs.
  - Treat life-threatening illness/injuries.
  - Transport considerations: Transport in a position of comfort.
- Focused history and physical exam/secondary assessment
  - Obtain SAMPLE history and chief complaint (OPQRST).

Management
- Administer oxygen at 15 L/min via nonrebreathing mask.
- Assess blood glucose level.
- Monitor vital signs.
- Apply cardiac monitor.

Cushing Syndrome

Pathophysiology

Cushing syndrome results from excessive levels of corticosteroid hormone (cortisol), either from excessive use of corticosteroid drugs or from a pituitary tumor that causes the adrenal glands to enlarge. Patients are characterized by their appearance, such as a "moon face" or a buildup of fat between the collar bones, causing a "buffalo hump" appearance.

Signs and Symptoms

- Obesity
- Thin skin that is easily bruised
- Weak bones
- Skin disorders
- Increase in facial hair and body hair
- Depression
- Diabetes

Assessment

- Scene size-up
  - Ensure BSI.
- Initial/primary assessment
  - Assess LOC.
  - Manage ABCs.
  - Treat life-threatening illness/injuries.
  - Transport considerations: Transport in a position of comfort.
- Focused history and physical exam/secondary assessment
  - Obtain SAMPLE history and chief complaint (OPQRST).

Management

- Administer oxygen at 15 L/min via nonrebreathing mask.
- Assess blood glucose level.
- Monitor vital signs.
- Apply cardiac monitor.

Addison's Disease

Pathophysiology

Addison's disease is a disorder characterized by insufficient production of the corticosteroid hormone. Episodes often occur as a result of stress, hypothermia, infection, trauma, and other circumstances in which cortisol would normally be produced to cope with the stress but is not produced. Blood glucose levels decrease, and the body loses its ability to regulate the levels of sodium, potassium, and water. This leads to dehydration and loss of muscle tone. Ultimately, blood pressure falls, along with blood volume.

Signs and Symptoms

- Weakness
- Hypotension
- Hyponatremia
- Hyperkalemia
- Increased skin pigmentation
- Weight loss
- Increased gastrointestinal motility

Assessment

- Scene size-up
  - Ensure BSI.
- Initial/primary assessment
  - Assess LOC.
  - Manage ABCs.
  - Treat life-threatening illness/injuries.
  - Transport considerations: Transport in a position of comfort.
- Focused history and physical exam/secondary assessment
  - Obtain SAMPLE history and chief complaint (OPQRST).

Management

- Administer oxygen at 15 L/min via nonrebreathing mask.
- Assess blood glucose level.
- Monitor vital signs.
- Apply cardiac monitor.

Vital Vocabulary

adrenal cortex The outer part of the adrenal glands that produces corticosteroids.

adrenal medulla The inner portion of the adrenal glands that synthesizes, stores, and eventually releases epinephrine and norepinephrine.

androgens Hormones that are involved in the development of male sexual characteristics but are also present in females.

calcitonin Hormone secreted by the thyroid gland; helps maintain normal calcium levels in the blood.

catecholamines Hormones produced by the adrenal medulla (epinephrine and norepinephrine) that assist the body in coping with physical and emotional stress by increasing the heart and respiratory rates and the blood pressure.

corticosteroids Hormones that regulate the body's metabolism, the balance of salt and water in the body, the immune system, and sexual function.

estrogen One of the major female hormones. At puberty, estrogen brings about the secondary sex characteristics.

glucagon Hormone produced by the pancreas that is vital to the control of the body's metabolism and blood glucose level. Glucagon stimulates the breakdown of glycogen to glucose.

hyperkalemia An increased level of potassium in the blood.

hypokalemia A low blood serum potassium level.

insulin Hormone produced by the pancreas that is vital to the control of the body's metabolism and blood glucose level. Insulin causes sugar, fatty acids, and amino acids to be taken up and metabolized by cells.

myxedema coma Decompensated hypothyroidism. Usually precipitated by a stressful event.

ovaries Female gonads; ovaries release eggs and secrete the female hormones.

parathyroid hormone (PTH) A hormone secreted by the parathyroids that acts as an antagonist to calcitonin. PTH is secreted when calcium blood levels are low.

progesterone One of the major female hormones.

testes Male gonads located in the scrotum that produce hormones called androgens.

testosterone The most important androgen in men.

thyrotoxicosis Excessive levels of circulating thyroid hormone.

thyroxine The body's major metabolic hormone. Thyroxine stimulates energy production in cells, which increases the rate at which the cells consume oxygen and use carbohydrates, fats, and proteins.

type 1 diabetes The type of diabetic disease that usually starts in childhood and requires daily injections of supplemental synthetic insulin to control blood glucose levels. Formerly known as juvenile or juvenile-onset diabetes.

type 2 diabetes The type of diabetic disease that usually starts later in life and often can be controlled through diet and oral medications. Formerly known as adult-onset diabetes.

CHAPTER 11

Medical Emergencies

General medical emergencies are a common, daily occurrence throughout the United States. As an ALS provider, these type of calls require you to obtain the pertinent history and ask the pertinent questions in an attempt to unravel exactly what is going on with the patient. This chapter discusses some of the various medical emergencies you may encounter:

- Syncope
- Allergic reactions and anaphylaxis
- Altered mental status
- Nausea and vomiting
- Seizures
- Headache
- Meningitis
- Dehydration
- Combative patients
- Electrolyte abnormalities

Syncope

Pathophysiology

<u>Syncope</u>, or fainting, is a transient state of unresponsiveness related to temporary inadequate perfusion of the brain.

Causes

- Cardiac arrhythmias
- Dehydration
- Hypoglycemia
- Vasovagal response
- Psychogenic reactions

Signs and Symptoms

- Light-headedness
- Dizziness
- Transient loss of consciousness
- Supine hypotension syndrome
- Orthostatic hypotension

Assessment

- Scene size-up
  - Ensure body substance isolation (BSI).
  - Ensure a safe scene for all responders.
- Initial/primary assessment
  - Assess level of consciousness (LOC).
  - Manage ABCs (airway, breathing, circulation).
  - Treat life-threatening illness/injuries.
  - Transport considerations: Transport patient in a position of comfort.

- Focused history and physical exam/secondary assessment
  – Obtain SAMPLE history and chief complaint (OPQRST).

Management

- Apply supplemental oxygen.
- Establish an intravenous line (IV) to keep open (TKO).
- Reassure patient.
- Monitor vital signs.
- Monitor orthostatic vital signs.
- Apply cardiac monitor.
- Provide supportive, symptomatic care.

Allergic Reactions and Anaphylaxis

Pathophysiology

An **allergic reaction** is an abnormal immune response to a substance that is generally harmless in other people, such as eggs, nuts, or medications. Certain **antigens** that enter the body cause the immune system to produce **antibodies** called IgE (immunoglobulin E), which then become sensitive to that particular antigen. These antibodies react by binding to the surface of mast cells in the body, where they wait for the next exposure to the antigen. On reexposure, the antigen binds to the antibodies on the mast cells, which then release histamines and leukotrienes. The effects of histamines are a runny nose, sneezing, watery eyes, and itching; leukotrienes cause bronchoconstriction.

Allergic reactions have two phases. The early phase begins within a few minutes of exposure and responds to most antihistamine medications. The late phase can take hours to manifest and results from migration of other cells into the zone of injury. The late phase is not dependent on histamine, so antihistamines are less effective.

Anaphylaxis is the most extreme form of allergic reaction. It usually involves more than one body system. Common causes of anaphylaxis include penicillin, aspirin, bee stings, shellfish, and nuts. When a person first comes into contact with a specific allergen, the body produces IgE antibodies that bind to the mast cells in tissues surrounding the blood vessels and to basophils (white blood cells). On subsequent contact with the same antigen, the IgE antibodies react with the antigen, causing the mast cells and basophils to degranulate or release chemical mediators such as leukotrienes (responsible for bronchoconstriction), eosinophils, prostaglandins, and histamines (responsible for vessel permeability). This results in vasodilation, increased capillary permeability, bronchoconstriction, and increased gastrointestinal motility (**Figure 11-1**).

Vasodilation causes hypotension by decreasing capacitance (mainly) and also negatively affects cardiac output by decreasing preload and stroke volume. Increased capillary permeability allows plasma and fluids to leak into the interstitial spaces and decreases the amount of systemic volume needed for the heart to pump effectively.

Signs and Symptoms

- Urticaria
- Wheezing
- Edema
- Itching
- Dyspnea
- Hypotension
- Agitation, anxiety
- Stridor
- Altered LOC

Tip

It should be remembered that syncope is a transient state and will resolve once the patient becomes supine. If the patient does not immediately regain consciousness, search for other causes because it is not syncope.

Tip

It is important to be able to distinguish an allergic reaction from true anaphylaxis. Typically, an allergic reaction will result in localized signs and symptoms, whereas anaphylaxis will present with systemic complaints that involve multiple organ systems. Anaphylaxis is a true life-threatening emergency.

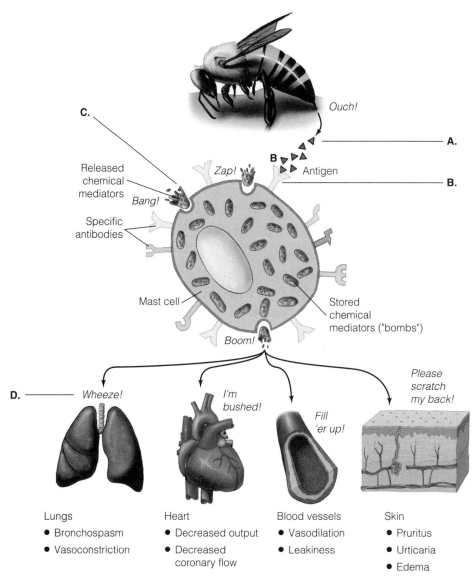

Figure 11-1 The sequence of events in anaphylaxis. **A.** The antigen is introduced into the body. **B.** The antigen-antibody reaction at the surface of a mast cell. **C.** Release of mast cell chemical mediators. **D.** Chemical mediators exert their effects on end organs.

- Vomiting
- Throat or chest tightness
- Difficulty swallowing
- Diarrhea

Assessment

- Scene size-up
  - Ensure BSI.
  - Ensure a safe scene for all responders.
- Initial/primary assessment
  - Assess LOC.
  - Manage ABCs.
  - Treat life-threatening illness/injuries.
  - Transport considerations: Transport patient in a position of comfort.

- Focused history and physical exam/secondary assessment
  - Obtain SAMPLE history and chief complaint (OPQRST).

Management

- Administer oxygen at 15 L/min via nonrebreathing mask.
- Establish IV, TKO.
- Monitor vital signs.
- Apply cardiac monitor.

Table 11-1 summarizes the treatment of allergic reactions.

Table 11-1 Initial Treatment of Allergic Reactions and Anaphylaxis

Treatment	Purpose	Initial Adult Dose	Initial Pediatric Dose
Oxygen	Increase cellular oxygenation	12-15 L/min via nonrebreathing mask	12-15 L/min via nonrebreathing mask
0.9% normal saline	Perfusion	IV: 250-500 mL titrated to a systolic blood pressure of 90 mm Hg or to maintain radial pulses	IV: 20 mL/kg
Methylprednisolone	Anti-inflammatory	IV/IM: 125 mg	IV: 1-2 mg/kg
Albuterol	Bronchodilation; adrenergic effects	Nebulizer: 2.5 mg	Nebulizer: 0.03 mg/kg
Ipratropium bromide	Bronchodilation; anticholinergic	Nebulizer: 500 μg	Safety and efficacy in children < 12 years not established for aerosol and solution
Levalbuterol	Bronchodilation	Nebulizer: 1.25 mg	Nebulizer: 0.625 mg
Epinephrine	Vasoconstriction of the peripheral and bronchial vessels; increase in contractility, rate, and overall cardiac output; smooth muscle relaxant	SQ: 0.3 mg IV: 0.3-0.5 mg	SQ: 0.15 mg IV: 0.15-0.03 mg
Diphenhydramine	Blocks histamines, causing vasoconstriction, decreased heart rate, hypotension, and decreased GI secretions and capillary permeability	IV/IM: 25-50 mg	IV/IM: 1-2 mg/kg

IV, intravenous; IM, intramuscular; SQ, subcutaneous.

Altered Mental Status

Pathophysiology

A patient with <u>altered mental status</u> (also called altered level of consciousness) does not respond appropriately to stimuli. Altered mental status results from dysfunction of the brain and/or brainstem (the reticular activating system is in the brainstem). Altered mental status can be caused by decreased perfusion, as in shock, or by medications, recreational drugs, head injury, stroke, hypoxia, metabolic problems, or any other condition that affects brain function. If it is not corrected in a timely fashion, the patient will enter into a comalike state. The most common concern with this patient is his or her chronic (baseline) status and whether or not this condition is an acute change.

> **Tip**
>
> A simple way to remember possible causes of decreased level of consciousness is AEIOU-TIPS:
> - Alcohol/Acidosis
> - Epilepsy
> - Insulin
> - Overdose
> - Uremia
> - Trauma
> - Infection
> - Psychosis
> - Stroke

Signs and Symptoms

- Confusion
- Decreased response to verbal or physical stimuli
- Inappropriate use of words or speech (aphasia)
- Hallucinations
- Poor memory
- Seizures
- Abnormal vital signs

Assessment

- Scene size-up
  - Ensure BSI.
  - Immobilize the cervical spine if trauma is suspected.
- Initial/primary assessment
  - Assess LOC.
  - Manage ABCs.
  - Treat life-threatening illnesses/injuries.
  - Transport considerations: Transport patient in a position of comfort.
- Focused history and physical exam/secondary assessment
  - Obtain SAMPLE history and chief complaint (OPQRST).

Management

- Be prepared to insert an oropharyngeal or nasopharyngeal airway adjunct based on patient presentation, Glasgow Coma Scale (GCS) score, and the ability to maintain a patent airway.
- Administer oxygen at 15 L/min via nonrebreathing mask.
- Assess blood glucose level.
- Reassure patient.
- Monitor vital signs.
- Apply cardiac monitor.
- Establish IV access.

Table 11-2 summarizes the treatment of altered mental status.

Table 11-2 Initial Treatment of Altered Mental Status

Treatment	Purpose	Initial Adult Dose	Initial Pediatric Dose
Oxygen	Increase cellular oxygenation	12-15 L/min via nonrebreathing mask	12-15 L/min via nonrebreathing mask
Oral glucose	Increase glucose levels in hypoglycemic conscious patients	PO: 12.5-25.0 g	PO: 6-12 g
Naloxone	Narcotic antagonist	IV: 0.4-2.0 mg	IV: 0.4-2.0 mg/kg
Romazicon	Benzodiazepine antagonist	IV: 0.2 mg	IV: 0.01 mg/kg
Thiamine	Used when alcohol abuse is suspected; vitamin B_1 complex needed for energy	IV: 100 mg	Not indicated for pediatric use
$D_{50}W$	Increase glucose levels in hypoglycemic unconscious adult patients	IV: 25 g	Not indicated for pediatric use
$D_{25}W$	Increase glucose levels in hypoglycemic unconscious pediatric patients	Not indicated for adult use	IV: 0.5 g/kg
PO, by mouth.			

Nausea and Vomiting

Pathophysiology

Nausea is a symptom and vomiting a sign associated with a variety of illnesses. They are not stand-alone conditions. Both may be chronic or episodic and may be associated with any medical condition or injury, minor or life threatening. Possible serious causes include:

- Increased intracranial pressure
- Stroke
- Hypertensive crisis
- Acute myocardial infarction
- Pericarditis
- Increased ocular pressure
- Gastrointestinal disorders
- Ovarian cyst
- Pregnancy
- Pneumonia
- Trauma
- Electrolyte imbalances
- Influenza
- Hypotension/shock

Assessment

- Scene size-up
  - Ensure BSI.
- Initial/primary assessment
  - Assess LOC.
  - Manage ABCs.
  - Treat life-threatening illnesses/injuries.
- Transport considerations: Transport patient in a position of comfort, ensuring airway patency.
- Focused history and physical exam/secondary assessment
  - Obtain SAMPLE history and chief complaint (OPQRST).

Management

- Administer oxygen at 15 L/min via nonrebreathing mask.
- Assess blood glucose level.
- Reassure patient.
- Monitor vital signs.
- Apply cardiac monitor.
- Establish IV access.

Table 11-3 summarizes treatment of nausea and vomiting.

Table 11-3 Initial Treatment of Nausea and Vomiting

Treatment	Purpose	Initial Adult Dose	Initial Pediatric Dose
Oxygen	Nausea/vomiting prevention	1-6 L/min via nasal cannula	1-6 L/min via nasal cannula
Promethazine	Nausea/vomiting prevention	SIVP: 12.5 mg IM: 25 mg	SIVP: 0.25 mg/kg
Ondansetron	Nausea/vomiting prevention	IV: 4 mg	IV: 0.1 mg/kg
SIVP, slow intravenous push.			

Seizures

Pathophysiology

Seizures are a result of disorganized electrical activity in the brain. If the abnormal activity spreads through the brain, the seizure becomes generalized. Seizures can cause **convulsions** but may also cause abnormal awareness, behaviors, or sensations. Seizures are caused by several conditions: infection, stroke, fever (in children), electrolyte imbalance, tumors, and others. First-time seizures in adults are often associated with very serious problems such as strokes and cancer. Febrile seizures in children are caused by the body's rapid change in temperature, not the temperature itself.

> **Tip**
>
> Many untrained people cannot distinguish a seizure from the onset of cardiac arrest.

Types of Seizures

Generalized Seizures

- Tonic-clonic (grand mal) seizure
  - Most commonly seen in prehospital setting
  - Bodywide rigidity
  - Jerky, uncontrolled rhythmic movements
  - Bowel or bladder incontinence
  - Eyes rolled back
  - Unresponsive
- Status epilepticus (two or more seizures with no intervening period of responsiveness)
  - Prolonged tonic-clonic type seizure episode(s)
  - Absence seizure
  - Often occurs in children
  - Abnormal behavior (staring into space, lip smacking, or blinking)
- Petit mal (absence) seizures
  - Brief, sudden lapse of conscious activity
  - Usually in children

Partial Seizures

- **Simple partial seizure (Jacksonian seizure):** Characterized by clonic activity (contraction and relaxation) in one particular body part. However, this type of seizure may progress into a grand mal type of seizure.
- **Complex partial seizure:** Marked by a change in behavior, beginning with an aura, followed by abnormal repetitive behavior. The patient regains consciousness within a minute, with no postictal period.

Febrile Seizures

Febrile seizures are brief, generalized tonic-clonic seizures that occur in children without underlying neurologic abnormalities and are triggered by a rise in body temperature. They occur mostly in children between the ages of 6 months and 3 years. A febrile seizure is the effect of a sudden rise in temperature to 39°C (102.0°F) or higher, rather than a fever that has been present for a prolonged length of time.

Signs and Symptoms

- Signs and symptoms vary, depending on the type of seizure the patient is experiencing.
- Prior to some seizures, patients have been known to experience an **aura** or headache.
- Postictal (postseizure) states can include lethargy, headache, dizziness, altered LOC, and confusion.

Assessment

- Scene size-up
  - Ensure BSI.
  - Protect the patient from further harm, and clear the immediate area of potential hazards.

- Initial/primary assessment
  - Assess LOC.
  - Manage ABCs.
  - Treat life-threatening illnesses/injuries.
  - Transport considerations: Transport patient in a position of comfort, ensuring airway patency.
- Focused history and physical exam/secondary assessment
  - Obtain SAMPLE history and chief complaint (OPQRST).
  - The family or bystanders can provide helpful information regarding the history of the seizure, preceding events, and other possible illnesses or causes.

Management

- Administer oxygen at 15 L/min via nonrebreathing mask.
- Assess blood glucose level.
- Reassure patient.
- Monitor vital signs.
- Apply cardiac monitor.
- Establish IV access.
- Observe the FACTS:
  - F = Focus/location of seizure activity
  - A = Activity/behavior
  - C = Color of skin
  - T = Time/duration of seizure
  - S = Secondary information/activity prior to seizure
- Do not restrain the patient, but move items out of the way to prevent injury.
- Obtain the patient's medication on hand or medication list because this may be helpful in determining whether the patient has a history of seizures. Be sure to take these medications to the emergency department with the patient.

Table 11-4 summarizes treatment of seizures.

Table 11-4 Initial Treatment of Seizures

Treatment	Purpose	Initial Adult Dose	Initial Pediatric Dose
0.9% normal saline	If hypotension develops, to maintain systolic BP of 90 mm Hg or radial pulses	Bolus: 250-500 mL	Bolus: 20 mL/kg
Diazepam	For increased presynaptic inhibition that causes seizures; skeletal muscle relaxer	IV: 2.5 mg-5.0 mg	IV: 0.1 mg/kg PR: 0.5 mg/kg
Lorazepam	For increased presynaptic inhibition that causes seizures; skeletal muscle relaxer	IV: 2-4 mg at 2 mg/min	IV: 0.05-0.1 mg/kg
Midazolam	For increased presynaptic inhibition that causes seizures; skeletal muscle relaxer	IV/IM/IN: 2.0-2.5 mg	IV: 0.1 mg/kg IM: 0.2 mg/kg
IN, intranasal.			

Headache

Pathophysiology

Most headaches are caused by tension, fever, or anxiety. Other causes include migraine, brain tumor, intracranial bleeding, hypertensive crisis, meningitis, poisoning, trauma, aneurysm, and stroke.

Signs and Symptoms

- Head pain
- Nausea
- Vertigo
- Stiff neck
- Elevated blood pressure
- Vomiting
- Neurologic deficit
- Visual disturbances
- Photophobia

Assessment

- Scene size-up
  - Ensure BSI.
- Initial/primary assessment
  - Assess LOC.
  - Manage ABCs.
  - Treat life-threatening illnesses/injuries.
  - Transport considerations: Transport patient in a position of comfort, ensuring airway patency.
- Focused history and physical exam/secondary assessment
  - Obtain SAMPLE history and chief complaint (OPQRST).

Management

- Administer appropriate level of oxygen based on the ventilatory status of the patient.
- Assess blood glucose level.
- Reassure patient.
- Monitor vital signs.
- Apply cardiac monitor.
- Establish IV access.
- Treatment of a headache will be mainly supportive.

Meningitis

Pathophysiology

<u>Meningitis</u> is an inflammation of the meninges (dura mater, arachnoid, and pia mater) that surround the brain and spinal cord. Pathogens, either viral or bacterial, trigger an inflammatory response in the brain and spinal cord. Often, inflammation begins in the pia mater and progresses to congestion of adjacent tissues, where exudates cause nerve cell destruction and increased intracranial pressure. This results in engorged blood vessels, disrupted blood supply, thrombosis, or rupture, and possibly cerebral infarction.

Signs and Symptoms

- Disorientation or lethargy
- Irritability
- Headache
- Nausea/vomiting
- **<u>Nuchal rigidity</u>**
- Chills, fever, malaise
- Muscle and joint pain
- Sore throat
- Rash (petechiae or purpura)

Tip

Thirty percent of children with meningitis develop permanent complications; 5% to 15% of children with bacterial meningitis die.

- Respiratory distress
- Dehydration
- Seizures
- **Kernig sign**

Assessment

- Scene size-up
  - Ensure BSI.
  - If you suspect meningitis, ensure that both you and your patient have a surgical mask on, preventing the spread of viral meningitis.
- Initial/primary assessment
  - Assess LOC.
  - Manage ABCs.
  - Treat life-threatening illnesses/injuries.
  - Transport considerations: Transport patient in a position of comfort, ensuring airway patency.
- Focused history and physical exam/secondary assessment
  - Obtain SAMPLE history and chief complaint (OPQRST).

Management

- Administer appropriate level of oxygen based on the ventilatory status of the patient.
- Assess blood glucose level.
- Reassure patient.
- Monitor vital signs.
- Apply cardiac monitor.
- Establish IV access.
- Treatment of a meningitis patient will be mainly supportive.

Tip

Be sure to take all universal and BSI precautions when handling meningitis patients.

Dehydration

Pathophysiology

Dehydration is a loss in the volume of fluid required by the body to maintain homeostasis. Excessive vomiting, diarrhea, and heat loss are common factors that lead to dehydration. Because children have a greater body proportion of fluid, they are more sensitive to the risk of dehydration. The standard treatment of this condition is to establish an IV and administer normal saline or lactated Ringer's solution.

Dehydration can be classified as isotonic, hypernatremic, and hyponatremic. These types are described in the following subsections.

General Signs and Symptoms

Mild Dehydration

- Thirst, warmth
- Poor skin turgor
- Dry mucous membranes
- Concentrated urine

Moderate Dehydration

- Irritability
- Intense thirst
- Diminished peripheral pulses
- Poor skin turgor
- Dry mucous membranes

- Cool body temperature
- Dark, sunken eyes
- Absent urination

Severe Dehydration
- Lethargy
- Possible unresponsiveness
- Tachycardia
- Hypotension
- Absent peripheral pulses
- Capillary refill time of longer than 2 seconds
- Intense thirst
- Poor skin turgor
- Very sunken eyes

Isotonic Dehydration

Pathophysiology
Isotonic dehydration results from excessive loss of sodium and water in equal amounts. Causes include severe or long-term vomiting or diarrhea, systemic infection, and intestinal obstruction.

Signs and Symptoms
- Dry mucous membranes
- Poor skin turgor
- Longitudinal wrinkles of the tongue
- Oliguria
- Anuria
- Acute weight loss
- Depressed/sunken fontanelle

Hypernatremic Dehydration

Pathophysiology
Hypernatremic dehydration is caused by water loss in excess of sodium loss. Causes include certain diuretics (loop diuretics, such as furosemide), profuse diarrhea, and insufficient water intake.

Signs and Symptoms
- Dry, sticky mucous membranes
- Flushed, doughy skin
- Intense thirst
- Oliguria
- Increased body temperature
- Altered mental status
- Hypotension

Hyponatremic Dehydration

Pathophysiology
Hyponatremic dehydration results from sodium loss in excess of water loss. It is caused by the use of some diuretics (such as thiazide), excessive perspiration, salt-losing renal disorders, and excessive water intake or use of water enemas.

Signs and Symptoms
- Abdominal or muscle cramps
- Seizures

- Rapid, thready pulse
- Diaphoresis
- Cyanosis

Assessment of Patients Who Are Dehydrated

- Scene size-up
  - Ensure BSI.
- Initial/primary assessment
  - Assess LOC.
  - Manage ABCs.
  - Treat life-threatening illnesses/injuries.
  - Transport considerations: Transport patient in a position of comfort, ensuring airway patency.
- Focused history and physical exam/secondary assessment
  - Obtain SAMPLE history and chief complaint (OPQRST).

Management of Patients Who Are Dehydrated

- Administer appropriate level of oxygen based on the ventilatory status of the patient.
- Assess blood glucose level.
- Reassure patient.
- Monitor vital signs.
- Apply cardiac monitor.
- Establish IV access.

Table 11-5 summarizes treatment of dehydration.

Table 11-5 Initial Treatment of Dehydration

Treatment	Purpose	Initial Adult Dose	Initial Pediatric Dose
0.9% normal saline	To restore intravasular volume	Bolus: 250-500 mL	Bolus: 20 mL/kg
Lactated Ringer's solution	To restore intravasular volume	Bolus: 250-500 mL	Bolus: 20 mL/kg

Combative Patients

Pathophysiology

Factors that contribute to violence or aggression include the following.

- **Biological/organic:** Medical conditions, medications, recreational drug use
- **Psychosocial:** Childhood trauma
- **Sociocultural:** The person's environment or life events

Signs and Symptoms

- Signs of violence
- Clenched teeth and/or fists
- Pacing back and forth
- Making threats
- Throwing objects
- Agitated, yelling and screaming

Assessment

- Scene size-up
  - Have a plan before you approach the patient. Is the scene safe to enter and remain in?
  - Is law enforcement present?

- Limit the number of people in the immediate area.
- Ensure the safety of rescuers and the patient at all times.
- Make sure additional resources are readily available.
- Ensure BSI.
- Initial/primary assessment
  - Assess LOC.
  - Manage ABCs.
  - Treat life-threatening illnesses/injuries.
  - Transport considerations: Transport patient in a position of comfort, ensuring airway patency, and in a position of safety for both patient and crew.
- Focused history and physical exam/secondary assessment
  - Obtain SAMPLE history and chief complaint (OPQRST).
    - Approach the patient slowly, respecting the patient's personal space.
    - Attempt to remove the patient from the situation.
    - Get the patient to express his or her feelings. Listen in an understanding manner.
    - Be honest and understanding with the patient.
    - Ask open-ended questions.
    - Maintain eye contact.
    - Never lie to combative patients or tell them that everything is going to be OK.

Management

- If needed, restrain the patient according to local protocols and document accordingly.
  - If restraints are necessary, monitor vital signs every 5 minutes.
- Administer appropriate level of oxygen based on the ventilatory status of the patient.
- Assess blood glucose level.
- Reassure patient.
- Monitor vital signs.
- Apply cardiac monitor.
- Establish IV access.

Electrolyte Abnormalities

Hypokalemia and Hyperkalemia

Pathophysiology

- **Hypokalemia** is a decreased level of blood potassium. Potassium (K^+) is the major positively charged ion in intracellular fluid. The body must maintain normal potassium levels for normal nerve, cardiac, and skeletal functioning. Hypokalemia may be caused by reduced dietary intake, increased gastrointestinal losses from vomiting or diarrhea, renal disease, adrenal problems, infusion of solutions poor in potassium, and excessive medication intake (mostly diuretics, but also steroids and theophylline).
- **Hyperkalemia** is an elevation in blood levels of potassium. It may be caused by acute or chronic renal failure, burns, crush injuries, severe infections, other conditions in which large amounts of potassium are released, excessive use of potassium salts, or a shift of potassium from the cells to the extracellular fluid, as with acidosis. Extreme elevation can lead to potentially life-threatening cardiac arrhythmias.

Signs and Symptoms

- Hypokalemia
  - Malaise
  - Skeletal muscle weakness
  - Cardiac conduction disturbances
    - Flattened T waves
    - U waves

- ST segment depression
- Prolonged QT interval
- Ventricular arrythmias or cardiac arrest
  - Delayed reflexes
  - Weak pulse
  - Faint, distant, or muffled heart tones
  - Shallow respirations
  - Hypertension
  - Anorexia
- Hyperkalemia
  - Lethal cardiac arrhythmias
  - Cardiac conduction disturbances
    - Widening QRS complex
    - Peaked T waves
    - Reduction in size of P wave
- Ventricular arrythmias or cardiac arrest
  - Irritability
  - Abdominal distention
  - Nausea
  - Diarrhea
  - Oliguria
  - Weakness (early sign)
  - Paralysis (late sign)

Other Electrolyte Imbalance Conditions

Pathophysiology
- **Hypocalcemia:** An electrolyte disturbance caused by an abnormally low level of calcium in the bloodstream. It can be caused by eating disorders, insufficient or low levels of parathyroid hormone, and medications.

Signs and Symptoms
- Paresthesia
- Tetany (muscle twitching)
- Abdominal cramps
- Neural excitability
- Personality changes
- Abnormal behavior
- Convulsions

Pathophysiology
- **Hypercalcemia:** An electrolyte disturbance caused by an elevated level of calcium in the bloodstream. It is typically caused by malignancy or hyperparathyroidism.

Signs and Symptoms
- Decreased muscle tone
- Renal stones
- Altered mental status
- Deep bone pain

Pathophysiology
- **Hypomagnesemia:** An electrolyte disturbance caused by an abnormally low level of magnesium in the bloodstream. It may be caused by chronic diarrhea, alcoholism, and diuretic usage.

Signs and Symptoms

  - Tremors
  - Nausea or vomiting
  - Diarrhea
  - Hyperactive deep reflexes
  - Confusion

Pathophysiology

- **Hypermagnesemia:** An electrolyte disturbance caused by an excessive level of magnesium in the bloodstream. Magnesium is normally excreted by the kidneys; hypermagnesemia is usually precipitated by renal failure. The second most common cause is iatrogenic overdose.

Signs and Symptoms

- Sedation
- Confusion
- Muscle weakness
- Respiratory paralysis
- Seizures
- Cardiac arrhythmias

Vital Vocabulary

allergic reaction An abnormal immune response the body develops when reexposed to a substance or allergen.

altered mental status A decrease from the baseline mental status, from conscious and alert, progressing to complete unresponsiveness.

anaphylaxis An extreme systemic form of an allergic reaction involving two or more body systems.

antibodies Proteins secreted by certain immune cells that bind antigens to make them more visible to the immune system.

antigens Agents that, when taken into the body, stimulate the formation of specific protective proteins called antibodies.

aura Sensations experienced by a patient before an attack occurs. Common in seizures and migraine headaches.

convulsions Involuntary contraction of the voluntary muscles.

dehydration Depletion of the body systemic fluid volume.

hyperkalemia An increased level of potassium in the blood.

hypokalemia A low blood serum potassium level.

Kernig sign Considered positive when the leg is fully bent at the hip and knee, and subsequent extension of the knee is painful. Often an indicator of meningitis.

meningitis An inflammation of the meningeal coverings of the brain and spinal cord, usually caused by a virus or bacterium.

nuchal rigidity Inability to flex the head forward and touch the chin to the chest as a result of rigidity of the neck muscles.

seizures Paroxysmal alterations in neurologic function (ie, behavioral and/or autonomic function).

syncope Fainting; brief loss of consciousness caused by transient and inadequate blood flow to the brain.

CHAPTER 12
Gastrointestinal Emergencies

Gastrointestinal Function and Anatomy

Gastrointestinal (GI) problems are relatively common and potentially life threatening. The functioning of the GI system begins in the mouth, where saliva helps to lubricate food for swallowing, and chewing helps to break up the food into pieces that are easier to digest. The enzymes in the saliva begin the process of breaking down complex carbohydrates into simple sugars usable by the body. Once food is swallowed, it progresses down the esophagus into the stomach, enters the small intestine (duodenum, jejunum, and ileum), and finally passes through the large intestine (ascending colon, transverse colon, descending colon, sigmoid colon, and rectum), exiting the body through the anus.

Table 12-1 shows the incidence and prevalence of GI disorders.

Pathophysiology

The following three major conditions are responsible for a significant amount of complaints regarding the GI tract:

- **Hypovolemia:** Caused by dehydration (due to vomiting, diarrhea, or bleeding). An example of this is loss of fluid volume and shock caused by trauma to an internal structure.
- **Infection:** Caused by ingestion of contaminated food, or internal damage or rupture. Signs and symptoms of infection may include malaise, weakness, chills, and fever as the body sends white blood cells to the site of infection.
- **Inflammation:** The body's natural defense against a pathogen, involving vasodilation, mobilization of white blood cells, and changes within the cellular metabolism that work together to ward off the offending agent.

Signs and Symptoms of Gastrointestinal Diseases

- Anorexia
- Chills
- Chest pain
- Dyspnea
- Abdominal pain (diffuse or localized)
- Reduced appetite
- Peritonitis signs, such as **guarding**
- Abdominal distention
- Fever
- Cough
- Diarrhea
- Nausea/vomiting
- **Hematemesis**
- **Hematochezia**, melena
- Signs and symptoms of hypovolemic shock

Table 12-1 Incidence and Prevalence of Gastrointestinal Disorders

Disorder	Incidence/Prevalence
All GI disorders	60-70 million (234,000 deaths per year)
Constipation	3.1 million
Crohn's disease	162 new cases/100,000 population
Diverticular disease (**diverticulosis**, diverticulitis)	2.5 million
Gallstones	20.5 million
Gastritis	3.7 million
GERD	20% of the US population
Hemorrhoids	8.5 million
Hepatitis A	8.5 million
Hepatitis B	31% of the US population
Hepatitis C	1.8% of the US population
Hepatitis D	15 million people worldwide; occurs in 5% of hepatitis B patients
Hepatitis E	Cases within the United States occur in people who have traveled to Central Asia, Southeast Asia, Africa, and Mexico
Infectious diarrhea	16 million new cases
Irritable bowel syndrome	2.1 million
Pancreatitis	17 new cases/100,000 population
Peptic ulcer disease	14.5 million
Ulcerative colitis	246 new cases/100,000 population

Signs and symptoms of GI disease and GI bleeding are shown in **Table 12-2** and **Table 12-3**, respectively. **Table 12-4** shows the common locations of pain associated with GI problems. Most abdominal pain begins diffusely or in the epigastric area, then localizes to the area of the involved organ.

Table 12-2 Gastrointestinal Diseases by Type of Condition and Presenting Problem

Disease	Type of Condition	Common Presenting Problems
Acute gastroenteritis	Infectious	Pain, diarrhea, dehydration
Acute hepatitis	Infectious or inflammatory	Pain, liver failure
Appendicitis	Acute inflammation	Pain, sepsis
Bowel obstruction	Infectious or inflammatory	Pain, sepsis
Cholecystitis	Acute inflammation	Pain
Colitis	Chronic inflammation	Pain, diarrhea, dehydration
Crohn's disease	Chronic inflammation	Pain, diarrhea, dehydration
Diverticulitis	Acute inflammation	Pain, sepsis
Esophageal varices	Hemorrhagic	Pain, hemorrhage
Gastroenteritis	Erosive	Pain, diarrhea, dehydration
Hemorrhoids	Hemorrhagic	Pain, hemorrhage
Pancreatitis	Acute inflammation	Pain, hemorrhage
Peptic ulcer disease	Erosive/infectious	Pain, hemorrhage

Table 12-3 Gastrointestinal Bleeding by Organ and Cause

Organ	Causes	Location	Substances
Esophagus	Inflammation (esophagitis) Varices (varicose veins) Tear (Mallory-Weiss syndrome) Cancer Dilated veins (cirrhosis, liver disease)	Upper GI	Melena, hematemesis
Stomach	Ulcers Cancer Inflammation (gastritis)	Upper GI	Melena, hematemesis, vomit with gross blood
Small intestine	Ulcer (duodenal) Cancer Inflammation (irritable bowel disease)	Upper or lower GI	Melena, hematemesis
Large intestine	Infections Inflammation (ulcerative colitis) Colorectal polyps Colorectal cancer Diverticular disease	Lower GI	Hematochezia
Rectum	Hemorrhoids	Lower GI	Hematochezia

Table 12-4 Signs, Symptoms, and Location of the Most Common Causes of Acute Abdominal Pain

Condition	Location	Signs/Symptoms
Cholecystitis	Right upper quadrant (RUQ)	Severe pain, nausea, vomiting, fever, jaundice, tachycardia
Gastroenteritis	Diffuse	Anorexia, nausea/vomiting, pain, diarrhea
Gastritis	Epigastric	Nausea/vomiting, mucosal bleeding, tenderness, melena
Diverticulosis	Left lower quadrant (LLQ)	Bleeding, bloating, pain, cramping, fatigue, dizziness, dyspnea
Appendicitis	Right lower quadrant (RLQ), just medial to iliac crest (McBurney's point)	Periumbilical pain, which localizes to RLQ; loss of appetite, fever, nausea, vomiting, increased urge to urinate
Peptic ulcer	LUQ/epigastric	Burning or gnawing pain in stomach that diminishes immediately after eating, then reemerges 2-3 hr later; nausea, vomiting, belching, heartburn, possibly hematemesis and melena
Chronic pancreatitis	Epigastric	Epigastric pain straight to the back; nausea/vomiting common

Table 12-4 Signs, Symptoms, and Location of the Most Common Causes of Acute Abdominal Pain (Continued)

Condition	Location	Signs/Symptoms
Acute pancreatitis	Epigastric, radiating to the back; usually severe	**Grey Turner sign**: Ecchymotic discoloration of the flank **Cullen sign**: Ecchymotic discoloration of the umbilicus Nausea, vomiting, diarrhea, fever, and chills
Bowel obstruction	Diffuse	Pain, distention, fecal vomiting, constipation
Esophageal varices	Epigastric	Hematemesis, nausea
Intra-abdominal hemorrhage	Diffuse	Cullen sign; hypotension
Pyelonephritis	Flank pain may radiate to the abdomen	Painful urination; nausea, vomiting
Cystitis	Periumbilical to suprapubic	Dysuria, nocturia, hematuria, and abnormal/foul-smelling urine
Renal calculi	LUQ	Pain starts in flank and radiates to groin; painful urination
Abdominal aortic aneurysm	Usually epigastric, radiating to back; may be LUQ	Sudden onset of sharp, tearing, or ripping pain that is constant and possibly radiating through to the back or flank; possible blood pressure discrepancy from one arm to the other; possible decrease or absence of femoral or carotid pulse on one side
Diverticulitis	LLQ	Fever, diarrhea, constipation, nausea, vomiting, abdominal cramping
Pelvic inflammatory disease	LLQ, RLQ, suprapubic	Vaginal discharge, fever, chills, painful intercourse, irregular menstrual bleeding
Ruptured spleen	LUQ	**Kehr sign**: Referred pain to the left shoulder, hypovolemia, tachycardia
Ulcerative colitis	Diffuse	Bloody diarrhea, abdominal cramping, nausea, vomiting
Hepatitis	LUQ	Malaise, muscle/joint aches, nausea, vomiting, diarrhea, headache, jaundice

Assessment of Abdominal Pain

- Scene size-up
  - Ensure body substance isolation (BSI) using personal protective equipment: gloves in the event of vomit, diarrhea, or soiled clothing; gowns can be helpful with incontinent patients; use masks for noxious odors.
- Initial/primary assessment
  - Noxious odors can be a sign of upper or lower GI bleeding.
  - Monitor patient's level of consciousness (LOC).
  - Manage ABCs (airway, breathing, circulation).

Table 12-5 Bowel Sounds

Sound Name	Description	Possible Causes
Normal	Soft gurgles or clicks occurring at 5 to 30/min	Normal movement of material through the intestines
Borborygmi	Loud gurgles heard without a stethoscope	Hyperperistalsis caused by the movement of gas through the bowels
Decreased	Quiet sounds occurring at less than 1 sound/15 to 20 sec	**Hypoperistalsis**, usually associated with inflammation, drugs, or injury
Absent	No sounds after 2 min of continuous listening	Bowel obstruction/intestinal paralysis (ileus)
Hyperactive and/or high-pitched	High-pitched or whistling >30 min	Bowel obstruction

- Obtain orthostatic vital signs to determine the extent of possible internal bleeding.
- Treat life-threatening illness/injuries; if patient is vomiting, maintain airway patency.
- Transport considerations: Transport the patient in a position of comfort.
- Focused history and physical exam/secondary assessment
  - Obtain SAMPLE history and chief complaint (OPQRST).
  - Perform thorough abdominal exam.
    - Protuberance: May be a sign of **ascites** (fluid buildup in abdomen), obesity, pregnancy, or organ enlargement.
    - **Scaphoid** (concave) abdomen: Decreased abdominal volume, usually associated with neonates with severe abdominal birth defects or patients with extreme weight loss (cathexia).
    - Listen for bowel sounds (**Table 12-5**).
    - Evaluate for pain (**Table 12-6**).

Table 12-6 Types of Abdominal Pain

Abdominal Pain Type	Origin	Description	Cause
Visceral pain	Hollow organs	Difficult to localize; described as burning, cramping, gnawing, or aching; usually felt superficially	Organ contracts too forcefully or is distended (stretched); any injury or inflammation of an organ (**visceral peritoneum**)
Parietal pain/rebound pain	Peritoneum	Steady, achy pain; more easy to localize than visceral. Pain increases with movement.	Inflammation of the **parietal peritoneum** (blood and/or infection)
Somatic pain	Peripheral nerve tracts	Well-localized pain, usually felt deeply	Irritation or injury to tissue, causing activation of peripheral nerve tracts
Referred pain	Peripheral nerve tracts	Pain originating in the abdomen and causing "pain" in distant locations; due to similar paths for the peripheral nerves of the abdomen and the distant location	Usually occurs after an initial visceral, parietal, or somatic pain

Management

- Administer oxygen at 15 L/min via nonrebreathing mask.
- Establish an intravenous line (IV) of normal saline or lactated Ringer's solution.
- Attach cardiac monitor.
- Administer nothing by mouth.
- Prepare to suction.
- Provide analgesia for pain control.
- Provide supportive, symptomatic care.

Types of Gastrointestinal Emergencies

- GI bleeding
- Peptic ulcer disease
- Pancreatitis
- Abdominal aortic aneurysm
- Infection/peritonitis

Gastrointestinal Bleeding

Pathophysiology

Hemorrhage anywhere in the GI tract, as a result of a lesion or lesions of the mucosa, is associated with a variety of conditions.

Bleeding within the GI tract is a symptom of another disease, not a disease itself. The differences between upper and lower GI bleeds are predominantly related to the consistency and characteristics of the vomit and stool that may be present. Upper GI bleeding is more common than lower GI bleeding.

- Upper GI bleeding:
  - **Peptic ulcer disease** and gastritis (inflammation of the lining of the stomach)
  - **Esophageal varices:** Dilation of submucosal veins in the esophagus; causes include alcoholism (cirrhosis of the liver) and liver disease (viral hepatitis)
  - **Esophagitis:** Inflammation of the esophagus; frequently caused by **gastroesophageal reflux disease (GERD)**, chemical inhalation, or esophageal trauma
  - **Mallory-Weiss syndrome:** A tear at the junction between the esophagus and the stomach; usually caused by severe retching, vomiting, or coughing
- Lower GI bleeding:
  - Diverticulitis
  - Tumors, hemorrhoids, polyps
    - **Hemmorrhoids:** Caused by inflammation of the blood vessels around the anus
    - **Polyps:** An abnormal growth of tissue present on a mucous membrane
  - **Ulcerative colitis:** Generalized inflammation of the colon; causes dilation of the colon, making it prone to tears

Signs and Symptoms

Upper GI bleeding may lead to bright red or "coffee ground" emesis or melena (black, tarry, foul-smelling stool). If bleeding is severe, the patient may pass bright red blood rectally. Lower GI bleeding may lead to bright red blood passed rectally. **Table 12-4** lists other signs and symptoms of GI bleeding.

Assessment of Gastrointestinal Bleeding

- Scene size-up
  - Ensure BSI.
- Initial/primary assessment
  - Monitor patient's LOC.

Tip

It has been thought that providing any form of analgesia (morphine, meperidine, or fentanyl) to a patient presenting with abdominal pain in the prehospital setting would mask the signs and symptoms, thus prohibiting the emergency department physician from performing a complete and rapid assessment. As with any field of medicine, the treatment of the abdominal pain patient has evolved, with an increasing number of physicians and medical directors requesting that pain management be accomplished prehospitally in the patient with acute abdominal pain. However, as a prehospital provider, you must take into consideration numerous factors:

1. Is it allowable by standing order to administer analgesia?
2. Is it in the patient's best interest to administer it?
3. Do I have an antagonist available, in case I accidently overdose the patient on the analgesic?

Remember: Do no harm. If your protocols allow you to administer analgesia to the acute abdominal pain patient, and you feel that it is clinically indicated, decrease that patient's pain and suffering by administering the analgesic.

- Manage ABCs: Airway obstruction is common as a result of vomiting. Have suction available.
- Treat life-threatening illness/injuries.
- Transport considerations: Transport the patient in a position of comfort. If patient is showing signs or symptoms of shock, place in the Trendelenburg position and rapidly transport.
- Note any history of bleeding.
- Note any pain or referred pain.
- Focused history and physical exam/secondary assessment
  - Obtain SAMPLE history and chief complaint (OPQRST).
  - Perform cardiac monitoring.

Management

- Establish a large-bore IV—preferably two—and administer fluid at appropriate rates to maintain radial pulses and blood pressure above 90 mm Hg.
- Administer oxygen at 15 L/min via nonrebreathing mask.
- Elevate feet 8" to 12" if patient is hypotensive and lung sounds are clear.
- Keep patient warm.
- Attach cardiac monitor.
- Administer nothing by mouth.
- If patient is actively vomiting, consider administration of an **antiemetic**, per local protocol.

Peptic Ulcer Disease

Pathophysiology

Peptic ulcer disease includes gastric ulcer and the more common duodenal ulcer. These lesions are caused by damage to the mucosal lining from acid and digestive enzymes. Most peptic ulcers are associated with *Helicobacter pylori* infection, which damages the protective mucous coating of the stomach and duodenum. Chronic nonsteroidal anti-inflammatory use is a common cause of ulcers because they block the protective effects of **prostaglandins**. Ulcers can cause bleeding, perforation, or obstruction of the GI tract.

Signs and Symptoms

- Classic sequence of burning or gnawing pain in the stomach that subsides or diminishes immediately after eating and then reemerges 2 to 3 hours later
- Nausea, vomiting, belching, and heartburn
- If erosion is severe, gastric bleeding can occur, resulting in hematemesis and melena.

Assessment

- Scene size-up
  - Ensure BSI.
- Initial/primary assessment
  - Monitor patient's LOC.
  - Treat life-threatening illnesses/injuries.
  - Transport considerations: Transport the patient in a position of comfort. If patient is showing signs or symptoms of shock, place in the Trendelenburg position and rapidly transport.
- Focused history and physical exam/secondary assessment
  - Obtain SAMPLE history and chief complaint (OPQRST). Ask patient about recent ingestion of alcohol, ibuprofen, and salicylates.

Management

The major focus for the prehospital management of patients with peptic ulcers is to accurately assess the extent of blood loss and prepare to manage any hypotension that is present. Ortho-static vital signs are critical in determining fluid needs and transportation/packaging issues.

Pancreatitis
Pathophysiology
Inflammation of the pancreas may be acute or chronic. Acute **pancreatitis** is a condition associated with tissue damage as a result of the inappropriate activation of enzymes. The mechanism that triggers this activation is unknown. However, it is associated with several conditions, most commonly biliary tract obstruction by gallstones and alcohol abuse. Alcohol stimulates pancreatic secretions.

Signs and Symptoms
- Mid-epigastric abdominal pain (may radiate to the patient's back)
- Fever (inflammation)
- Persistent vomiting and abdominal distention (**hypermotility**)
- Crackles at lung bases (heart failure)
- Left pleural effusion (circulation of pancreatic enzymes)
- Tachycardia (dehydration and possible hypovolemia)
- Cathexia (malabsorption)
- Malaise

Assessment
- Scene size-up
  - Ensure BSI.
- Initial/primary assessment
  - Monitor patient's LOC.
  - Manage ABCs.
  - Transport considerations: Transport the patient in a position of comfort.
- Focused history and physical exam/secondary assessment
  - Obtain SAMPLE history and chief complaint (OPQRST).

Management
- Establish an IV of normal saline or lactated Ringer's solution.
- If patient is actively vomiting, consider administration of an antiemetic, per local protocol. Consider analgesia (morphine, fentanyl, meperidine), per local protocol.
- Administer nothing by mouth.

Abdominal Aortic Aneurysm
Pathophysiology
An **abdominal aortic aneurysm** is a saclike widening in the abdominal aorta that is present in 2% to 4% of the population. Rupture results in a 35% mortality rate.

Signs and Symptoms
- May be asymptomatic until rupture
- Sudden onset of severe abdominal pain
- Pain radiating to back and scrotum
- Nausea/projectile vomiting
- Poor general health
- Pulsating mass in abdomen
- Diaphoresis
- Blue scrotum
- Weak, asymmetrical, or absent femoral pulse
- Distended, tender abdomen
- Signs and symptoms of shock

Assessment
- Scene size-up
  - Ensure BSI.

- Initial/primary assessment
  - Monitor patient's LOC.
  - Manage ABCs.
  - Transport considerations: Transport the patient in a position of comfort and use gentle handling.
- Focused history and physical exam/secondary assessment
  - Obtain SAMPLE history and chief complaint (OPQRST).
  - Refrain from palpating the abdomen if a pulsating mass is present.

Management
- Establish an IV—preferably two—of normal saline or lactated Ringer's solution.
- If patient is actively vomiting, consider administration of an antiemetic, per local protocol. Consider analgesia (morphine, fentanyl, meperidine), per local protocol.
- Administer nothing by mouth.

Infections
Peritonitis
- Peritonitis is the inflammation of the thin membrane (peritoneum) that lines the abdominal wall and covers the abdominal organs. This inflammation may be caused by bacterial or fungal infections. Peritonitis can be life threatening if not treated quickly.
- Signs and symptoms
  - Swelling and tenderness in the abdomen
  - Fever and chills
  - Nausea and vomiting
  - Thirst, loss of appetite

Appendicitis
- Appendicitis begins with the accumulation of material, usually feces, within the appendix. Once the normal flushing of this organ is obstructed, pressure may build within the appendix. This pressure decreases the flow of blood and lymph fluid, which in turn hinders the body's ability to fight infection. The combination of the bacteria within the feces and the body's decreased ability to fight any local infection provides an environment ripe for the bacteria's uncontrolled reproduction. If left unchecked, overpressurization of the appendix may eventually result in rupture, peritonitis, sepsis, and death.
- Signs and symptoms
  - Patients classically present with **periumbilical** (around the navel) pain that migrates to the right lower quadrant. The duration of the pain is usually less than 48 hours.
  - As the condition progresses, the pain will change characteristics. Rebound tenderness is a sign of perforation of the appendix with resultant peritonitis.
  - Patients often develop anorexia, nausea, and fever.
- Management
  - Monitor patient for septicemia and shock.
  - Volume resuscitation may not be adequate to restore blood pressure; be prepared to use dopamine if crystalloids are not effective.
  - Administer pain medications.

Diverticulitis
- In patients who consume a limited amount of fiber, the consistency of the normal stool becomes more solid. This hard stool takes more contractions and subsequently increases pressure within the colon to move. In this environment, small defects within the colonic wall that would otherwise not pose a problem now fail, resulting in bulges in the wall. These small outcroppings eventually turn into pouches, called diverticula.

- Fecal matter becomes trapped within these pouches. When bacteria grow there, they cause localized inflammation and infection.
- As the body attempts to manage this infection, scarring can occur, along with adhesions and fistulas. A fistula is an abnormal connection between two cavities. In the case of diverticulitis, fistulas are typically between the colon and the bladder, increasing their vulnerability to infection.
- Signs and symptoms
  - The presentation of diverticulitis is abdominal pain, which tends to be localized to the left side of the lower abdomen.
  - Classic signs of infection include fever, malaise, body aches, chills, nausea, and vomiting.
  - Bleeding is rare.
- Management
  - Examine the patient closely to ensure that severe infection is not present, as sepsis can occur easily in conjunction with fistulas to the urinary bladder.
  - Administer large amounts of fluids and/or dopamine to maintain blood pressure.

Vital Vocabulary

abdominal aortic aneurysm A saclike widening in the abdominal aorta that is present in 2% to 4% of the population. Rupture results in a 35% mortality rate.

antiemetic Medication that relieves nausea, to prevent vomiting.

ascites Abnormal accumulation of fluid in the peritoneal cavity.

Cullen sign Ecchymotic discoloration of the umbilicus—a sign of intraperitoneal hemorrhage.

diverticulosis Irritation or bleeding of the diverticula of the large intestine, thought to be caused by increased pressure within the colon.

gastroesophageal reflux disease (GERD) Also known as acid-reflux disease. Abnormal reflux in the esophagus, which results in persistent symptoms and may ultimately cause damage to the esophageal lining.

guarding Muscles of the abdomen wall contract and remain tense, to protect inflamed internal organs from external pressure.

Grey Turner sign Ecchymosis of the flanks.

hematemesis Vomit with blood. Can either be like coffee grounds in appearance, indicating partially digested blood, or contain bright red blood, indicating current active bleeding.

hematochezia The passage of stools containing blood.

hypermotility Overactivity of the gastrointestinal tract.

hypoperistalsis Decreased bowel movement.

Kehr's sign Left shoulder pain that may indicate a ruptured spleen.

Mallory-Weiss syndrome A tear at the junction between the esophagus and the stomach, usually caused by severe retching, vomiting, or coughing. Additional causes include chronic alcoholism as well as eating disorders.

pancreatitis Inflammation of the pancreas, which may be acute or chronic. Acute pancreatitis is a condition associated with tissue damage as a result of the inappropriate activation of enzymes.

parietal peritoneum The membrane that lines the abdominal wall and the pelvic cavity.

peptic ulcer disease Abrasion of the stomach or small intestine.

periumbilical Around the navel.

prostaglandins A group of lipids that act as chemical messengers.

scaphoid A concave shape of the abdomen. This can be caused by evisceration.

visceral peritoneum The portion of the peritoneum that covers the internal organs and forms the outer layer of most of the intestinal tract.

Toxicology: Poisoning and Substance Abuse

A **poison** is any substance taken into the body that interferes with normal physiologic function. Poisons can make people ill; they can also be fatal. A legal or illegal substance becomes a poison when taken in excess. A *toxin* is a poison that is the product of a living organism.

General Poisoning

Pathophysiology

Poisons may enter the body via four routes, with each method of entry having both acute and delayed effects.

- **Ingestion:** Most common route; poison is absorbed largely in the small intestine.
- **Inhalation:** Through the nose or mouth, moving into the lungs. Poison may damage tissue, causing respiratory distress, or enter cells, causing systemic toxicity.
- **Absorption:** Through the skin, into the bloodstream. Some chemicals are absorbed more easily into fat and are more likely to induce poisoning.
- **Injection:** Through the skin by needle or sting.

Signs and Symptoms

- Altered mental status
- Abdominal or muscle pain
- Numbness, tingling, or weakness
- Blurred vision
- Increased secretions
- Nausea and vomiting
- Itchy skin
- Respiratory distress
- Tachycardia or bradycardia
- Cardiac dysrhythmia
- Wheezing or stridor
- Change in body temperature
- Change in pupil size or reactivity
- Flushed or cyanotic skin

> **Tip**
>
> In cases of poisonings, the best reference for treatment is your local poison control center. Never hesitate to contact this resource for guidance.

> **Cyanide Poisoning**
>
> The antidote for cyanide poisoning is amyl nitrite ampules, sodium nitrite, and sodium thiosulfate. Amyl nitrate and sodium nitrite are the first part of the antidote for cyanide poisoning. They convert hemoglobin into methemoglobin, which binds with the cyanide to minimize its toxic effects.
>
> Sodium thiosulfate, the second part of the antidote, converts cyanide into thiocyanate, a nontoxic substance, which is then excreted in the urine.

Table 13-1 lists the main classes of toxins, their common signs, causative agents, and treatments.

Assessment

- Scene size-up
  - Ensure body substance isolation (BSI).
  - Ensure a safe scene for all responders.
- Initial/primary assessment
  - Assess level of consciousness (LOC).
  - Manage ABCs (airway, breathing, circulation).
  - Treat life-threatening illness/injuries.
  - Transport considerations: Transport the patient in a position of comfort.
- Focused history and physical exam/secondary assessment
  - Obtain SAMPLE history and chief complaint (OPQRST).

Table 13-1 Classes of Poison

Toxin	Common Signs	Causative Agents	Specific Treatment
Anticholinergics	Remember DUMBELS: D - Diarrhea U - Urination M - Miosis B - Bronchiospasm E - Emesis L - Lacrimation S - Salivation	Belladonna alkaloids Tricyclic antidepressants Synthetic anticholinergics Organophosphates Carbonate insecticides Nerve agents	Atropine Pralidoxime (2-PAM chloride) Diazepam (Valium) Activated charcoal
Benzodiazepines	Decreased level of consciousness, respiratory depression	Benzodiazepines Diazepam Midazolam	Flumazenil
Beta-blockers	Cardiac arrhythmias, hypotension, decreased level of consciousness, respiratory depression, seizures, hypoglycemia	Esmolol Propanolol Labetalol	Glucagon Alpha- and beta-agonists such as epinephrine and isoprenaline; may need high doses
Calcium channel blockers	Hypotension, cardiac arrhythmias, respiratory depression, pulmonary edema, acidosis, hyperglycemia, hyperkalemia	Dihydropyridines Nifedipine Amlodipine Benzothiapines Diltiazem Phenylalkylamines Verapamil	10% calcium chloride Calcium gluconate
Digoxin	Cardiac arrhythmias	Digoxin	Digibind
Hallucinogens	Visual illusions, delusions, bizarre behavior, respiratory and central nervous system depression	LSD, PCP, mescaline, some mushrooms, marijuana, jimsonweed, nutmeg, mace, some amphetamines	Minimal sensory stimulation and calming measures Diazepam Haloperidol
Opioids	Euphoria, hypotension, respiratory depression, nausea, pinpoint pupils, seizures, coma	Heroin Morphine Codeine Meperidine propoxyphene Fentanyl	Naloxone Nalmefene (Revex)
Sympathomimetics	Delusions, paranoia, cardiac arrhythmias, acute myocardial infarction, hypertension, diaphoresis, seizures, hypotension	Cocaine Amphetamines Methamphetamines Over-the-counter decongestants	Minimal sensory stimulation and calming measures Benzodiazepines
Tricyclic antidepressant overdose	Nausea, vomiting, dry mouth, drowsiness, hypotension, hallucinations, seizures, cardiac dysrhythmias	Amitriptyline Nortriptyline Desipramine Amoxapine	Sodium bicarbonate Benzodiazepines

Management

- Administer oxygen at 15 L/min via nonrebreathing mask.
- Establish intravenous (IV) access.
- Reassure patient.

- Remove contaminated clothing.
- Monitor vital signs.
- Apply cardiac monitor.
- For poisoning by ingestion:
  - Consider administration of activated charcoal via nasogastric or orogastric (NG/OG) tube, if recent ingestion.
- For poisoning through inhalation:
  - Remove patient to open air.
  - Provide ventilatory support.
- For poisoning by absorption:
  - Brush off dry toxins.
  - Remove patient's contaminated clothing.
  - Flush affected area with water for a minimum of 20 minutes.
- For injected poisons:
  - For patients displaying respiratory depression, administer naloxone.

Table 13-2 summarizes the treatment of general poisoning.

Table 13-2 Initial Treatment of General Poisoning

Treatment	Purpose	Initial Adult Dose	Initial Pediatric Dose	Notes
Activated charcoal	Adsorbs toxins that enter the GI tract	1-2 g/kg	1-2 g/kg	Via NG/OG or PO
Amyl nitrate	Treats cyanide poisoning by converting hemoglobin into methemoglobin to attract cyanide and prevent toxic effects	Inhaled: 20 sec crushed pearl, 40 sec O_2	Inhaled: 20 sec crushed pearl, 40 sec O_2	N/A
Atropine	Anticholinesterase; treats organophosphate poisoning; increases heart rate; blocks cholinergic receptors in parasympathetic nervous system	IV: 2-4 mg every 3-5 min until symptom reversal	0.2 mg/kg	In severe cases of organophosphate poisoning, pralidoxime may need to be administered.
Diazepam	Anticonvulsant and sedative/relaxant	IV: 5-10 mg/kg	IV: 0.2-0.5 mg/kg or per Broselow tape	N/A
Flumazenil	Treats benzodiazepine overdose by blocking the effect/receptors of benzodiazepines	IV: 0.2 mg	Not recommended	Use caution when administering to patients with a history of seizures.
Oxygen	Treats carbon monoxide poisoning	15 L/min via nonrebreathing mask	15 L/min via nonrebreathing mask	Needed to replace oxygen in hemoglobin

Continues

Table 13-2 Initial Treatment of General Poisoning (Continued)

Treatment	Purpose	Initial Adult Dose	Initial Pediatric Dose	Notes
Pralidoxime (2-PAM)	Organophosphate poisoning; inhibits anticholinesterase	IV: 1-2 g	IV: 20-40 mg/kg	Used in conjunction with atropine
Sodium bicarbonate	Hydrogen ion buffers	IV: 1 mEq/kg	IV: 1 mEq/kg	Alkalizes urine; treats metabolic acidosis
Sodium nitrate	Treats cyanide poisoning by converting hemoglobin into methemoglobin to attract cyanide and prevent toxic effects	IV: 10 mL of 3%	IV: 0.33 mL/kg	N/A
Sodium thiosulfate	Treats cyanide poisoning by converting cyanide to thiocyanate	IV: 50 mL of 25% over 10 min	IV: 1.65 mL/kg	N/A
IV, intravenous; PO, by mouth.				

Toxic Gases

Pathophysiology

Toxic gases are absorbed by inhalation. They include carbon monoxide (CO), chlorine gas, and hydrocarbons. Several factors determine the effects of toxic gases, including their water solubility or water insolubility. Water-soluble gases are absorbed by saliva and mucus and cause damage to the upper airway. Water-insoluble gases pass through the upper airway, displacing oxygen or interfering with its absorption and use by the body. Some gases cause metabolic changes. Irritant gases have immediate, delayed, and chronic effects.

There are three categories of toxic gases:

- **Inert:** Displace oxygen, resulting in asphyxiation
- **Irritant:** Water-soluble; irritate mucous membranes of the upper airway
- **Water-soluble:** Deposit on the bronchioles/alveoli and cause extensive tissue damage and systemic poisoning of the cells, leading to severe dysfunction

Signs and Symptoms

- Altered LOC
- Abnormal lung sounds
- Tachypnea
- Flushed or cyanotic skin
- Cherry red skin
- Tachycardia
- Nausea/vomiting
- Runny nose
- Itchy, watery, burning eyes and skin
- Distress, anxiety
- Chest pain
- Dyspnea

- Headache, drowsiness
- Confusion
- Pulmonary edema

Assessment

- Scene size-up
  - Ensure BSI.
  - Ensure a safe scene for all responders.
- Initial/primary assessment
  - Assess LOC.
  - Manage ABCs.
  - Treat life-threatening illness/injuries.
  - Transport considerations: Transport the patient in a position of comfort.
- Focused history and physical exam/secondary assessment
  - Obtain SAMPLE history and chief complaint (OPQRST).

Management

- Administer oxygen at 15 L/min via nonrebreathing mask.
- Establish IV access.
- Reassure patient.
- Remove contaminated clothing.
- Monitor vital signs.
- Apply cardiac monitor.

Carbon Monoxide Poisoning

Pathophysiology

<u>Carbon monoxide</u> (CO) is a colorless, odorless, flavorless gas that has an affinity for hemoglobin 200 times more than that of oxygen and binds to hemoglobin in red blood cells, preventing oxygen from binding to it. Thus, cells are not oxygenated properly, and gas exchange does not occur.

Signs and Symptoms

- Chest pain
- Altered LOC
- Headache
- Cherry red skin
- Abnormal lung sounds
- Blisters
- General malaise
- Nausea/vomiting
- Drowsiness
- Lack of responsiveness

Assessment

- Scene size-up
  - Ensure BSI.
  - Ensure a safe scene for all responders.
- Initial/primary assessment
  - Assess LOC.
  - Manage ABCs.
  - Treat life-threatening illness/injuries.
  - Transport considerations: Transport the patient in a position of comfort.

- Focused history and physical exam/secondary assessment
  - Obtain SAMPLE history and chief complaint (OPQRST).

Management

- Administer oxygen at 15 L/min via nonrebreathing mask.
- Establish IV access.
- Reassure patient.
- Remove contaminated clothing.
- Monitor vital signs.
- Apply cardiac monitor.
- Monitor CO levels, if technology is available.
- Transport to a facility with a hyperbaric chamber, if available.

> **Carbon Monoxide Monitoring With the Rad-57**
>
> The Rad-57, manufactured by Massimo, analyzes more than 7+ wavelengths of light to accurately measure carboxyhemoglobin and methemoglobin percent levels in the blood noninvasively and continuously. Operating under the same premise as pulse oximetry, the Rad-57 allows prehospital providers to quickly and accurately diagnose cases of CO poisoning.

It is important to remember that patients experiencing CO exposure may present with a normal Spo_2 reading. This is because pulse oximetry reads "something" bound to the hemoglobin molecules. In this case, the CO is bound, not oxygen.

Table 13-3 summarizes the treatment of CO poisoning.

Table 13-3 Treatment of Carbon Monoxide Poisoning

Treatment	Purpose	Adult Dose	Pediatric Dose
Oxygen	Replaces CO in the hemoglobin	15 L/min via nonrebreathing mask	15 L/min via nonrebreathing mask

Overdose: Narcotics and Sedative-Hypnotics

Pathophysiology

Narcotics are drugs that have sedating and analgesic properties, similar to opiates. Opiates are natural and synthetic substances that are used primarily for their pain-relieving qualities. With repeated use of narcotics, tolerance and dependence develop. The development of tolerance is characterized by a shortened duration and a decreased intensity of analgesia, euphoria, and sedation, which creates the need to administer progressively larger doses to attain the desired effect. Common opiates are morphine, codeine, oxycodone, and methadone. Heroin is an illegal opiate.

Sedative-hypnotic drugs are used for induction of sleep and to reduce anxiety. Benzodiazepines and barbiturates are examples.

Signs and Symptoms

- Altered LOC
- Pupillary constriction (pinpoint)
- Hypotension
- Respiratory depression
- Bradycardia
- Pulmonary edema

Assessment

- Scene size-up
  - Ensure BSI.
  - Ensure a safe scene for all responders.

- Initial/primary assessment
  - Assess LOC.
  - Manage ABCs.
  - Treat life-threatening illness/injuries.
  - Transport considerations: Transport the patient in a position of comfort.
- Focused history and physical exam/secondary assessment
  - Obtain SAMPLE history and chief complaint (OPQRST).

Management

- Administer oxygen at 15 L/min via nonrebreathing mask.
- Establish IV access.
- Reassure patient.
- Monitor vital signs.
- Apply cardiac monitor.
- Prepare intubation equipment if significant respiratory depression is present.

Table 13-4 summarizes the treatment of overdoses of narcotics and opiates.

Table 13-4 Initial Treatment of Narcotic and Opiate Overdose

Treatment	Purpose	Initial Adult Dose	Initial Pediatric Dose
Normal saline	Increase blood pressure	IV: 250-mL bolus	IV: 20 mL/kg
Naloxone	Binds with narcotic receptors to block or reverse the effects of narcotic drugs	IV/IM/IN: 0.4-2.0 mg/min	IV/IM/IN: 0.1 mg/kg
Flumazenil	Binds with benzodiazepine receptors to block the effects of benzodiazepines	IV: 0.2 mg/min	IV: 0.01 mg/kg/min
IM, intramuscular; IN, intranasal.			

Overdose: Tricyclic Antidepressants

Pathophysiology

Once commonly prescribed for depression, tricyclic antidepressants (TCAs) have a very narrow therapeutic index. Because of this narrow window, TCAs are not as commonly prescribed any longer. They work by blocking the reuptake of serotonin and dopamine.

Signs and Symptoms

- Agitation
- Tachycardia
- Dilated pupils
- Hyperthermia
- Warm, dry skin
- Hypotension
- Respiratory depression
- Cardiac dysrhythmias (ie, tachycardia, prolonged QRS)
- Nausea/vomiting
- Drowsiness
- Seizures

- Blurred vision
- Dry mouth
- Hallucinations
- Confusion
- Inability to void

Assessment

- Scene size-up
  - Ensure BSI.
  - Ensure a safe scene for all responders.
- Initial/primary assessment
  - Assess LOC.
  - Manage ABCs.
  - Treat life-threatening illness/injuries.
  - Transport considerations: Transport the patient in a position of comfort.
- Focused history and physical exam/secondary assessment
  - Obtain SAMPLE history and chief complaint (OPQRST).

Management

- Administer oxygen at 15 L/min via nonrebreathing mask.
- Establish IV access.
- Reassure patient.
- Monitor vital signs.
- Apply cardiac monitor.

Table 13-5 summarizes the treatment of overdose of TCAs.

Table 13-5 Initial Treatment of Tricyclic Antidepressant Overdose

Treatment	Purpose	Initial Adult Dose	Initial Pediatric Dose
0.9% normal saline	Increase blood pressure	IV: 250-mL bolus	IV: 20 mL/kg
Sodium bicarbonate	Alkalizes urine; treats metabolic acidosis	IV: 1 mEq/kg	IV: 1 mEq/kg

Ethanol Poisoning (Alcoholism)

Pathophysiology

Alcoholism is the chronic use of alcohol as a result of alcohol dependence; alcohol abuse is excessive alcohol consumption. The following chronic conditions may be caused by alcoholism:

- Cirrhosis of the liver
- Hepatitis
- Pancreatitis
- Esophageal varices
- Gastrointestinal (GI) bleeding
- Poor balance and coordination
- Jaundice

- Edema
- Diabetic ketoacidosis
- Head injury
- Meningitis
- Hypoglycemia
- Hypoxia

Alcoholism may also be associated with the abuse of other drugs. Beware of other conditions that may mimic alcohol intoxication, such as diabetic ketoacidosis, cerebrovascular accident, head injury, and seizures. Excessive intake of alcohol can be fatal due to direct toxic effects or due to sedation and airway obstruction.

Signs and Symptoms

- Altered LOC
- Slurred speech
- Nausea/vomiting
- Abnormal behavior
- Odor of alcohol
- Hypotension
- Seizures
- Labored, slow respiration
- Signs of GI bleeding
- Alcohol withdrawal
  - Elevated blood pressure
  - Bloodshot eyes
  - Alcohol withdrawal seizures: grand mal within 24 to 48 hours
  - **Delirium tremens**: Can occur within 12 to 48 hours
  - Fever
  - Tachycardia
  - Hypertension

Assessment

- Scene size-up
  - Ensure BSI.
  - Ensure a safe scene for all responders.
- Initial/primary assessment
  - Assess LOC.
  - Manage ABCs.
  - Treat life-threatening illness/injuries.
  - Transport considerations: Transport the patient in a position of comfort.
- Focused history and physical exam/secondary assessment
  - Obtain SAMPLE history and chief complaint (OPQRST).

Management

- Administer oxygen at 15 L/min via nonrebreathing mask.
- Establish IV access.
- Reassure patient.
- Monitor vital signs.
- Apply cardiac monitor.

Table **13-6** summarizes the treatment of ethanol poisoning.

Table 13-6 Initial Treatment of Ethanol Poisoning

Treatment	Purpose	Adult Dose	Pediatric Dose
Dextrose 50%	To restore a functioning blood glucose level, if below 60 mg/dL	IV: 25 g	Not indicated for pediatric use
Dextrose 25%	To restore a functioning blood glucose level, if below 60 mg/dL	Not indicated for adult use	0.5-1.0 g/kg
Thiamine (vitamin B_{12} complex)	Given due to possible malnutrition and to prevent **Wernicke encephalopathy**	IV/IM: 100 mg	IV/IM: 10-25 mg

Vital Vocabulary

absorption The process by which a substance's molecules are moved from the site of entry or administration into the body and into systemic circulation.

carbon monoxide A chemical asphyxiant that results in cellular respiratory failure; this gas binds to hemoglobin to the extent that oxygen in the blood becomes inaccessible to the cells.

delirium tremens A severe withdrawal syndrome seen in people with alcoholism who are deprived of ethyl alcohol; characterized by restlessness, fever, sweating, disorientation, agitation, and seizures.

ingestion Eating or drinking materials for absorption through the gastrointestinal tract.

inhalation The process by which a substance enters the body through the nose or mouth, moving into the lungs.

injection When the skin is pierced, and foreign material is deposited into the skin.

poison A substance whose chemical action could damage structures or impair function when introduced into the body.

Wernicke encephalopathy An acute disease of the brain caused by thiamine deficiency.

CHAPTER 14

Hematology and the Immune System

As an ALS provider, you will rarely be called upon to respond to a hematologic emergency, but when you are, your quick actions may save the patient's life. To provide appropriate interventions, you should have a basic understanding of blood, its components, and the immune system.

Blood and Its Components

Functions of Blood

- **Transportation:** Blood transports oxygen from the lungs to the tissues and carbon dioxide from the tissues to the lungs. It carries nutrients to the cells and waste products (metabolic wastes, excessive water, and ions) away from the cells.
- **Regulation:** Blood carries hormones to the organs and excess internal heat to the surface of the body, regulating body temperature.
- **Protection:** The blood's clotting mechanism protects against blood loss. Leukocytes (white blood cells) provide immunity against many disease-causing agents, as well as protect from infection.

Components of Blood

The average adult has about 5 liters (about 5,000 mL) of blood. Blood consists of the following (**Figure 14-1**):

- Formed elements
  - Red blood cells (**erythrocytes**)
  - White blood cells (**leukocytes**)
  - Platelets (**thrombocytes**)
- Plasma
  - Water
  - Dissolved solutes

Red Blood Cells (RBCs)

- Also known as erythrocytes
- Do not have a nucleus and cannot reproduce (average lifespan about 120 days)
- Transport hemoglobin (each RBC has about 280 million hemoglobin molecules)

Erythropoiesis **Erythropoiesis** is the formation of erythrocytes. This process takes place mainly in the bone marrow of the sternum, ribs, vertebral processes, and skull bones in adults. The erythrocyte starts as a stem cell (hemocytoblast), and over 2 million new RBCs must be produced every second.

Oxygen levels regulate the rate of erythrocyte production as follows:

- Hypoxia (lower-than-normal oxygen levels) is detected by cells in the kidneys.
- Kidney cells release the hormone erythropoietin into the blood.
- Erythropoietin stimulates erythropoiesis in the bone marrow.

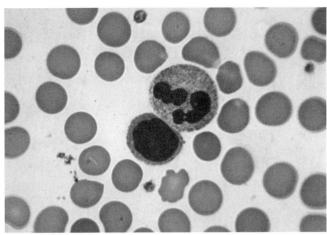

Figure 14-1 The components of blood include red blood cells, white blood cells, platelets, and plasma.

Hemoglobin

- <u>Hemoglobin</u> is an iron-based protein in RBCs that binds with oxygen and transports it to body cells. It is called *oxyhemoglobin* when it is bound with oxygen molecules. The combination of oxygen and hemoglobin gives blood its red color. Each molecule of hemoglobin can carry four molecules of oxygen.

White Blood Cells (WBCs)

- Also known as leukocytes
- Have nuclei and contain no hemoglobin
- Typical concentration in the blood is 4,500 to 11,000 per cubic millimeter
- There are two types of WBCs:
  - Granular WBCs, which include <u>neutrophils</u> (50%–70%), <u>eosinophils</u> (1%–4%), and <u>basophils</u> (less than 1%)
  - Agranular (or nongranular) WBCs, which include <u>lymphocytes</u> (25%–40%) and <u>monocytes</u> (2%–8%)

Granular White Blood Cells

- Contain lobed nuclei
- Produced in the bone marrow
- Have numerous granules in the cytoplasm
- Three types of granular WBCs:
  - Neutrophils
    - Most abundant type of WBC
    - Very mobile and quickly localize at areas of infection
    - Perform <u>phagocytosis</u> (eating or engulfing a foreign substance to destroy it)
  - Eosinophils
    - Develop and mature in bone marrow
    - Assist in fighting infections and parasites
  - Basophils
    - Least common type of WBC
    - Synthesize and store histamine (substance released during inflammation) and heparin (an anticoagulant)
    - Current studies in mice indicate that basophils may control the activities of T cells and mediate the scale of the secondary immune response

Agranular White Blood Cells

- Nucleus is round, with no granules in the cytoplasm
- Produced in lymph nodes

- Monocytes
  - Perform phagocytosis in tissues, where they are known as macrophages
  - Present antigens to T lymphocytes to develop immunity
- Lymphocytes
  - Major function is immunity.
  - There are many different forms of lymphocytes, all with different functions.
  - B lymphocytes produce plasma cells, which form antibodies to antigens (humoral immune response); T lymphocytes produce suppressor cells, helper cells, and cytotoxic killer cells.

Platelets

- Also known as thrombocytes
- Formed in the bone marrow from cells called megakaryocytes
- Responsible for hemostasis (the body's natural blood-clotting ability)
- Contain no nucleus
- Can secrete a variety of substances
- Have the ability to contract because they contain actin and myosin
- Normal concentration in the blood is about 250,000 per cubic millimeter
- Removed from the blood by macrophages in the spleen and liver
- Are attracted to damaged areas of blood vessels
- Accumulate at the damaged area and form a clot to stop bleeding

Plasma

Plasma is composed largely of water (92%), which transports heat as well as the following materials:

- Proteins produced by the liver
  - Albumins
    - 60%–80% of plasma proteins; most important in maintenance of osmotic balance
  - Globulins
    - Alpha and beta (transport materials through the blood; have some clotting factors)
    - Gamma globulins (immunoglobulins, or antibodies, produced by lymphocytes)
  - Fibrinogen
    - Important in clotting
- Inorganic constituents (1% of plasma)
  - Sodium, chloride, potassium, and calcium
- Nutrients
  - Glucose, amino acids, lipids, and vitamins
- Waste products
  - Include nitrogenous wastes such as urea
- Dissolved gases
  - Oxygen and carbon dioxide
- Hormones

Hemostasis

Hemostasis is the process by which bleeding is stopped. This involves changing the blood from a liquid form to a solid form. There are three steps in the clotting process.

1. Vasoconstriction of the damaged blood vessel: Contraction of the smooth muscle in the wall of the vessel causes vasospasms. These spasms reduce blood flow but do not stop blood loss.
2. A platelet plug is formed at the site. When the platelets are exposed to collagen, a protein in the connective tissue just outside the blood vessel, the platelets release adenosine diphosphate and thromboxane, which cause the surfaces of nearby platelets to become sticky, accumulate, and plug the damaged site.

3. Clotting or coagulation occurs when the circulating protein fibrinogen is converted to threads of fibrin during the **coagulation cascade**. Fibrinogen is converted to fibrin during the coagulation cascade, where a series of proteins (clotting factors I–XIII) interact.

Bleeding Disorders

Hemophilia is an inherited disorder in which the blood does not clot normally. Although it is rare for women to have either hemophilia A (factor VIII deficiency) or hemophilia B (factor IX deficiency), which are both sex-linked disorders, women can be symptomatic carriers and have bleeding episodes that are just as severe as those with "true" hemophilia. Thrombocytopenia is characterized by an abnormally low platelet count. In most cases, thrombocytopenia is idiopathic; in others, it occurs as the result of an autoimmune disease.

Blood Typing

Blood type is determined by the presence of antigens, or proteins that can stimulate an immune response. The main blood groups are the ABO and Rh groups, but about 30 lesser groups are known. These lesser known groups can also lead to a transfusion reaction.

ABO System

The process of blood transfusion relies primarily on the ABO system of classifying blood types to ensure compatibility. This system is based on the presence or absence of the antigens A and B on the surface of the RBCs. Blood containing RBCs with type A antigen has antibodies against type B. If a person with type A blood receives a transfusion of type B blood, a transfusion reaction results.

Type O blood is the most common blood type, followed by type A, type B, and the least common type, AB. Type O is called the "universal donor" blood type because it can be given to people with any of the other blood types. People with type AB ("universal recipient") can receive any of the other types.

Antibodies
- Produced even if blood antigen is not present
- Produced because common intestinal bacteria have A- and B-like antigens (some antigen must be present)
- Produced by about 6 months of age

Table 14-1 lists the corresponding antigen and antibody for each blood type.

Table 14-1 Blood Types

Blood Type	Antigen	Antibody
A	A	Anti-B
B	B	Anti-A
AB	A and B	Neither
O	Neither	Both anti-A and anti-B

Rh System

A secondary antigen on RBCs is the Rh antigen, or Rh factor.
- **Rh positive:** Rh antigen present on RBCs (and no antibodies)
- **Rh negative:** No Rh antigen, and antibodies will be produced if exposure occurs

The blood type of a person with A and Rh antigens is A positive (A+); without the RH antigen, it would be A negative (A–).

Erythroblastosis fetalis, also called Rh disease, may occur when an Rh-negative mother and Rh-positive father have an Rh-positive child. Rh disease occurs when the mother's antibodies to Rh factor attack the fetus' Rh+ red cells. The disease does not affect the mother's first child. During the first childbirth, some of the fetus' blood enters the mother's circulation and she develops antibodies to the Rh factor (active immunity). During subsequent pregnancies, those antibodies attack the fetus' blood, causing Rh disease. RhoGAM is given to the Rh⁻ mother immediately after childbirth. RhoGAM contains antibodies to Rh factor. By binding with fetal Rh antigen in the mother's system, RhoGAM prevents the formation of active immunity and prevents Rh disease in subsequent pregnancies.

The Immune System

Immunity is the body's ability to resist or eliminate potentially harmful foreign materials or abnormal cells. Responsible for combating infection, the **immune system's** primary component is WBCs. Its activities include:

- Defense against invading pathogens (viruses and bacteria)
- Removal of worn-out cells (eg, old RBCs) and tissue debris (eg, from injury or disease)
- Identification and destruction of abnormal or mutant cells (primary defense against cancer)
- Rejection of "foreign" cells (eg, organ transplant)
- Inappropriate responses: allergy (response to normally harmless substances), autoimmune diseases

Major Targets of Body Defense System

- **Bacteria** cause tissue damage and disease by releasing enzymes or toxins that physically injure or functionally disrupt affected cells and organs.
- **Viruses** can reproduce only in host cells. They cause cellular damage or death by:
  - Destroying essential cellular components
  - Producing substances toxic to the cell
  - Mutating normal cells into cancer cells
  - Inducing destruction of cells because infected cells are no longer recognized as "normal-self" cells

The Immune Response

The first time an antigen is encountered in the body, it elicits a *nonspecific immune response*. Defense mechanisms include inflammation, **interferon**, natural killer cells, and the complement system.

If the body encounters the same antigen again, the immune system "remembers" it and a *specific immune response* occurs. Two classes of specific immune response are humoral immunity and cell-mediated immunity.

Nonspecific Immune Response
Inflammation
Inflammation is a response to tissue injury. Its function is to destroy invaders and prepare the affected area for healing and repair:

- Release of histamine by mast cells (plus chemotaxins by damaged cells)
- Arterial vasodilation and increased capillary permeability
- Increased blood flow to tissue and accumulation of fluid
- Increased number of phagocytes and more clotting factors into surrounding tissues
- "Walling off" of inflamed area

The causes of inflammation include:

- Microbial infections (eg, bacteria)
- Physical agents (burns, trauma, etc.)
- Insufficient blood flow, causing tissue necrosis

The signs and symptoms of inflammation are as follows:

- **Pain:** Caused by tissue stretching and distortion from the pus and edema at the site
- **Redness:** Inflamed tissue resulting from vessel dilation within the damaged area
- **Swelling:** Results from edema (accumulation of fluid in the extravascular space)
- **Heat:** Caused by increased blood flow to the area as a result of vascular dilation

Interferon

Interferon is a family of similar proteins that interfere with the replication of the same or unrelated viruses in other host cells. Its mechanism of action is as follows:

1. A virus enters a cell.
2. The cell releases interferon.
3. Interferon binds with receptors on uninvaded cells.
4. The uninvaded cells produce enzymes capable of breaking down viral mRNA.
5. The virus enters previously uninvaded cells (now with interferon).
6. Virus-blocking enzymes are activated.
7. The virus is unable to multiply in the newly invaded cells.

Natural Killer Cells

Natural killer cells are an important first line of defense against newly arising malignant cells and cells infected with viruses. They form a distinct group of lymphocytes with no immunologic memory. Their specific function is to kill infected and cancerous cells by lysing their membranes on first exposure. Their mode of action is similar to that of cytotoxic T cells (but the latter can attack only cells to which they have been previously exposed).

The Complement System

The **complement system**, also known as the complement cascade system, is activated by invading organisms (it complements the action of antibodies). Complement becomes toxic to invading organisms once activated. Antibodies that bind to a foreign cell also bind to complement, which then becomes activated. Complement consists of 11 plasma proteins produced by the liver. Each protein has a specialized job acting on the next molecule in line.

The mechanisms of the complement system are as follows:

- Some complement proteins bind to channel proteins in the membrane of an invading cell. This results in an influx of water, which causes lysis (or bursting) of the invading cell.
- **Chemotaxins** are released and attract more WBCs to the area of inflammation.
- **Opsonins** bind with microbes, thereby enhancing their phagocytosis.
- Vasodilation and increased vascular permeability increase blood flow to the invaded area.
- Stimulation causes release of histamine from mast cells, which enhances vascular changes characteristic of inflammation.
- **Kinins** reinforce vascular changes induced by histamine and act as powerful chemotaxins.

Specific Immune Response

A specific immune response occurs if there has been a prior exposure to the specific antigen. The two classes of specific immune response are:

- **Humoral immunity:** Production of antibodies by B lymphocytes (B cells)
- **Cell-mediated immunity:** Activated by T lymphocytes (T cells)

Lymphocytes originate as stem cells in the bone marrow. Some migrate to the thymus and develop into T cells; others remain in the bone marrow and develop into B cells. Both B and T cells then migrate to lymphoid tissue. B cells are most effective against bacteria, their toxins, and a few viruses, whereas T cells recognize and destroy body cells such as viral and cancer cells. Each B and T cell has receptors on its surface for binding with a particular antigen.

Humoral or Antibody-Mediated Immunity

B cells bind with an antigen and differentiate into plasma cells and memory cells.

- Plasma cells begin to produce IgG antibodies (up to 2,000 per second). The **primary response** occurs several days after exposure to an antigen; peak antibody production may occur a week or two after exposure.
- Memory cells remain dormant until reexposure to the same antigen. The **secondary response** is rapid, so infection is typically prevented. They form the basis for long-term immunity.

Figure 14-2 illustrates the mechanics of the primary and secondary response.

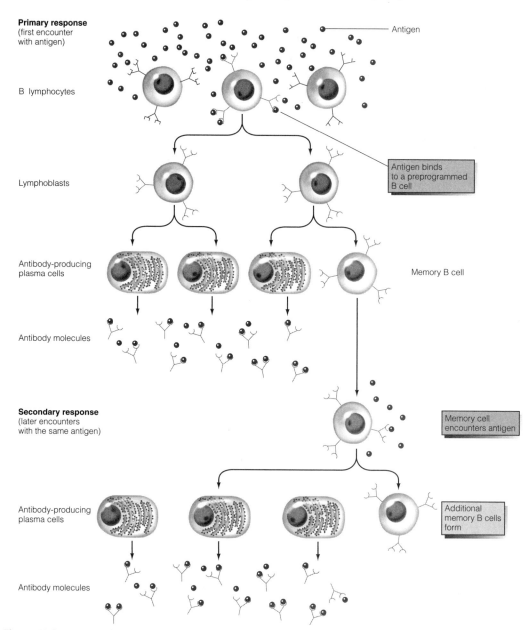

Figure 14-2 Humoral immunity: primary and secondary responses.

Antibodies Antibodies are grouped into five subclasses:

- **IgG:** Most abundant antibody; produced in large numbers. Remembers an antigen and recognizes any repeated exposures.
- **IgM:** Cell surface receptor for antigen attachment; secreted early in an immune response.
- **IgE:** Mediator for common allergic responses (hay fever, asthma, and hives). People with allergies generally have excess amounts of IgE.
- **IgA:** Found in secretions of digestive, respiratory, urinary, and reproductive systems, as well as in breast milk and in tears.
- **IgD:** Found on the surface of many B cells; acts as an antigen receptor.

Antibodies protect by one of the following actions:

- Neutralization
  - Binding with bacterial toxins to prevent them from harming susceptible cells; may also bind with viruses and prevent them from entering body cells
- Agglutination
  - The clumping of cells such as bacteria or RBCs in the presence of an antibody
- Triggering other defense systems:
  - Complement system
  - Phagocytosis
  - Killer cells

Active Immunity Versus Passive Immunity Active, or natural, immunity is the production of antibodies resulting from exposure to an antigen. Passive immunity is acquired by receiving antibodies via maternal circulation or via injection with antibodies that have been created outside the body. An example of passive immunity is the prevention of hepatitis A or B by giving injections of immunoglobulin to people who have been exposed to hepatitis, but before the disease occurs. Another example is immunity that newborns receive from the antibodies in their mother's milk. Generally, passive immunity lasts from days to months. Active immunity is humoral immunity and lasts for years or an entire lifetime.

Cell-Mediated Immunity

Cell-mediated immunity is provided by T cells, which attack antigens directly rather than producing antibodies. These cells defend against invaders inside the cells that are unreachable by the complement system or antibodies. They are activated by a foreign antigen only when present on the surface of a cell that also has self-antigens.

There are three types of T cells:

- **Helper T cells:** Enhance development of B cells into antibody-secreting cells and enhance activity of cytotoxic and suppressor T cells
  - **B cell growth factor:** Enhances antibody-secreting ability of B cells
  - **Interleukin 2:** Enhances activity of cytotoxic T cells, suppressor T cells, and other helper T cells
  - **Chemotaxins:** Attract neutrophils and macrophages
  - **Macrophage:** Migration-inhibiting factor inhibits migration and creates "angry macrophages"
- **Regulatory T cells:** Suppress B-cell antibody production and cytotoxic and helper T-cell activity; effects are primarily the result of chemicals called *cytokines* (or *lymphokines*)
  - Limit responses of other cells (B and T cells)
  - Make immune response self-limiting
  - Prevent excessive immune response, which might be detrimental to the body
  - May also prevent immune system from attacking the body's own cells and tissues (immune tolerance)

- **Cytotoxic (killer) T cells:** Destroy host cells bearing foreign antigen (eg, host cells invaded by viruses and cancer cells)

<u>Autoimmunity</u> is an abnormal immune response in which the immune system attacks the body itself. It may arise in several ways, including:

- Reduction in suppressor T-cell activity
- Normal self-antigens modified by drugs, environmental chemicals, viruses, or mutations
- Exposure to antigens very similar to self-antigens

Sickle Cell Disease

Pathophysiology

Sickle cell disease is an inherited blood disorder that affects RBCs in blacks as well as people of Mediterranean descent. It is less common among whites. Patients with sickle cell disease have hemoglobin S, an abnormal type of hemoglobin. RBCs become sickle-shaped and have difficulty passing through small blood vessels, causing blockage to that part of the body (**Figure 14-3**).

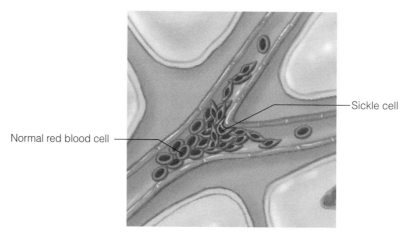

Normal red blood cell — — Sickle cell

Figure 14-3 Normal red blood cells and sickle cells.

The patient experiences what is called a *sickle cell crisis* or *pain crisis*. The lack of circulation to the affected body parts damages tissues and cells; without intervention, the tissues eventually die. Oxygen is critical to restoring sickle cells to normal RBCs, which are soft and round and can squeeze through tiny blood vessels. Normally, RBCs live for about 120 days before being replaced. However, in patients with sickle cell disease, the RBCs live about 16 days.

Causes of sickle cell crisis include:

- Infection
- Hypoxia (such as at high altitude)
- Dehydration
- Cold water
- Stress
- Alcohol intoxication

Signs and Symptoms

- Anemia
- Jaundice
- Gallstones (if gallbladder has not been removed)
- Pain crisis in joints, chest, abdomen
- Stroke

- Priapism
- Abdominal pain
  - Splenic sequestration (occurs when large amounts of RBCs are trapped in the spleen, resulting in sudden worsening of anemia and shock; this condition usually occurs in the first few years of life)
- Acute chest syndrome (pneumonia symptoms due to occlusion of pulmonary capillaries)
- Swollen hands and feet

Assessment

- Initial/primary assessment
  - Ensure body substance isolation (BSI).
  - Monitor patient's level of consciousness (LOC).
  - Manage ABCs (airway, breathing, circulation).
  - Transport considerations: Transport the patient in a position of comfort.
  - Treat life-threatening illness/injuries.
- Focused history and physical exam/secondary assessment
  - Obtain SAMPLE history and chief complaint (OPQRST).

Management

- Administer oxygen at 15 L/min via nonrebreathing mask.
- Monitor vital signs.
- Establish intravenous (IV) line.
- Perform cardiac monitoring.

Table 14-2 summarizes the treatment for sickle cell disease.

Table 14-2 Treatment for Sickle Cell Disease

Treatment	Purpose	Adult Dose	Pediatric Dose
Morphine	Pain management	SIVP: 2-5 mg	SIVP: 0.1 mg/kg
Fentanyl	Pain management	SIVP: 0.5-1.0 µg/kg	SIVP: 0.25-0.5 µg/kg
Demerol	Pain management	IV: 25 mg IV or IM: 50-100 mg	SIVP or IM: 1-2 mg/kg
Ketorolac	Pain management, anti-inflammatory	IV/IM: 30 mg	IV/IM: 15 mg
Normal saline	Dilutant	Infusion: 250-mL bolus	Infusion: 20 mL/kg
Oxygen	Increases oxygen saturation to prevent sickling	15 L/min via nonrebreathing mask	15 L/min via nonrebreathing mask
SIVP, slow intravenous push; IV, intravenous; IM, intramuscular.			

Leukemia

Pathophysiology

Leukemia is cancer of the blood or bone marrow, characterized by abnormal production of blood cells, usually WBCs. The most common types of leukemia are:

- Acute lymphocytic leukemia
- Acute myelogenous leukemia
- Chronic lymphocytic leukemia
- Chronic myelogenous leukemia
- Hairy cell leukemia

Treatments such as radiation therapy, chemotherapy, and bone marrow transplants have resulted in extended remission of certain types of leukemias.

Signs and Symptoms

- Moderate to severe anemia
- Jaundice
- Gallstones (if gallbladder has not been removed)
- Pain
- Abdominal pain
- Weakness
- Pallor
- Anorexia

Assessment

- Initial/primary assessment
  - Ensure BSI.
  - Monitor patient's LOC.
  - Manage ABCs.
  - Transport considerations: Transport the patient in a position of comfort.
  - Treat life-threatening illness/injuries.
- Focused history and physical exam/secondary assessment
  - Obtain SAMPLE history and chief complaint (OPQRST).

Management

- Administer oxygen at 15 L/min via nonrebreathing mask.
- Monitor vital signs.
- Establish IV.
- Perform cardiac monitoring.
- Administer analgesics if indicated.

Anemia

Pathophysiology

Anemia is an abnormally low number of RBCs or inadequate hemoglobin within the RBCs. Anemia, typically defined as having a hematocrit below 40% in men and 36% in women, is one of the most common diseases affecting the RBCs. Anemia is actually not itself a disease, but rather a sign of an underlying disease that destroys the RBCs or prevents the manufacturing of RBCs or hemoglobin. Anemia may also be defined as a hemoglobin level less than 12 in women and less than 14 in men.

Signs and Symptoms

- Dyspnea
- Fatigue
- Syncope
- Headache
- Dizziness
- Pallor
- Tachycardia

Assessment

- Initial/primary assessment
  - Ensure BSI.
  - Monitor patient's LOC.
  - Manage ABCs.

– Transport considerations: Transport the patient in a position of comfort.
– Treat life-threatening illness/injuries.
- Focused history and physical exam/secondary assessment
  – Obtain SAMPLE history and chief complaint (OPQRST).

Management

- Administer oxygen at 15 L/min via nonrebreathing mask.
- Monitor vital signs.
- Establish IV; administer fluid bolus if signs of dehydration are present.
- Perform cardiac monitoring.

Polycythemia

Pathophysiology

Polycythemia is defined as an abnormally high hematocrit due to an excess production of RBCs. Although a relatively rare disorder, it typically occurs in patients older than 60 years of age.

Signs and Symptoms

- Bleeding abnormalities
- Dizziness
- Itching
- Headache
- Congestive heart failure

Assessment

- Initial/primary assessment
  – Ensure BSI.
  – Monitor patient's LOC.
  – Manage ABCs.
  – Transport considerations: Transport the patient in a position of comfort.
  – Treat life-threatening illness/injuries.
- Focused history and physical exam/secondary assessment
  – Obtain SAMPLE history and chief complaint (OPQRST).

Management

- Administer oxygen at 15 L/min via nonrebreathing mask.
- Monitor vital signs.
- Establish IV.
- Perform cardiac monitoring.

Disseminated Intravascular Coagulation

Pathophysiology

Disseminated intravascular coagulation is a coagulation disorder caused by the systemic activation of the coagulation cascade. This disorder leads to the formation of small blood clots inside the blood vessels throughout the body. As the small clots consume all the available coagulation proteins and platelets, normal coagulation is disrupted and abnormal bleeding occurs from the skin, the digestive tract, the respiratory tract, and wounds. The small clots also disrupt normal blood flow to organs (such as the kidneys), which may malfunction as a result. This disorder most commonly results from sepsis, hypotension, tissue injury, cancer, and transfusion reactions.

Signs and Symptoms

- Bleeding abnormalities
- Purpuric rash
- Decreased LOC
- Shock

Assessment

- Initial/primary assessment
  - Ensure BSI.
  - Monitor patient's LOC.
  - Manage ABCs.
  - Transport considerations: Transport the patient in a position of comfort.
  - Treat life-threatening illness/injuries.
- Focused history and physical exam/secondary assessment
  - Obtain SAMPLE history and chief complaint (OPQRST).

Management

- Administer oxygen at 15 L/min via nonrebreathing mask.
- Monitor vital signs.
- Establish IV; administer fluid boluses if patient is hypotensive.
- Perform cardiac monitoring.

Vital Vocabulary

autoimmunity The production of antibodies or T cells that work against the tissues of a person's own body, producing autoimmune disease.

bacteria Small organisms that can grow and reproduce outside the human cell in the presence of the proper temperature and nutrients, and that cause disease by invading and multiplying in the tissues of the host.

basophils White blood cells that work to produce chemical mediators during an immune response.

cell-mediated immunity Immune process by which T-cell lymphocytes recognize antigens and then secrete cytokines (specifically, lymphokines) that attract other cells or stimulate the production of cytotoxic cells that kill the infected cells.

chemotaxins Components of the activated complement system that attract leukocytes from circulation to help fight infections.

coagulation cascade A series of biochemical activities involving clotting factors that result in the formation of the fibrin clot.

complement system A group of plasma proteins whose function is to do one of three things: attract leukocytes to sites of inflammation, activate leukocytes, and directly destroy cells.

eosinophils Cells that make up approximately 1% to 3% of the leukocytes; they play a major role in allergic reactions and bronchoconstriction in an asthma attack.

erythrocytes Red blood cells.

erythropoiesis The formation of erythrocytes, taking place mainly in the marrow of the sternum, ribs, vertebral processes, and skull bones in adults.

hemoglobin An iron-containing protein within red blood cells that has the ability to combine with oxygen.

hemophilia A bleeding disorder that is primarily hereditary, in which clotting does not occur or occurs insufficiently.

hemostasis The stoppage of bleeding.

humoral immunity The use of antibodies dissolved in the plasma and lymph to destroy foreign substances.

immune system The body system that includes all of the structures and processes designed to mount a defense against foreign substances and disease-causing agents.

immunity The body's ability to protect itself from acquiring a disease.

inflammation A reaction by tissues of the body to irritation or injury, characterized by pain, swelling, redness, and heat.

interferon Protein produced by cells in response to viral invasion. Interferon is released into the bloodstream or intercellular fluid to induce healthy cells to manufacture an enzyme that counters the infection.

kinins A group of polypeptides that mediate inflammatory responses by stimulating visceral smooth muscle and relaxing vascular smooth muscle to produce vasodilation.

leukocytes White blood cells.

lymphocytes The white blood cells responsible for a large part of the body's immune protection.

monocytes Mononuclear phagocytic white blood cells derived from myeloid stem cells. They circulate in the bloodstream for about 24 hours and then move into tissues to mature into macrophages.

natural killer cells A distinct group of lymphocytes with no immunologic memory. Their specific function is to kill infected and cancerous cells by lysing their membranes on first exposure.

neutrophils Cells that make up approximately 55% to 70% of the leukocytes responsible in large part for the body's protection against infection. They are readily attracted by foreign antigens and destroy them by phagocytosis.

opsonins Antibodies that cause bacteria and other foreign cells to become more susceptible to phagocytosis.

phagocytosis Process in which one cell eats or engulfs a foreign substance to destroy it.

primary response The first encounter with the foreign substance to begin the immune response.

secondary response The body's reaction when it is exposed to an antigen for which it already has antibodies, in which it responds by killing the invading substance.

thrombocytes Platelets.

thrombocytopenia Reduction in the number of platelets.

viruses Small organisms that can only multiply inside a host, such as a human, and cause disease.

CHAPTER
15

Environmental Emergencies

Environmental emergencies occur when a medical condition is caused or exacerbated by environmental factors, such as weather, temperature, terrain, or atmospheric pressure, to a point at which the body is no longer able to compensate. For example, conditions such as heat exposure, cold exposure, high altitudes, diving, and water emergencies can cause an environmental emergency.

Predisposing risk factors include the following:

- Age
- Health: Medical conditions and medications
- Dehydration
- Fatigue
- Obesity
- Physical activity

Tip

Medications can affect the body temperature by decreasing thirst and sweating and increasing the production of heat.

Temperature Regulatory Mechanisms

The body has three types of heat regulatory mechanisms.

1. The hypothalamus gland is responsible for temperature regulation. Thermoreceptors in the body detect the amount of heat loss and heat gain and send signals to the hypothalamus, which in turn responds with appropriate efferent signals to decrease heat loss and increase heat production, or increase heat loss and decrease heat production. Peripheral thermoreceptors are located in the skin and mucous membranes; central thermoreceptors are located in the abdomen and along the spinal cord.
2. The control of blood flow is another way the body regulates temperature. If the body gets too hot, it will attempt to dissipate heat through the skin by dilating some blood vessels and constricting others to shunt blood to the periphery. When the body gets too cold, it will shunt warm blood away from the peripheral arteries to the core arteries to supply the vital organs.
3. The body will adjust its metabolic rate to maintain the core body temperature by generating heat. The basal metabolic rate, also called the resting metabolic rate, is the amount of energy expended in a resting state.

Mechanisms of Heat Gain and Loss

Heat Gain
- Heat generation, or **thermogenesis**, is a result of muscular activity (ie, exercise, shivering) and metabolic reactions.
- Ambient air temperature determines the rate at which body heat can be exchanged in regulatory processes to maintain normal body temperature.

General Heat Loss
- Perspiration/evaporation (not effective when humidity is greater than 75%)
- Increased respiratory rate to aid in evaporation
- Vasodilation: Heat is lost through the skin
- Increase in cardiac output to aid vasodilation

Tip

Normal body temperature is 37°C (98.6°F).

<u>Radiation</u> is the transmission of heat through space. Factors important in radiant heat loss are the surface area and the temperature gradient.

<u>Convection</u> refers to the loss of heat that takes place when moving air picks up heat and carries it away (ie, air moving across the body surface picks up heat and carries it away).

<u>Evaporation</u> occurs when water is converted from a liquid to a gas (eg, perspiration, sweating, and even respiration).

<u>Conduction</u> occurs through direct contact between objects as the molecular transference of heat energy. Because water is denser than air, it conducts heat away from the body quicker. Therefore, keep the patient dry.

<u>Respiration</u> is actually a combination of radiation, convection, and evaporation. Heat is expelled during normal breathing activity and replaced with cool oxygen, and the moisture created is evaporated in the lungs.

Local Cold Injuries

Frostbite or Frostnip

Pathophysiology

Frostbite and frostnip are conditions that occur more commonly in the fingers, toes, ears, nose, and face after exposure to very cold temperatures. They are caused by the formation of ice crystals within tissues. In frostbite, these crystals damage the blood vessels and tissue, resulting in tissue necrosis. In frostnip, no tissue damage occurs if the skin is warmed soon and the ice crystals melt rapidly. Predisposing factors include poor peripheral circulation and history of cold injury, which may render the tissues more susceptible to further damage from the cold.

Signs and Symptoms

- Pale, mottled skin may appear white, waxy, or yellowish; skin may also appear to be flushed, purple, or cyanotic
- Loss of feeling and sensation in the injured area
- Tingling sensation when rewarmed
- Firm or frozen feeling on palpation
- Swelling and blisters

Assessment

- Scene size-up
  - Ensure body substance isolation (BSI).
  - Assess the environment.
  - Assess risk to rescuers.
- Initial/primary assessment
  - Manage ABCs (airway, breathing, circulation).
  - Monitor patient's level of consciousness (LOC).
  - Treat life-threatening illness/injuries.
  - Transport considerations: Transport the patient in a position of comfort; prevent further injury to frozen areas
- Focused history and physical exam/secondary assessment
  - Obtain SAMPLE history and chief complaint (OPQRST).
  - Handle patient gently.
  - Do not give anything by mouth.

Management

- Establish an intravenous (IV) line of a warmed crystalloid solution, to keep open.
- Administer warm, humidified oxygen (O_2) at 15 L/min via nonrebreathing mask.

- Perform cardiac monitoring.
- Remove victim from the cold environment.
- Protect the cold extremities from further injuries.
- Remove restrictive clothing and all jewelry before swelling, if possible.
- Splint the extremity and cover the injury with a dry sterile dressing.
- Do not reexpose the area to cold environment.
- Do not break blisters.
- Do not rub or massage the area.
- Do not apply heat to or actively rewarm the area.
- Do not allow the patient to walk on the affected extremity.

Hypothermia

Pathophysiology

Hypothermia is a condition in which the core or internal body temperature is less than 35°C (95°F) as a result of either decreased heat production or increased heat loss from the body. Hypothermia depresses the central nervous system. Exposure to cold results in peripheral vasoconstriction, decreased heart rate, and shunting of the blood to the core. This reduces the flow of oxygenated blood to vital organs. Shivering, produced by rapid contractions of the muscles, is the body's way of generating heat and increasing the metabolic rate.

Signs and Symptoms

Signs and symptoms differ according to body temperature, as follows:

- 32.2° to 35°C (90° to 95°F)—mild hypothermia
    - Extreme cold
    - Normal to slightly elevated blood pressure
    - Increased heart rate
    - Increased respiratory rate
    - Pupils equal and reactive
    - Shivering and vasoconstriction
    - Mild alteration of LOC
    - Loss of fine motor control
    - Lack of coordination
- 27.8° to 32.2°C (82° to 90°F)—moderate hypothermia
    - Tense muscles
    - Muscular rigidity and stiffness
    - Confusion
    - Decreased respiratory rate
    - Slow, irregular, and barely palpable pulse
    - Lethargy
    - Blood pressure may be low and difficult to detect
    - Glassy stare with marked change in mental status and responsiveness
    - Skin pale and cyanotic, stiff and hard
    - Pupils may be sluggish
- Less than 27.8°C (82°F)—severe hypothermia
    - Patient usually unresponsive
    - Deep coma
    - Rigidity of pupils, or pupils fixed and dilated

Assessment

- Scene size-up
    - Ensure BSI.
    - Maintain horizontal position.

Tip

Remember: When assessing a person with a potential hypothermic condition, the person is not dead until he or she is warm and dead!

Tip

The patient may appear to be pulseless and apneic. Check for pulse for a minimum of 30 to 45 seconds.

- Initial/primary assessment
  - Monitor patient's LOC.
  - Manage ABCs.
  - Treat life-threatening illness/injuries.
  - Transport considerations: Transport the patient in a position of comfort.
- Focused history and physical exam/secondary assessment
  - Obtain SAMPLE history and chief complaint (OPQRST).

Management
- Administer warm, humidified oxygen at 15 L/min via nonrebreathing mask.
- Establish IV with warm fluids; use a large-bore macro drip with normal saline or lactated Ringer's solution, infusing a 125- to 250-mL bolus bilaterally.
- Handle patient gently (rough handling can cause cardiac dysrhythmia).
- Perform cardiopulmonary resuscitation, if patient is in cardiopulmonary arrest.
- Defibrillate if indicated (maximum: three shocks).
- Attempt, confirm, and secure airway.
- Ventilate with warm, humidified oxygen.
- Turn up heat in the patient compartment of the unit.
- Remove wet clothes and maintain the patient in a warm environment.
- Do not rewarm the patient's extremities. Rewarming extremities will cause vasodilation, resulting in a bolus of cold blood flowing into the central circulation.
- Passive rewarming: Mild hypothermia is reversed with passive rewarming. This technique relies on the patient's own metabolism to rewarm the body. Once wet clothing is removed and the skin is dried, the patient is covered with blankets and placed in a warm room in an attempt to increase the core temperature. Monitor temperature via rectal thermometer, if available.
- Active rewarming: Add heat to the patient's body using warmed oxygen and heat pads (39° to 40°C, or 102° to 104°F) placed at the groin, armpits, neck, and head. Active rewarming should be used in the following situations:
  - Cardiovascular collapse or instability
  - Patient core temperature of less than 32.2°C (90°F)
  - Insufficient rewarming with passive methods
  - Adrenal insufficiency, hypopituitarism, hypothyroidism
  - Severe metabolic acidosis (lactic acidosis, ketoacidosis)
  - Peripheral vasodilation (due to drugs, neurologic disease, or spinal cord transection)
  - Comorbid conditions causing impaired thermoregulation
  - Comorbid conditions resulting in increased heat loss
  - Patient is an infant
- Monitor for cardiac arrhythmias.

Heat-Related Illnesses

The body's cooling system allows heat to escape through conduction, convection, evaporation, radiation, and respiration. If these mechanisms are impaired, the body may not be able to cool itself, leaving the person at risk for heat-related illness. If not treated promptly, death may result.

Heat Cramps
Pathophysiology
- Heat cramps are caused by dehydration and overexertion in a warm environment and are one of the most common forms of heat-related injury.

Signs and Symptoms
- Fluid loss; depletion of vital electrolytes such as calcium and sodium
- Abdominal/extremity cramping
- Weakness
- Nausea
- Muscle fatigue
- Muscle twitch/spasm
- Diaphoresis
- Tachycardia
- Hypotension
- Vomiting

Assessment
- Scene size-up
  - Ensure BSI.
- Initial/primary assessment
  - Remove patient from warm environment.
  - Manage ABCs.
  - Monitor patient's LOC.
  - Treat life-threatening illness/injuries.
  - Transport considerations: Transport the patient in a position of comfort.
- Focused history and physical exam/secondary assessment
  - Obtain SAMPLE history and chief complaint (OPQRST).

Management
- Administer oxygen at 15 L/min via nonrebreathing mask.
- Establish an IV of a crystalloid solution, to keep open.
- Give patient cool liquid to sip; do not give solid foods.
- Have suction available if needed.
- Gently stretch the cramped muscle.

Heat Exhaustion

Pathophysiology
Heat exhaustion is a more severe form of fluid loss, usually following exertion in hot, humid weather. Those individuals more susceptible to heat exhaustion are children, the elderly, and anyone taking diuretics or suffering from a prolonged illness with vomiting, diarrhea, thirst, and fever.

Signs and Symptoms
- Extreme thirst
- Weakness
- Headaches
- Fatigue
- Pale skin
- Profuse sweating
- Diaphoresis
- Tachycardia
- Hypotension
- Vomiting

Assessment
- Scene size-up
  - Ensure BSI.

- Initial/primary assessment
  - Remove patient from warm environment.
  - Manage ABCs.
  - Monitor patient's LOC.
  - Treat life-threatening illness/injuries.
  - Transport considerations: Transport the patient in a position of comfort.
- Focused history and physical exam/secondary assessment
  - Obtain SAMPLE history and chief complaint (OPQRST).

Management
- Establish an IV of a crystalloid solution, to keep open.
- Administer oxygen at 15 L/min via nonrebreathing mask.
- Perform cardiac monitoring.
- Have suction available, if needed.

Heatstroke
Pathophysiology
Heatstroke is a life-threatening condition caused by the body's failure to cool itself as a result of a severe disturbance in the body's thermoregulation mechanism.

Signs and Symptoms
- Markedly elevated temperature
- Nausea
- Shortness of breath
- Anxiety
- Fatigue
- Altered LOC
- Absence of sweating
- Reddened skin that feels hot and dry
- Signs of shock—decompensated (late sign)
- Tachycardia
- Tachypnea
- Vomiting
- Collapse

Assessment
- Scene size-up
  - Ensure BSI.
- Initial/primary assessment
  - Remove patient from warm environment.
  - Manage ABCs.
  - Monitor patient's LOC.
  - Treat life-threatening illness/injuries.
  - Transport considerations: Transport the patient in a position of comfort.
- Focused history and physical exam/secondary assessment
  - Obtain SAMPLE history and chief complaint (OPQRST).

Management
- Administer oxygen at 15 L/min via nonrebreathing mask.
- Remove patient's clothing.
- Spray the patient with tepid water while fanning.
- Apply ice packs to axillary region, groin, and neck.
- Start an IV line, give normal saline, and check the blood glucose level. Remember to be careful with fluids; watch for pulmonary edema.
- Be prepared to treat seizures.

- Perform cardiac monitoring.
- Have suction available, if needed.

Bites and Stings

Bites and stings from any insect or animal can cause intense pain, swelling, and/or death. Even the human bite can be injurious because the mouth carries a wide variety of potentially dangerous bacteria.

Tip

How to remember which coral snakes found in the United States are poisonous: "Red on yellow will kill a fellow; red on black, venom will lack."

Bites and Stings

Pathophysiology

Arthropods with potentially harmful bites or stings include the following:

- Brown recluse spiders
- Black widow spiders
- Ticks
- Tarantulas
- Scorpions
- Bees and wasps
- Centipedes
- Ants

Signs and Symptoms

- Pain
- Swelling
- Redness
- Hives/urticaria
- Weakness
- Anxiety
- Headache
- Breathing difficulties
- Nausea/vomiting
- Diarrhea
- Anaphylactic shock

Assessment

- Scene size-up
  - Ensure BSI.
  - Ensure crew and patient safety.
- Initial/primary assessment
  - Manage ABCs.
  - Monitor patient's LOC.
  - Treat life-threatening illness/injuries.
  - Transport considerations: Transport the patient in a position of comfort.
- Focused history and physical exam/secondary assessment
  - Obtain SAMPLE history and chief complaint (OPQRST).

Management

- Bees and wasps
  - Remove the stinger by scraping with a knife, credit card, or fingernail. *Do not use tweezers*. This may squeeze the venom sac located on the stinger, causing more venom to be injected into the skin.
- Spiders
  - Black widow spider affects the nervous system, causing muscle cramps, a rigid, nontender abdomen, breathing difficulties, sweating, nausea, and vomiting.

- The brown recluse spider generally produces localized rather than systemic problems; however, local tissue damage around the bite can be severe and can lead to an ulcer and severe tissue necrosis.
- Other bites or stings
  - Treat any other bites by washing the area, and transport the patient to a hospital. In case of allergic reaction or anaphylaxis, treat accordingly.

Snakes

Four types of poisonous snakes found in the United States are as follows:

- Coral snakes
- Rattlesnakes
- Copperheads
- Water moccasins (cottonmouths)

Assessment

- Scene size-up
  - Ensure BSI.
  - Ensure crew and patient safety.
- Initial/primary assessment
  - Manage ABCs.
  - Monitor patient's LOC.
  - Treat life-threatening illness/injuries.
  - Transport considerations: Transport the patient in a position of comfort.
- Focused history and physical exam/secondary assessment
  - Obtain SAMPLE history and chief complaint (OPQRST).

Management

- Keep affected extremity below the level of the heart.
- Do not give stimulants such as caffeinated products or tobacco.
- Do not use any salves or ointments that would impede seepage of the venom.
- Do not freeze the site, wrap the limb in ice, or apply ice directly to the skin.
- *For arm or leg:* Place two constricting bands 1 to 2 fingerbreadths above and below the bite. If you have only one band on hand, place it between the bite and the heart, making sure not to place the constricting band directly over a joint.
- *For hand or foot:* Place one band above the wrist or ankle just tight enough to slow the flow of venous blood near the skin, but not so tight that it cuts arterial circulation off completely.
- Place the bands above and below the swollen area. If the swelling continues past the band, adjust it accordingly. If possible, avoid removing the band already in place and place a new band outside the area of swelling.

Drowning

Pathophysiology

<u>Drowning</u> is defined as suffocation by submersion in water or other fluids. There are several different types of drowning episodes.

- **Secondary drowning** is a recurrence of respiratory distress (usually in the form of pulmonary edema or aspiration pneumonia) after successful recovery from an immersion incident. It can occur from a few minutes to up to 4 days after the incident.
- **Near drowning** is defined as near suffocation by submersion in water or other fluids with survival (even if temporary).
- **Dry drowning** is caused by anoxia as a result of a laryngospasm, which prevents the entrance of water, as well as air, into the lungs. In a drowning incident, the victim struggles to hold his or her breath for as long as possible. However, because the

respiratory center of the brain still functions to ensure that the body is well oxygenated, the victim eventually inhales and the aspiration of water causes laryngospasms in the throat. In approximately 10% to 15% of drowning victims, the laryngospasm prevents any water from entering the lungs, hence the term *dry drowning*. In other cases, water enters both the lungs and the stomach, and vomiting and aspiration can occur.

The type of water also determines the effect drowning has on the body. Drowning in fresh water is more common than in salt water, even in coastal areas.

- **Freshwater drowning:** Fresh water is a hypotonic solution. When it enters the lungs, it washes surfactant out of the alveoli. Surfactant helps keep alveoli open and aids in air exchange. Collapse (atelectasis) of alveolar segments occurs, with a resultant shunting of blood to functional areas and hypoxia.
- **Saltwater drowning:** Salt water is hypertonic. Because of osmotic gradients, fluid is shifted from the bloodstream into the alveoli. Pulmonary edema results, with shunting and profound hypoxia.

Signs and Symptoms
- Progressive shortness of breath
- Wheezing or other adventitious sounds
- Tachycardia
- Cyanosis
- Chest pains or altered mental status
- Coma, respiratory arrest, or possible cardiac arrest

Assessment
When assessing victims of near drowning, it is important to note that they may appear asymptomatic. Victims must be assessed for the following:

- Airway obstruction
- Cardiac arrest
- Signs of heart attack
- Injuries to the head and neck
- Internal injuries
- Hypothermia
- Substance abuse

Management
- Ensure the safety of all rescue personnel.
- Suspect spinal injury if the patient was diving or if diving cannot be ruled out.
- If spinal injury is suspected, use in-line immobilization and removal from the water with a backboard.
- If there is no suspected spinal injury, place patient on his or her left side to allow water, vomitus, and secretions to drain from the upper airway.
- Resuscitate the patient if necessary.
- Establish and maintain an open airway. Suction as needed.
- Administer supplemental oxygen via nonrebreathing mask.
- In cold-water drowning consider the length of time submerged. Any pulseless, nonbreathing patient who has been submerged in cold water should be resuscitated.
- Consider hypothermia:
  – Hypothermia often accompanies near drownings.
  – It may help protect organs in cold-water near drownings.

Tip

Children survive near-drowning accidents more often than adults.

Mammalian Dive Reflex

The colder the water, the greater the chance for survival during an immersion incident. This is because of the following two factors:

1. Bradycardia is the first response to submersion. Immediately upon facial contact with cold water, the human heart rate slows down 10% to 25%.
2. Next, peripheral vasoconstriction sets in. When under high pressure induced by deep diving, capillaries in the extremities start closing off, stopping blood circulation to those areas.

Tip

A patient involved in an immersion incident of unknown etiology should be managed as a trauma patient.

Tip

Remember: When assessing and managing victims of cold-water drowning, the patient is not dead until he or she is warm!

- Always treat hypoxia first.
- Treat all near-drowning patients for hypothermia.
- If gastric distention interferes with artificial ventilation, turn the patient on his or her left side. With suction immediately available, place your hand over the epigastric area of the abdomen and apply firm pressure to relieve the distention. This procedure should only be done if the gastric distention interferes with the ability to artificially ventilate the patient effectively.
- If protocols permit, insert a nasogastric tube to facilitate gastric decompression.
- Be aware of postresuscitation complications.
  - Adult respiratory distress syndrome or renal failure often occurs after resuscitation.
  - Symptoms may not appear for 24 hours or more.
  - All near-drowning patients should be transported for evaluation.

Diving Emergencies

Pathophysiology

Diving with self-contained underwater breathing apparatus is a popular sport. Scuba diving equipment is completely carried by the diver and is not connected to the surface. Although diving emergencies are relatively uncommon (about 90 deaths are reported each year), they do occur.

Most diving emergencies are caused by ascending too rapidly from depth. As a diver descends, pressure increases and more gas dissolves in plasma and body tissues. Most of the oxygen we breathe is metabolized and used by the cells, so only a small amount actually dissolves. Nitrogen, on the other hand, is an inert gas and is not used by the body, so a larger quantity can be dissolved in the blood. As a diver ascends, this additional gas must be released. If the ascent is controlled, the gas can be released gradually through respiration. If the diver ascends too rapidly, however, the gases are released and can form bubbles in the blood, brain, muscles, and joints. Once bubbles have formed, it is difficult for the body to remove them.

> **Pressure and Gases**
>
> People live in an atmosphere of air. At sea level, air is a mixture of gases, including nitrogen (78%), oxygen (21%), and carbon dioxide, water vapor, and other trace gases (less than 1%). These elements combine to exert a pressure of about 760 mm Hg at sea level. This pressure is known as *atmospheric pressure* and varies depending on the particular point above or below sea level at which it is measured. Ascending to an altitude of 1 mile above sea level will decrease the atmospheric pressure by 17%, whereas descending 33 feet into the ocean increases this pressure by twice the amount.

Classification of Diving Emergencies

The potential for a diving emergency exists throughout all phases of a dive—on the surface, during descent, on the bottom, and during ascent. On the surface, divers may become cold or tired, become entangled in kelp, or be injured by boats in the area. On descent, the diver may experience injuries caused by the increase in pressure. For example, the diver may not be able to equilibrate the pressure in the ears or sinuses. This can cause ear pain, headaches, and dizziness. In extreme cases, the increased pressure can cause the eardrum to rupture. At the bottom, the diver may experience nitrogen narcosis or run out of breathable air. The most serious injuries can occur during ascent and include decompression illness, pulmonary overpressurization syndrome, arterial gas embolism (AGE), and nitrogen narcosis.

Decompression Sickness

Pathophysiology

Decompression sickness, or "the bends," occurs when a diver ascends too rapidly and excess gases (usually nitrogen) form bubbles in the diver's body. This occurs in the joints, tendons, spinal cord, skin, brain, and inner ear. The bubbles increase pressure in the various body parts and can occlude circulation in the smaller blood vessels.

Signs and Symptoms

- Abdominal pain (the hallmark symptom)
- Joint pain
- Fatigue
- Paresthesias (numbness, tickling, or burning sensations)
- Central nervous system disturbances
- Disorientation

Assessment

- Scene size-up
  - Ensure BSI.
- Initial/primary assessment
  - Manage ABCs.
  - Monitor patient's LOC.
  - Treat life-threatening illness/injuries.
  - Transport considerations: Transport the patient in a position of comfort.
- Focused history and physical exam/secondary assessment
  - Obtain SAMPLE history and chief complaint (OPQRST).

Management

- Administer high-flow oxygen. Patients who receive early oxygen therapy have a better outcome.
- Place patient in the supine position.
- Treat for shock.
- Initiate IV therapy.
- Transport to the emergency department, preferably one with hyperbaric capabilities.

Pulmonary Overpressurization Syndrome

Pathophysiology

Pulmonary overpressurization syndrome is the most common diving emergency and commonly occurs at shallow depths of less than 6 feet. This accident occurs when the lungs are overinflated as a result of rapid ascent. As the pressure decreases during ascent, the volume of air in the lungs increases. If the air is trapped in the lungs, the alveolar membranes can rupture, producing a pneumothorax. Air can be trapped in the lungs by breath holding, bronchospasm, or mucous plugs.

Signs and Symptoms

- Respiratory distress
- Substernal chest pain
- Diminished breath sounds
- Subcutaneous emphysema

Assessment

- Scene size-up
  - Ensure BSI.
- Initial/primary assessment
  - Manage ABCs.
  - Monitor patient's LOC.

Application of Gas Laws

Being familiar with the following gas laws will help you to understand how air pressure affects patients involved in diving accidents. The behavior of all gases is affected by three factors: the temperature of the gas, the pressure of the gas, and the volume of the gas.

- **Boyle's law:** The volume of a gas is inversely proportional to its pressure if the temperature is kept constant. This relates to the changes in the volume of a gas to changes in pressure (depth) and defines the relationship between pressure and volume in breathing gas supplies.

- **Dalton's law:** The total pressure of a mixture of gases is equal to the sum of the partial pressures of the individual gases. In a gas mixture, the portion of the total pressure contributed by a single gas is called the partial pressure of that gas. This means that although the total pressure of the air will change as altitude or depth varies, the proportion of the component gases remains constant.

- **Henry's law:** The amount of gas dissolved in a given volume of fluid is proportional to the pressure of the gas above it. This law simply states that, because a large percentage of the human body is water, more gas will dissolve into the blood and body tissues as depth increases, until the point of saturation is reached. The gas will remain in the solution as long as pressure is maintained. For example, when a bottle of carbonated soda is opened, there is a sudden release of pressure. The gases come out of the solution and form bubbles. This is similar to what happens if a diver ascends to the surface too quickly.

Tip

Definitive care for decompression illness is typically hyperbaric oxygen therapy (HBO). In HBO, the patient is subjected to oxygen at a higher pressure than normal to force the excess nitrogen to redissolve. The patient is then gradually decompressed to allow the nitrogen to be released without forming bubbles.

- Treat life-threatening illness/injuries.
- Transport considerations: Transport the patient in a position of comfort.
- Focused history and physical exam/secondary assessment
  - Obtain SAMPLE history and chief complaint (OPQRST).

Management
- Treatment for this type of injury is the same as for pneumothorax of any etiology.
- Rest and supplemental oxygen can help ease the symptoms, but HBO is not usually required.

Arterial Gas Embolism
Pathophysiology
This condition occurs secondary to pulmonary overpressure injuries. When the alveoli rupture as a result of increased pressure, a large bubble of gas may escape into circulation. This AGE can enter the central circulation via the left atrium, travel to various parts of the body, and occlude small blood vessels. This obstructed blood flow can result in cardiac, pulmonary, and cerebral compromise.

Signs and Symptoms
The signs and symptoms of AGE usually appear within 10 minutes of surfacing (most commonly within 2 minutes) and may vary according to the organ system that is primarily affected. The most common presentation is similar to cerebrovascular accident (stroke). Specific signs and symptoms include the following:
- Vertigo
- Confusion
- Loss of consciousness
- Visual disturbances
- Paralysis, stroke signs

Assessment
- Scene size-up
  - Ensure BSI.
- Initial/primary assessment
  - Assess ABCs.
  - Place the patient in the supine position.
  - Treat as you would for a near-drowning victim and according to any other symptoms you find on assessment.
  - Transport to a recompression chamber as rapidly as possible. The best treatment for AGE may be immediate HBO.
  - Attempt to keep the patient at or below the altitude of the injury during transport.
- Focused history and physical exam/secondary assessment
  - Obtain SAMPLE history and chief complaint (OPQRST).

Management
- Administer high-flow oxygen.

Nitrogen Narcosis
Pathophysiology
Nitrogen narcosis occurs when excess nitrogen dissolves in the bloodstream under pressure. The nitrogen acts as an anesthetic and causes intoxication and impaired judgment. It most commonly occurs at depths of 70' to 100'. The primary danger comes from accidents that result from this impaired judgment.

Signs and Symptoms
- Intoxication, impaired judgment
- Altered LOC

Assessment

- Scene size-up
  - Ensure BSI.
  - Ensure crew and patient safety.
- Initial/primary assessment
  - Manage ABCs.
  - Monitor patient's LOC.
  - Treat life-threatening illness/injuries.
  - Transport considerations: Transport the patient in a position of comfort.
- Focused history and physical exam/secondary assessment
  - Obtain SAMPLE history and chief complaint (OPQRST).

Management

- Nitrogen narcosis is self-resolving on controlled ascent, so a return to shallow depths should eliminate the symptoms. To prevent nitrogen narcosis, divers usually breathe a mixture of oxygen and helium during deep dives.

Other Diving-Related Illnesses

Less common illnesses and injuries that can occur as a result of diving include the following:

- **Hyperventilation:** Hyperventilation may result in decreased LOC, and muscle cramps and spasm.
- **Contaminated gases:** "Bad air" injuries include carbon dioxide excess, carbon monoxide (CO) poisoning, and oil vapor inhalation. These injuries occur if the diver inhales contaminated gases when faulty air compressors leak harmful CO fumes into the diver's air tank. Contaminated gases increase the risk of hypoxia, narcosis, and accidental injury.
- **Oxygen toxicity:** Oxygen toxicity is usually seen only with prolonged exposure or an excess concentration of oxygen. Symptoms of oxygen toxicity include muscle twitching, nausea and vomiting, dyspnea, and mental status changes or seizures.
- **Hypercapnia:** Hypercapnia is defined as increased carbon dioxide levels and can result from inadequate breathing or faulty equipment. Hypercapnia can lead to unconsciousness.

Altitude Illness

Pathophysiology

In contrast to diving emergencies, high-altitude illnesses occur as a result of decreased atmospheric pressure, resulting in hypoxia. High altitude is essentially a low-oxygen environment. Exposure to high altitudes may exacerbate chronic medical conditions, such as angina, congestive heart failure, chronic obstructive pulmonary disease, and hypertension, even without inducing altitude illness.

High-altitude illnesses usually occur at altitudes higher than 8,000' above sea level and can affect otherwise healthy individuals.

Types of high-altitude illnesses include the following:

- **Acute mountain sickness (AMS)**, or altitude sickness, occurs most commonly in unacclimatized people who ascend rapidly to an altitude of 8,000' or greater. The condition occurs due to hyperventilation that results in respiratory alkalosis and subsequent electrolyte imbalance.
- **High-altitude pulmonary edema (HAPE)** occurs when the air spaces of the lungs fill with fluid from leaking pulmonary blood vessels, making breathing and oxygenation difficult. It develops from increased pulmonary artery pressure that develops in response to hypoxia.

Preventive measures include the following.

- **Gradual ascent:** By ascending gradually, the body adjusts to the lower concentration of oxygen. This acclimatization occurs by resetting ventilation to accommodate the decrease in oxygen, increasing the heart rate to deliver more oxygen to the body's tissues, constricting the peripheral veins, which causes the blood to concentrate, and producing more red blood cells to carry oxygen.

- **Limited exertion:** Avoiding exertion can help minimize the effects of oxygen deprivation.

- **Decreased sleeping altitude:** The hypoxia that results from high altitude can result in disrupted sleep patterns. Descending to a lower altitude to sleep improves sleep and allows the body to recover, but can interfere with acclimatization.

- **High-carbohydrate diet:** Carbohydrates provide quick energy, and some believe this can be helpful in acclimatizing to high altitude.

- **Medications:** Certain medications can help limit the development of high-altitude illnesses, including the following:
  - Acetazolamide, which speeds acclimatization and decreases incidence of AMS
  - Nifedipine, which is used solely by those with a previous history of HAPE to prevent recurrence on ascent

- **High-altitude cerebral edema (HACE)** is the most severe form of altitude illness and results in fluid retention in the brain tissue and increased intracranial pressure. The exact cause of HACE is unknown. Progression from mild AMS to HACE usually takes 1 to 3 days, although symptoms can occur in as little as a few hours. HACE rapidly progresses to coma and death without treatment.

- Both HAPE and HACE are more common in people who ascend too rapidly and who continue to sleep at higher altitudes despite having had symptoms of AMS at lower elevations. Both conditions are gradually progressive and tend to occur over days.

Signs and Symptoms

Symptoms of **AMS** usually develop within 4 to 6 hours and may range from mild to severe; they include the following:

- Dizziness
- Headache
- Irritability
- Breathlessness
- Euphoria

Symptoms of **HAPE** typically develop 24 to 72 hours after exposure and include the following:

- Shortness of breath with fluid in the lungs
- Cough (with or without frothy sputum)
- Generalized weakness
- Altered mental status

Patients with **HACE** have a progressively worsening LOC, confusion, and disorientation. Other symptoms include:

- Malaise
- Anorexia
- Headache
- Sleep disturbances
- Respiratory distress that increases with exertion

Assessment

- Scene size-up
  - Ensure BSI.
- Initial/primary assessment
  - Manage ABCs.
  - Monitor patient's LOC.
  - Treat life-threatening illness/injuries.
  - Transport considerations: Transport the patient in a position of comfort.
- Focused history and physical exam/secondary assessment
  - Obtain SAMPLE history and chief complaint (OPQRST).

Management

- Descend to a lower altitude.
- Administer oxygen at 15 L/min via nonrebreathing mask.
- Transport to a facility that is capable of providing HBO support.
- Administer medications according to medical direction. The following medications may be used to treat altitude illnesses:
  - Acetazolamide for AMS, HAPE, or HACE
  - Nifedipine for HAPE only
  - Steroids for severe AMS or HACE only
  - Prochlorperazine for AMS or HACE

Vital Vocabulary

acute mountain sickness (AMS) An altitude illness characterized by headache, dizziness, irritability, breathlessness, and euphoria.

Boyle's law At a constant temperature, the volume of gas is inversely proportional to its pressure (if you double the pressure on a gas, you halve its volume); written as $PV = K$, where P = pressure, V = volume, and K = a constant.

conduction Transfer of heat to a solid object or a liquid by direct contact.

convection Mechanism by which body heat is picked up and carried away by moving air currents.

Dalton's law Each gas in mixture exerts the same partial pressure that it would exert if it were alone in the same volume, and the total pressure of a mixture of gases is the sum of the partial pressures of all the gases in the mixture.

drowning The process of experiencing respiratory impairment from submersion or immersion in liquid.

evaporation The conversion of a liquid to a gas.

Henry's law The amount of gas dissolved in a liquid is directly proportional to the partial pressure of the gas above the liquid.

high-altitude cerebral edema (HACE) An altitude illness in which there is a change in mental status and/or ataxia.

high-altitude pulmonary edema (HAPE) An altitude illness characterized by dyspnea at rest, cough, severe weakness, and drowsiness that may eventually lead to central cyanosis, audible rales or wheezing, tachypnea, and tachycardia.

radiation Emission of heat from an object into surrounding, colder air.

respiration The exchange of gases between a living organism and its environment.

thermogenesis The production of heat in the body.

CHAPTER 16

Obstetric and Gynecologic Emergencies

<u>Gynecology</u> is the branch of medicine that deals with the health maintenance and diseases of women, primarily of the reproductive system. <u>Obstetrics</u> deals specifically with the care of women throughout pregnancy. A basic understanding of normal full-term childbirth and possible complications as well as certain gynecologic emergencies will help you to more effectively manage care for these female patients.

Normal Childbirth

Obtain History

Tip

Naegele's rule is used to calculate the due date. Add 9 months and 1 week (40 weeks total) to the date of the first day of the last menstrual period (LMP). If the first day of the LMP is June 1, 2008, counting forward 9 months and 1 week gives a due date of March 8, 2009. You can also go back 3 months, add 1 week, and change the year. Another easy method is to change the dates into numbers. If the LMP began on 11/25/2008, subtract 3 months and add 7 days to get 9/2/2008, then change the year. The estimated due date is 9/2/2009.

- Determine the estimated date of confinement, or due date. **Gestation** is the period from conception to birth, during which the fetus develops in the uterus. The average gestation time is 266 days.
- Determine the patient's gravida/para status (**Table 16-1**).
- Any problems or complications with past pregnancies?
- Any expected problems or complications with this pregnancy?
- Contractions: When did they start? How far apart are they?
  - Contractions less than 3 minutes apart implies that delivery is imminent.
- Ruptured membranes: Has the water broken?
- Any spotting or "bloody show"?
- Any urge to push or feeling the need to have a bowel movement?
  - Implies that delivery is imminent.

Assessment for the Patient With an Imminent Delivery

- Scene size-up
  - Ensure body substance isolation (BSI) and use the obstetrics (OB) kit.
- Initial/primary assessment
  - Assess level of consciousness (LOC).
  - Manage ABCs (airway, breathing, circulation).
  - Treat life-threatening illness/injury.
  - Visually check for <u>crowning</u>.
  - Feel for uterus contractions.
  - Time the contractions.
  - Assess vital signs.

Management

- Administer oxygen at 15 L/min via nonrebreathing mask.
- Establish intravenous (IV) access with lactated Ringer's solution.
- Place a gloved hand over the baby's cranium to prevent an explosive delivery.
- Support the baby's head as it delivers.
- If the baby is still enclosed in the amniotic sac, tear or cut the sac open. Gently slide your finger along the head and neck to ensure that the umbilical cord is not wrapped around the baby's neck.

Table 16-1 Gravida/Para Status: G/P T-P-A-L

Gravida (G)	Para (P)	Full-Term Infants (T)	Preterm Infants (P)	Number of Abortions (A)	Number of Living Children (L)
Total number of pregnancies, including the current pregnancy	Total number of deliveries after 20 weeks' gestation	Number of delivered full-term infants	Number of delivered preterm infants	Number of abortions, both spontaneous (miscarriage) and induced	Number of currently living children

- Suction the mouth, and then the nose (**Figure 16-1**). Keep the head lower than the chest to allow drainage. If meconium is present, use a suction trap or meconium aspirator to suction the hypopharynx. If the possibility of aspiration is present, tracheal suctioning via endotracheal tube may be required.
- Assist in delivering the upper shoulder by gently guiding the baby's head downward (**Figure 16-2**).
- Assist in delivering the lower shoulder by gently guiding the head upward (**Figure 16-3**).
- Support the baby's trunk and feet as they deliver.
- Place the baby on its side, level with the vagina, with the head slightly downward to allow fluids to drain.
- Suction the baby's mouth and nose again.
- Keep the baby at the level of the vagina to prevent over- or undertransfusion of blood from the cord. Palpate the umbilical cord to ensure that pulsating has stopped.
- Apply the first clamp approximately 10 cm from the baby and the second 5 cm from the first, and cut in between.
- Dry and wrap the neonate in warm blankets to prevent heat loss.

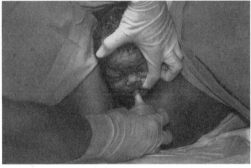

Figure 16-1 Suction the baby's mouth.

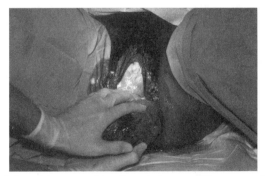

Figure 16-2 Guide the baby's head downward to allow delivery of the upper shoulder.

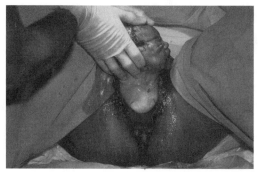

Figure 16-3 Guide the baby's head upward to allow delivery of the lower shoulder.

- Assess the Apgar score (**Table 16-2**) at 1 minute and again at 5 minutes after birth.
- Allow the mother to hold the baby, and encourage breastfeeding.
- Reassess the mother's vital signs.
- Deliver the placenta and transport in a biohazard bag.

Special Management Considerations

Postpartum Hemorrhage

- Place a sanitary napkin over the vagina. *Do not place anything inside the vagina!*
- Lower the mother's knees and keep them together.
- Massage the uterus to assist in contraction and control bleeding.
- Palpate the uterus in a circular motion.
- Mix 20 units oxytocin in 1,000 mL of lactated Ringer's solution and infuse wide open.

Neonatal Resuscitation

- If the baby is apneic (ie, has a 20-sec or longer respiratory pause) or has a pulse rate less than 100 beats/min after 30 sec of drying and stimulation and supplemental free-flow (blow-by) oxygen, begin positive-pressure ventilation (PPV) by bag-mask device.
- If the infant's pulse rate is less than 60 beats/min after 30 sec of adequate ventilation by PPV with 100% oxygen via a bag-mask device, begin chest compressions.
- For neonatal bradycardia despite 30 seconds of ventilations, administer epinephrine via IV or use an endotracheal tube with 0.01 to 0.03 mg/kg per dose.
- Naloxone is not recommended during the primary stage of neonatal resuscitation. Avoid giving naloxone to babies whose mothers have had long-term exposure to opioids because it can cause withdrawal symptoms in the baby.

Table 16-2 The Apgar Score

Condition	Description	Score
Appearance, skin color	Completely pink Body pink, extremities blue Centrally blue, pale	2 1 0
Pulse rate	> 100 < 100, > 0 Absent	2 1 0
Grimace, irritability	Cries Grimaces No response	2 1 0
Activity, muscle tone	Active motion Some flexion of extremities Limp	2 1 0
Respiratory, effort	Strong cry Slow and irregular Absent	2 1 0

- Consider volume expanders in the following situations:
  - Neonate does not respond to resuscitative efforts.
  - Neonate appears hypovolemic.
    - Administer 10 mL/kg of normal saline, lactated Ringer's solution, or O-negative blood over 10 minutes.

Supine Hypotensive Syndrome

Pathophysiology

<u>Supine hypotensive syndrome</u> usually occurs in the third trimester of pregnancy. Also known as vena cava syndrome, supine hypotensive syndrome usually occurs when the gravid uterus compresses the inferior vena cava when the mother is in a supine position, but can also occur with the mother in a seated position. It is characterized by the inadequate return of venous blood to the heart, reduced cardiac output, and lowered blood pressure.

Signs and Symptoms

- Occurs late in pregnancy
- Dizziness, caused by decreased return of blood to the right atrium and consequent lowering of cardiac output, leading to a decrease in blood pressure
- Nausea
- Tachycardia
- Possible recent hemorrhage or fluid loss

Assessment

- Scene size-up
  - Ensure BSI/Use OB kit.
- Initial/primary assessment
  - Assess LOC.
  - Manage ABCs.
  - Treat life-threatening illness/injury.
  - Transport considerations: Rapid, gentle transport to the nearest facility, with the mother in a left lateral recumbent position or with the right hip elevated. If unable to position the patient on her left side, you can perform manual displacement of the uterus.
- Focused history and physical exam/secondary assessment
  - Obtain SAMPLE history and chief complaint (OPQRST).
  - Assess for fluid depletion.

Management

- Have the mother lay on her left side. If the low blood pressure does not resolve, then:
  - Administer oxygen at 15 L/min via nonrebreathing mask.
  - Establish IV of lactated Ringer's solution.
  - Reassure the patient.
  - Perform cardiac monitoring.
  - Monitor vital signs frequently.
  - Check for orthostatic pressure changes (a decrease in blood pressure and increase in heart rate when rising from the supine position).

Uterine Rupture

Pathophysiology

Uterine rupture is a life-threatening medical emergency in which the wall of the uterus ruptures and the fetus floats in the abdomen. It occurs most commonly after the onset of labor and as a prehospital emergency following a traumatic event such as a car accident. Contractions stop after the mother experiences severe abdominal pain. Risk factors include a history of uterine surgery, trauma, prolonged or obstructed labor, previous cesarean section, overdistention of the uterus, multiparity greater than 4, previous rupture, and abnormal fetal presentation. The mortality rate for both mother and fetus is high. Fetal complications include hypoxia, acidosis, anoxia, and death. It is critical that these patients be transported rapidly to an appropriate trauma center.

Signs and Symptoms

- Continuous sharp, severe abdominal pain
- Nausea
- Signs and symptoms of hypovolemic shock
- Anxiety
- Tearing sensation in the abdomen
- Minimal vaginal bleeding
- Easily palpated fetus in abdomen
- Onset of severe pain mimicking a contraction followed by a cessation of contractions
- Tachycardia
- Tachypnea
- Distended abdomen

Assessment

- Scene size-up
  - Ensure BSI/Use OB kit.
- Initial/primary assessment
  - Assess LOC.
  - Manage ABCs.
  - Treat life-threatening illness/injury.
  - Transport considerations: Rapid, gentle transport to the nearest facility with the mother in a left lateral recumbent position or with the right hip elevated.
- Focused history and physical exam/secondary assessment
  - Obtain SAMPLE history and chief complaint (OPQRST).

Management

- Administer oxygen at 15 L/min via nonrebreathing mask.
- Establish IV of lactated Ringer's solution.
- Monitor vital signs.
- Reassure the patient.
- Gently palpate the fetus in the mother's abdomen.
- Place patient in the left lateral recumbent position.
- Uterine contractions can be encouraged with the infusion of 20 units of oxytocin in 1,000 mL of lactated Ringer's solution and may lessen bleeding via blood vessel constriction.

Prolapsed Umbilical Cord

Pathophysiology

A **prolapsed umbilical cord** is an umbilical cord that precedes the fetus during delivery, resulting in diminishing or absent fetal circulation from the placenta. It occurs in 1 of every 250 pregnancies. Risk factors include multiple gestations, preterm delivery, and breech presentation.

Signs and Symptoms

- Umbilical cord protruding from the vagina
- Fetal bradycardia

Assessment

- Scene size-up
  - Ensure BSI/Use OB kit.
- Initial/primary assessment
  - Assess LOC.
  - Manage ABCs.
  - Treat life-threatening illness/injury.
  - Transport considerations: Transport in a position of comfort; remove pressure of fetus from the umbilical cord by elevating the mother's hips.
- Focused history and physical exam/secondary assessment
  - Obtain SAMPLE history and chief complaint (OPQRST).

Management

- Administer oxygen at 15 L/min via nonrebreathing mask.
- Establish IV of lactated Ringer's solution.
- Check vital signs.
- Elevate the fetus off the cord. With a gloved hand, insert two fingers into the vagina, forming a "V," with one finger on either side of the cord to help keep pressure off the cord.
- Position the mother in the knee-chest or Trendelenburg position.
- Cover the cord with moistened gauze or cloth. Monitor cord for pulsation.
- Cover the mother with a blanket.
- Do not attempt or encourage delivery.
- Do not pull on the cord or attempt to push the cord or fetus back in.
- Instruct the patient to pant with each contraction to prevent bearing down.

Limb Presentation

Pathophysiology

In this condition, which often occurs in preterm deliveries, the presenting parts may be the fetus' arms or legs. This is a high-risk delivery that is best delivered in the hospital. However, it may be necessary to manage a limb presentation prehospitally.

Signs and Symptoms

- Limb presenting

Assessment

- Scene size-up
  - Ensure BSI/Use OB kit.
- Initial/primary assessment
  - Assess LOC.
  - Manage ABCs.
  - Treat life-threatening illness/injury.
  - Transport considerations: Transport rapidly to an appropriate hospital, communicating the situation to the hospital in a timely manner. Transport the patient with the hips elevated or on her knees.
- Focused history and physical exam/secondary assessment
  - Obtain SAMPLE history and chief complaint (OPQRST).

Management

- Administer oxygen at 15 L/min via nonrebreathing mask.
- Establish IV of lactated Ringer's solution.
- Monitor vital signs.
- Insert two gloved fingers to hold the fetus off the cord, if prolapse is suspected.

Breech Presentation

Pathophysiology

In a **breech presentation**, you will note buttocks "crowning." It is important in this type of birth to provide an airway for the fetus. Breech presentations occur in 3% to 4% of all term pregnancies and have a morbidity rate three to four times that of **cephalic deliveries**.

Signs and Symptoms

- Increased pain
- Buttocks showing at the vaginal opening

Assessment

- Scene size-up
  - Ensure BSI/Use OB kit.
- Initial/primary assessment
  - Assess LOC.
  - Manage ABCs.
  - Treat life-threatening illness/injury.
  - Transport considerations: Rapidly transport to an appropriate hospital with high-risk obstetric capabilities; notify the hospital of estimated time of arrival.
- Focused history and physical exam/secondary assessment
  - Obtain SAMPLE history and chief complaint (OPQRST).

Management

- Administer oxygen at 15 L/min via nonrebreathing mask.
- Monitor vital signs.
- Do not push the fetus back into the vagina or pull on the fetus.
- Allow the body to deliver with contractions.
- Support the baby's legs and trunk.
- Allow the baby to deliver until you can visualize the umbilicus. At this point you may need to gently extract approximately 5" of umbilical cord to allow further delivery and decrease traction on the cord. Be careful not to compress the cord during this procedure.
- Gently rotate the fetus so that the shoulders are in an anterior-posterior position.
- Continue with gentle traction until the underarm is visible.
- Guide the infant upward to deliver the posterior shoulder.
- Guide the infant downward to deliver the anterior shoulder.
- Gently facilitate delivery of the head through the birth canal.
- If the head does not deliver, place a gloved hand in the vagina with the palm toward the fetus' face. Form a "V" with your index and middle finger on either side of the fetus' nose to provide an airway and push the vaginal wall away from the fetus' face until the head is delivered. If the head still does not deliver, maintain this position during transport, thus maintaining an airway.
- Establish an IV of lactated Ringer's solution in the mother.

Hypertensive Emergencies

Preeclampsia and Eclampsia

Pathophysiology

Pregnancy-induced hypertension, which includes preeclampsia and eclampsia, occurs in approximately 5% of all pregnancies. **Preeclampsia** is a progressive disorder that is usually categorized as mild or moderate. **Eclampsia**, the most severe form, is characterized by seizures. Known risk factors include age older than 35 years or younger than 15 years, history of preeclampsia, multiparity, preexisting renal or cardiovascular disease, diabetes, family history, and African American descent.

Preeclampsia is the most common hypertensive disorder seen in pregnant women and occurs in 6% to 8% of all live births. There is a higher incidence among primigravidas (women who are pregnant for the first time), particularly teenagers or in women older than 35 years of age. Others at increased risk are women with diabetes, women with a history of preeclampsia, and women carrying multiple fetuses.

Preeclampsia is defined as an increase in systolic blood pressure by 30 mm Hg and/or a diastolic increase of 15 mm Hg over baseline on at least two occasions at least 6 hours apart. Maternal blood pressure normally drops during pregnancy, so a woman may be hypertensive at 120/80 if her baseline in early pregnancy was 90/60. If there is no baseline blood pressure available, a reading higher than 140/90 is considered hypertensive.

Preeclampsia is most commonly seen in the last 10 weeks of gestation, during labor, or in the first 48 hours postpartum. The exact cause is unknown. It is thought to be caused by abnormal vasospasm, which results in increased maternal blood pressure and other associated symptoms. Additionally, the vasospasm causes decreased placental perfusion, contributing to fetal growth retardation and chronic fetal hypoxia.

Mild preeclampsia is characterized by hypertension, edema, and protein in the urine. Severe preeclampsia progresses rapidly, with maternal blood pressures reaching 160/110 or higher, generalized edema, visual disturbances, right upper quadrant (RUQ) pain, and a significant increase in the amount of protein in the urine. Other common signs and symptoms in the severe state include headache, hyperactive reflexes, and the development of pulmonary edema, along with a dramatic decrease in urine output.

Because a large percentage of their body fluid is edema fluid in the tissues, patients who are preeclamptic experience intravascular volume depletion. Those who develop severe preeclampsia and eclampsia are at increased risk for cerebral hemorrhage, pulmonary embolism, abruptio placentae, and renal failure.

Eclampsia is the most serious level of pregnancy-induced hypertension. It is characterized by grand mal (major motor) seizure activity. It is often preceded by visual disturbances, such as flashing lights or spots before the eyes. Epigastric pain or pain in the RUQ often indicates impending seizure. Eclampsia can be distinguished from epilepsy by the history and physical appearance of the patient. Eclamptic patients are usually grossly edematous and have markedly elevated blood pressure, whereas epileptic patients usually have a history of seizures and are usually taking anticonvulsant medications. The development of eclampsia greatly increases the risk of death for both the mother and fetus. The risk of fetal mortality increases by 10% with each maternal seizure.

Hypertension

Closely monitor the pregnant patient who has elevated blood pressure without edema or other signs of preeclampsia. Record the fetal heart tones and the mother's blood pressure level.

Chronic Hypertension

Chronic hypertension should be considered when the maternal blood pressure is higher than 140/90 before pregnancy or prior to the 20th week of gestation, or if high blood pressure persists for more than 42 days postpartum. As a general rule, if the diastolic pressure exceeds 90 mm Hg during the second trimester, chronic hypertension is likely.

Preeclampsia

Signs and Symptoms

- Elevated blood pressure
- Excessive weight gain: 3 pounds or more in a month during the second trimester or 1 pound or more in a week during the third trimester
- Headaches
- Sudden weight gain of 4 to 5 pounds per week any time
- Visual disturbance (blurred/double vision)
- Change in mental status
- Epigastric or RUQ pain
- Protein in the urine
- Decreased urine output
- Pulmonary edema

Assessment

- Scene size-up
  - Ensure BSI/Use OB kit.
- Initial/primary assessment
  - Assess LOC.
  - Manage ABCs.
  - Treat life-threatening illness/injury.
  - Transport considerations: Rapid, gentle transport to the nearest facility with obstetric capabilities.
- Focused history and physical exam/secondary assessment
  - Obtain SAMPLE history and chief complaint (OPQRST).

Management

- Administer oxygen at 15 L/min via nonrebreathing mask.
- Monitor vital signs.
- Establish IV of lactated Ringer's solution.
- Keep the patient calm.

Table 16-3 summarizes the management of a patient with preeclampsia.

Table 16-3 Management of a Patient With Preeclampsia

Treatment	Purpose	Adult Dose
Hydralazine	Antihypertensive	IM: 5 mg
Morphine sulfate	Decrease pulmonary edema by increasing venous capacitance	IV: 2-5 mg
Furosemide	Decrease pulmonary edema by decreasing fluid overload	IV: 0.5-1.0 mg/kg
IV, intravenous; IM, intramuscular.		

Eclampsia

Signs and Symptoms

- Elevated blood pressure
- Excessive weight gain: 3 pounds or more in a month during the second trimester or 1 pound or more in a week during the third trimester

- Headaches
- Sudden weight gain of 4 to 5 pounds per week any time
- Visual disturbance (blurred/double vision)
- Irritability or change in mental status
- Epigastric or RUQ pain
- Protein in the urine
- Decreased urine output
- Pulmonary edema
- Seizures

Assessment
- Scene size-up
  - Ensure BSI/Use OB kit.
- Initial/primary assessment
  - Assess LOC.
  - Manage ABCs.
  - Treat life-threatening illness/injury.
  - Transport considerations: Immediately transport the patient (lying on her left side) to a hospital with surgical obstetric and neonatal care availability. Notify the receiving facility of patient status and estimated time of arrival.
- Focused history and physical exam/secondary assessment
  - Obtain SAMPLE history and chief complaint (OPQRST).

Management
- Administer oxygen at 15 L/min via nonrebreathing mask.
- Establish IV of lactated Ringer's solution.
- Monitor vital signs.
- Administer anticonvulsants as needed.
- Maintain a patent airway.
- Protect patient from injury.

Table 16-4 summarizes the management of a patient with eclampsia.

Tip

Seizures in an eclamptic patient usually occur during the third trimester.

Table 16-4 Management of a Patient With Eclampsia

Treatment	Purpose	Adult Dose
Magnesium sulfate	Anticonvulsant	IV: 2 g
Diazepam	Skeletal muscle relaxer that treats increased presynaptic inhibition that causes seizures	IV: 2.5-5.0 mg
Hydralazine	Antihypertensive	IM: 5 mg
Morphine sulfate	Decrease pulmonary edema	SIVP: 2.5-5.0 mg
Furosemide	Decrease pulmonary edema	IV: 0.5-1.0 mg/kg
SIVP, slow intravenous push.		

Spontaneous Abortion

Pathophysiology

A **spontaneous abortion**, or *miscarriage*, is an unexpected expulsion of the fetus prior to viability. It usually occurs during the first trimester but can occur up to week 20 of gestation. After week 20, fetal loss is referred to as *intrauterine fetal demise*, or *stillbirth*.

Signs and Symptoms
- Abdominal pain
- Abdominal cramping

- Anxiety
- Vaginal bleeding or spotting with clots
- Possible signs and symptoms of shock
- Orthostatic hypotension

Medications that raise the risk of miscarriage include illegal drugs and nonsteroidal anti-inflammatory drugs such as aspirin and ibuprofen.

Assessment

- Scene size-up
  - Ensure BSI/Use OB kit.
- Initial/primary assessment
  - Assess LOC.
  - Manage ABCs.
  - Treat life-threatening illness/injury.
  - Transport considerations: Transport in a position of comfort.
- Focused history and physical exam/secondary assessment
  - Obtain SAMPLE history and chief complaint (OPQRST).

Management

- Administer oxygen at 15 L/min via nonrebreathing mask.
- Provide emotional support.
- Monitor vital signs.
- Establish IV of lactated Ringer's solution.
- Keep patient warm.
- Treat for shock.
- Salvage any large clots or fetal tissue to give to hospital staff.

Tip

Often in a miscarriage, the placenta does not detach, and the fetus is suspended by the umbilical cord. In such a case, place the umbilical clamps from the OB kit on the cord and cut it. Carefully wrap the fetus in linen or other suitable material and transport it to the hospital with the mother.

Ruptured Ectopic Pregnancy

Pathophysiology

The fertilized egg is normally implanted in the endometrial lining of the uterine wall. The term **ectopic pregnancy** refers to the abnormal implantation of the fertilized egg outside the uterus. In most cases, the egg is implanted in the fallopian tube. Occasionally, it is implanted in the abdominal cavity. This condition is generally detected between the 2nd and 12th weeks of pregnancy. The emergency occurs when the growing egg sac ruptures the fallopian tube or a vessel in the abdominal cavity and can cause severe bleeding. This is the leading cause of maternal death during the first trimester.

Predisposing factors in the development of ectopic pregnancy include scarring of the fallopian tubes as a result of pelvic inflammatory disease, a previous ectopic pregnancy, or previous pelvic or tubal surgery, such as a tubal ligation. Other factors include endometriosis or use of an intrauterine device for birth control.

Signs and Symptoms

- Weakness
- Dizziness
- Abdominal pain that starts as diffuse pain, then localizes as a sharp pain in the lower abdomen; pain and tenderness may become generalized again
- Nausea, vomiting
- Referred pain to shoulder (25% of cases) on the affected side
- Last menstrual period: 4 to 6 weeks prior
- Syncope
- Vaginal bleeding or spotting (rare)

Assessment

- Scene size-up
  - Ensure BSI/Use OB kit.
- Initial/primary assessment
  - Monitor patient's LOC.
  - Manage ABCs.
  - Treat life-threatening illness/injury.
  - Transport considerations: Transport rapidly in a position of comfort to a facility with surgical capabilities.
- Focused history and physical exam/secondary assessment
  - Obtain SAMPLE history and chief complaint (OPQRST).

Management

- Administer oxygen at 15 L/min via nonrebreathing mask.
- Establish IV of lactated Ringer's solution.
- Monitor vital signs.

Tip

Assume that any female of childbearing age with lower abdominal pain is experiencing an ectopic pregnancy, and provide rapid transport to an appropriate medical facility.

Placenta Previa

Pathophysiology

<u>Placenta previa</u> is a condition in which the placenta partially or completely covers the cervical opening (**Figure 16-4**). Vaginal bleeding can occur after the seventh month of the pregnancy as the lower uterus begins to dilate in preparation for the onset of labor. This process pulls the placenta away from the uterine wall, causing painless, bright red vaginal bleeding. Placenta previa is classified as complete, partial, or marginal, depending on whether the placenta covers all or part of the cervical opening or is merely in close proximity to the opening. During labor the placenta may be the presenting part and will detach from the uterus. *Danger to the fetus can develop if the placenta detaches and delivers first, depriving the fetus of oxygen and nutrients.*

Although the exact cause of placenta previa is unknown, predisposing factors include a previous history of placenta previa, multiparity, a rapid succession of pregnancies,

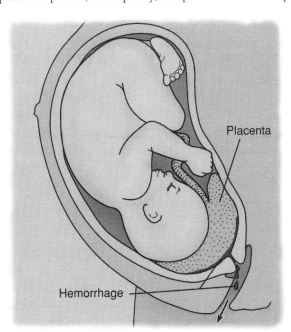

Figure 16-4 In placenta previa, the placenta covers the cervix either partially or completely (as shown here).

and maternal age over 35 years. Smoking doubles the risk, as do cocaine use, multifetal gestations, and previous cesarean sections or curettage. Another contributing factor is the defective development of blood vessels in the uterine wall.

Do not perform a vaginal examination, which could puncture the placenta and cause fatal hemorrhaging.

Signs and Symptoms

- Painless, bright red vaginal bleeding (acute onset)
- Placenta known to be in abnormal position
- Soft uterus
- Possible false contractions

Assessment

- Scene size-up
  - Ensure BSI/Use OB kit.
- Initial/primary assessment
  - Monitor patient's LOC.
  - Manage ABCs.
  - Treat life-threatening illness/injury.
  - Transport considerations: Transport in a shock position.
- Focused history and physical exam/secondary assessment
  - Obtain SAMPLE history and chief complaint (OPQRST).

Management

- Administer oxygen at 15 L/min via nonrebreathing mask.
- Establish IV of lactated Ringer's solution.
- Monitor vital signs.
- Place a bulky dressing or sanitary napkin over the vagina.
- Save all blood-soaked dressings so blood loss can be estimated.
- Monitor vital signs and fetal heart tones.

Table 16-5 summarizes the treatment of placenta previa.

Table 16-5 Treatment of Placenta Previa

Treatment	Purpose	Adult Dose
Normal saline	Perfusion/hydration	Infusion: 250 mL to maintain systolic BP of 90 mm Hg or radial pulses
Lactated Ringer's solution	Perfusion/hydration	Infusion: 250 mL to maintain systolic BP of 90 mm Hg or radial pulses

Abruptio Placentae

Pathophysiology

Abruptio placentae is the premature detachment of a normally situated placenta from the uterine wall. Detachment may be complete or partial and can occur at any stage of pregnancy, but most often during the third trimester. It occurs in about 0.83% of all deliveries.

Partial abruptions can be marginal or central. *Marginal abruptio placentae* is characterized by vaginal bleeding but no increase in pain. In *central abruptio placentae*, the placenta separates centrally and the bleeding is trapped between the placenta and the uterine wall, or concealed, so there is no vaginal bleeding. In *complete abruptio placentae*, there is massive vaginal bleeding and profound maternal hypotension. If the patient is in labor at the time of the abruption, separation of the placenta from the uterine wall progresses rapidly, with fetal distress versus fetal demise dependent on the percentage of separation.

Risk Factors

- History of preeclampsia
- Chronic or gestational hypertension
- Trauma
- Multiple pregnancies
- History of abruptio placentae
- Smoking
- Cocaine use
- Increasing maternal age (older than 35 years)
- Uterine scarring from surgeries
- Infection

Signs and Symptoms

Signs and symptoms vary, depending on the extent and character of the abruption.
- Sudden, severe, constant lower abdominal pain
- Abdominal tenderness and a contracting uterus
- Dizziness
- Anxiety
- Tachypnea
- Tachycardia
- Dark vaginal bleeding
- Signs and symptom of shock
- Vaginal bleeding not necessarily present
- Sharp, tearing pain

Assessment

- Scene size-up
  - Ensure BSI/Use OB kit.
- Initial/primary assessment
  - Assess LOC.
  - Manage ABCs.
  - Treat life-threatening illness/injury.
  - Transport considerations: Transport rapidly, with patient in a shock or left lateral recumbent position, to an appropriate hospital (surgical obstetric and high-risk neonatal care) with timely communication to emergency department personnel.
- Focused history and physical exam/secondary assessment
  - Obtain SAMPLE history and chief complaint (OPQRST).

Management

- Administer oxygen at 15 L/min via nonrebreathing mask.
- Establish IV access. Two large-bore IVs are preferred.
- Monitor vital signs.
- Place a bulky dressing or sanitary napkin over the vagina.
- Save all blood-soaked dressings.

> **Tip**
>
> Abruptio placentae is a life-threatening obstetric emergency. Immediate intervention to maintain maternal oxygenation and perfusion is imperative. Place two large-bore IV lines and begin fluid resuscitation. Position the patient in the left lateral recumbent position. Transport immediately, with timely communication, to a hospital with available surgical obstetric and high-risk neonatal care.

Preterm Labor

Preterm labor is defined as frequent uterine contractions resulting in progressive cervical dilation between weeks 20 and 37. Occurring in approximately 10% to 15% of all pregnancies, it complicates 8% to 12% of all births.

Risk Factors

- Premature rupture of the amniotic membranes
- Smoking
- Cocaine usage
- Previous preterm delivery
- Infections
- Sexually transmitted diseases, such as chlamydia, gonorrhea, and syphilis

Signs and Symptoms

- Mild abdominal cramps, with or without diarrhea
- Frequent, regular contractions (every 10 minutes or more)
- Vaginal bleeding or a change in the type or amount of vaginal discharge
- Dull ache in lower back
- Pelvic pressure

Assessment

- Scene size-up
  - Ensure BSI/Use OB kit.
- Initial/primary assessment
  - Assess LOC.
  - Manage ABCs.
  - Treat life-threatening illness/injury.
  - Transport considerations: Rapidly transport in a left lateral recumbent position to appropriate hospital (surgical obstetrics and high-risk neonatal care) with timely communication to emergency department personnel.
- Focused history and physical exam/secondary assessment
  - Obtain SAMPLE history and chief complaint (OPQRST).

Management

- Administer oxygen at 15 L/min via nonrebreathing mask.
- Establish IV of lactated Ringer's solution.
- Monitor vital signs.
- Prepare for delivery.

Gestational Diabetes

Gestational diabetes is defined as those cases of diabetes that initially manifest during pregnancy. Occurring in approximately 1% to 15% of all pregnancies, it mimics type II diabetes.

Risk Factors

- Maternal obesity
- Previous large birth weight infant
- Preeclampsia
- Excessive weight gain

Signs and Symptoms

- Altered mental status
- Tachycardia
- Pale, diaphoretic skin
- Confirmed hyperglycemia

Assessment

- Scene size-up
  - Ensure BSI.
- Initial/primary assessment
  - Assess LOC.
  - Manage ABCs.
  - Treat life-threatening illness/injury.
  - Transport considerations: Transport in a position of comfort.
- Focused history and physical exam/secondary assessment
  - Obtain SAMPLE history and chief complaint (OPQRST).

Management

- Administer oxygen at 15 L/min via nonrebreathing mask.
- Establish IV of lactated Ringer's solution.
- Monitor vital signs.
- If blood glucose level is below 60 mg/dL, administer 25 g of dextrose 50%.

Gynecologic Problems

Pelvic Inflammatory Disease

Pathophysiology

Pelvic inflammatory disease is an acute infection of the female upper reproductive organs (uterus, ovaries, and fallopian tubes) that can be caused by a bacteria, virus, or fungus. It is one of the most common causes of nontraumatic abdominal pain among sexually active women. It occurs most commonly in women aged 15 to 24 years with infections caused by *Neisseria gonorrhoeae* or *Chlamydia*.

Signs and Symptoms

- Fever
- Chills
- Nausea
- Vomiting
- Septic shock
- Foul-smelling vaginal discharge
- Irregular menses
- Midcycle bleeding
- Shuffling gait when walking (most noticeable sign)
- Slightly increased pulse rate

Assessment

- Scene size-up
  - Ensure BSI.
- Initial/primary assessment
  - Assess LOC.
  - Manage ABCs.

- Treat life-threatening illness/injury.
  - Transport considerations: Transport in a position of comfort.
- Focused history and physical exam/secondary assessment
  - Obtain SAMPLE history and chief complaint (OPQRST).

Management
- Monitor vital signs.
- Place patient in a position of comfort.
- Establish an IV if patient has inadequate perfusion or dehydration.

Ruptured Ovarian Cyst
Pathophysiology
__Ovarian cysts__ are fluid-filled pockets that form on or in an ovary. When an egg is released from the ovary, a corpus luteum cyst is sometimes left in its place. Occasionally the cyst ruptures, spilling a small amount of blood into the abdomen, which irritates the peritoneum and causes pain.

Signs and Symptoms
- Complaints of pain radiating to the back
- History of irregular bleeding, dyspareunia, or late periods

Assessment
- Scene size-up
  - Ensure BSI/Use OB kit.
- Initial/primary assessment
  - Assess LOC.
  - Manage ABCs.
  - Treat life-threatening illness/injury.
  - Transport considerations: Transport in a position of comfort.
- Focused history and physical exam/secondary assessment
  - Obtain SAMPLE history and chief complaint (OPQRST).

Management
- Administer oxygen at 15 L/min via nonrebreathing mask.
- Monitor vital signs.
- Place patient in a position of comfort.
- Establish an IV if patient has inadequate perfusion or dehydration.

Endometritis
Pathophysiology
__Endometritis__ is an infection of the uterine lining resulting from miscarriage, childbirth, or gynecologic procedures.

Signs and Symptoms
- Mild to severe lower abdominal pain
- Bloody, foul-smelling discharge
- Fever
- Onset of symptoms usually 48 to 72 hours after procedure or miscarriage
- Signs and symptoms of infection (fever, chills, malaise)

Assessment
- Scene size-up
  - Ensure BSI/Use OB kit.
- Initial/primary assessment
  - Assess LOC.
  - Manage ABCs.

- Treat life-threatening illness/injury.
  - Transport considerations: Transport in a position of comfort.
- Focused history and physical exam/secondary assessment
  - Obtain SAMPLE history and chief complaint (OPQRST).

Management
- Monitor vital signs.
- Place patient in a position of comfort.
- Establish an IV if patient has inadequate perfusion or dehydration.

Endometriosis

Pathophysiology

Endometriosis is a condition in which endometrial tissue grows outside the uterus, most commonly in the abdomen and pelvis. It is usually seen in women aged 30 to 40.

Signs and Symptoms
- Dull, cramping pelvic pain
- Painful bowel movements
- Pain is usually worse during menstrual periods

Assessment
- Scene size-up
  - Ensure BSI/Use OB kit.
- Initial/primary assessment
  - Assess LOC.
  - Manage ABCs.
  - Treat life-threatening illness/injury.
  - Transport considerations: Transport in a position of comfort.
- Focused history and physical exam/secondary assessment
  - Obtain SAMPLE history and chief complaint (OPQRST).

Management
- Administer oxygen at 15 L/min via nonrebreathing mask.
- Monitor vital signs.
- Place patient in a position of comfort.
- Establish an IV if patient has inadequate perfusion or dehydration.

Vital Vocabulary

abruptio placentae A premature separation of the placenta from the wall of the uterus.

breech presentation A delivery in which the buttocks come out first.

cephalic delivery Fetus delivers head first.

crowning The appearance of the infant's head at the vaginal opening during labor.

eclampsia The most severe form of pregnancy-induced hypertension, characterized by seizures.

ectopic pregnancy A pregnancy in which the ovum implants somewhere other than the uterine endometrium.

endometriosis A condition in which endometrial tissue grows outside the uterus.

endometritis An inflammation of the endometrium that often is associated with a bacterial infection.

gestation Period of time from conception to birth. For humans, the full period is normally 9 months.

gynecology The branch of medicine that deals with the health maintenance and diseases of women, primarily of the reproductive system.

obstetrics The branch of medicine that deals specifically with the care of women throughout pregnancy.

ovarian cysts Fluid-filled pockets that form on or in an ovary.

pelvic inflammatory disease An infection of the female upper organs of reproduction, specifically the uterus, ovaries, and fallopian tubes.

placenta previa A condition in which the placenta develops over and covers the cervix.

preeclampsia A condition of late pregnancy that involves the gradual onset of hypertension, headache, visual changes, and swelling of the hands and feet, also called pregnancy-induced hypertension or toxemia of pregnancy.

prolapsed umbilical cord When the umbilical cord presents itself outside the uterus while the fetus is still inside; an obstetric emergency during pregnancy or labor that acutely endangers the life of the baby; can happen when the water breaks and the cord comes along with the gush of water.

spontaneous abortion Expulsion of the fetus that occurs naturally; also called miscarriage.

supine hypotensive syndrome Low blood pressure resulting from compression of the inferior vena cava by the weight of the pregnant uterus when the mother is supine.

Special Populations

CHAPTER 17

Pediatric Emergencies

Pediatric patients differ from adults in many important ways, including the kinds of illnesses and injuries they sustain. This chapter reviews some of these conditions, the differences between pediatric and adult patients, and how to tailor your assessment and management procedures to young patients.

Anatomic Differences Between Children and Adults

Children typically have healthier organs than adults. Because their tissues are softer and more flexible, they are generally more resilient and have a greater ability to compensate. Specific differences are outlined below.

Head

- Proportionately larger relative to the body
- Fontanelles must be examined
  - Anterior: Diminishes after 6 months, closes between 9 and 18 months
  - Posterior: Closes by 4 months
- Trauma: Should be held in the neutral position
- Medical: Should be held in the sniffing position to align pharynx and trachea

Airway

- Larynx at C3-C4 extends to the pharynx
- Cricoid ring is the narrowest part of the airway
- Epiglottis extends 45° into airway
- Trachea is softer, flexible, and funnel-shaped when compared to an adult
- Manual maneuvers to maintain a patent airway should be attempted prior to attempting an oropharyngeal airway or nasopharyngeal airway, because of the increased potential for swelling and trauma in an already narrow passage
- Infants up to 4–6 months of age are obligate nose breathers and become obstructed more easily than adults

Chest and Lungs

- Depend more on the diaphragm to breathe
- Prone to gastric distention
- Soft, pliable ribs
- Lungs prone to pneumothorax following barotraumas

Abdomen

- Frequent liver and spleen damage because these organs occupy a relatively greater percentage of a child's abdomen
- Higher risk of multiple organ damage as a result of compactness of organs

Skin and Body Surface Area

- Skin thinner than adults (less subcutaneous fat)
- Larger body surface area relative to weight
  - More sensitive to exposure

Pediatric Development and Common Illnesses/Injuries

Pediatric patients can be classified by age into neonates (newborn to 1 month), infants (1 to 12 months), toddlers (12 to 36 months), preschoolers (3 to 6 years), school age, and adolescents.

Neonates

- **Development:** Limited behaviors—sleeping, eating, and crying
- **Common illnesses:** Meningitis, jaundice, vomiting, and respiratory distress

Infants, 1 to 5 Months

- **Development:** Birth weight doubles and muscle control develops
- **Common illnesses:** Sudden infant death syndrome (SIDS), vomiting, dehydration, meningitis, child abuse, and household accidents

Infants, 6 to 12 Months

- **Development:** Oral fixations
- **Common illnesses:** SIDS, foreign body airway obstruction (FBAO), febrile seizures, vomiting, diarrhea, dehydration, bronchiolitis, motor vehicle collisions (MVCs), croup, child abuse, poisoning, falls, and meningitis

Toddlers

- **Development:** Fine motor development
- **Common illnesses:** FBAO, febrile seizures, vomiting, diarrhea, dehydration, bronchiolitis, MVCs, croup, child abuse, poisoning, falls, choking, meningitis, and respiratory syncytial virus (RSV) infections

Preschoolers

- **Development:** Increase in fine and gross motor development and language skills; temperamental
- **Common illnesses:** Epiglottitis and croup

Primary Assessment

Your actions depend on your across-the-room assessment. **Figure 17-1** shows the Pediatric Assessment Triangle, a tool that will help you form a rapid initial assessment of a pediatric patient's condition. It comprises three elements—appearance, work of breathing, and circulation—that together help assess the level of acuity of the child's illness.

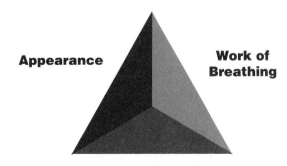

Figure 17-1 The Pediatric Assessment Triangle.

Used with permission of the American Academy of Pediatrics, Pediatric Education for Prehospital Professionals, © American Academy of Pediatrics, 2000.

Assessing Vital Signs

Table 17-1 shows normal rates for pulse, respirations, and blood pressure in children. *An abnormally low pulse indicates hypoxia and imminent cardiac arrest.*

Table 17-1 Vital Signs at Various Ages

Age	Pulse Rate (beats/min)	Respirations (beats/min)	Blood Pressure (mm Hg)	Temperature (°C)
Newborn (0 to 1 month)	90 to 180	30 to 60	50 to 70	36.6 to 37.7
Infant (1 month to 1 year)	100 to 160	25 to 50	70 to 95	36 to 37.5
Toddler (1 to 3 years)	90 to 150	20 to 30	80 to 100	36 to 37.5
Preschool age (3 to 5 years)	80 to 140	20 to 25	80 to 100	36
School age (5 to 12 years)	70 to 120	15 to 20	80 to 110	36
Adolescent (12 to 18 years)	60 to 100	12 to 16	90 to 110	36
Early adult (19 to 40 years)	70	12 to 20	90 to 140	36
Middle adult (41 to 60 years)	70	12 to 20	90 to 140	36
Late adult (61 and older)	Depends on health	Depends on health	Depends on health	36

Glasgow Coma Scale

The **Glasgow Coma Scale** is a method for assessing mental status and neurologic function. **Table 17-2** shows the values used with pediatric patients.

Table 17-2 Pediatric Glasgow Coma Scale

Eyes		Verbal		Motor	
Spontaneous	4	Happy, coos	5	Spontaneous	6
Open to speech	3	Consolable	4	Localizes pain	5
Open to pain	2	Weak cry	3	Withdraws (pain)	4
None	1	Moans	2	Flexion (decorticate)	3
		None	1	Extension (decerebrate)	2
				None	1

Common Causes of Altered Mental Status

AEIOU–TIPS
- **A** – Alcohol, anoxia
- **E** – Encephalitis, epilepsy
- **I** – Insulin (diabetes)
- **O** – Overdose
- **U** – Uremia
- **T** – Trauma
- **I** – Infection
- **P** – Psychiatric
- **S** – Stroke (cardiovascular)

Assessing the Newborn

The **Apgar score** is a tool for assessing the condition of a newborn and determining whether the newborn requires resuscitation (**Table 17-3**). It is performed at 1 minute and 5 minutes after delivery. If the 5-minute score is lower than 7, the newborn is reassessed again every 5 minutes until 20 minutes after birth.

Table 17-3 The Apgar Score

	0 (Absent)	1 (Some)	2 (Lively)
Appearance	Cyanotic	Acrocyanosis	Pink, lively
Pulse	Absent	Central/no peripherals; < 100 beats/min	Strong; > 100 beats/min
Grimace, irritability	Absent	Some	Lively cry
Activity, muscle tone	Absent	Some flexion	Active movement
Respirations	Absent	Weak/irregular	Strong

Respiratory Distress/Cyanosis in the Newborn

Pathophysiology

Prematurity is the most common factor in respiratory distress. The term *premature* refers to any baby born prior to 37 weeks of gestation or with a birth weight of 0.6 to 2.2 kg. A fetus is generally considered viable after 28 weeks. Respiratory distress frequently occurs in infants who weigh less than 1 kg (2 lb) and are born prior to 30 weeks.

Signs and Symptoms

- Accessory muscle use
- Nasal flaring
- Retractions
- Increased work of breathing
- Cyanosis
- Increased air intake
- Tachycardia
- Bradycardia (a sign of severe hypoxia and impending cardiac arrest)
- Altered level of consciousness (LOC)

Assessment

- Scene size-up
  - Ensure body substance isolation (BSI).
- Initial/primary assessment
  - Assess LOC.
  - Manage ABCs (airway, breathing, circulation).
  - Treat life-threatening illness/injuries.
  - Transport considerations: Transport in a position of comfort.
- Focused history and physical exam/secondary assessment
  - Obtain SAMPLE history and chief complaint (OPQRST).

Management

- Apply supplemental oxygen.
- Suction, as needed.
- Establish intravenous (IV) access.
- Reassure patient.
- Monitor vital signs.
- Apply cardiac monitor.
- Provide supportive, symptomatic care.
- Maintain body temperature.
- Ventilate if the heart rate is less than 100 beats/min and the patient is cyanotic.
- Perform chest compressions if the heart rate is less than 60 beats/min.

Upper Airway Emergencies

Four upper airway conditions that commonly affect children are croup, epiglottitis, bacterial tracheitis, and FBAO.

Croup (Laryngotracheobronchitis)

Pathophysiology

<u>Croup</u> is a viral infection of the upper airway. It is characterized by inflammation and spasm of the upper airway and usually occurs following an upper respiratory infection with a low-grade fever. The inflammation of the larynx causes primary symptoms. This illness is most common in children between 3 months and 3 years of age. Croup usually resolves without significant breathing problems.

As a general rule, if there is stridor but no fever, be particularly concerned about the possibility of FBAO. If both stridor and fever are present, suspect croup or epiglottitis.

Signs and Symptoms

- Respiratory distress
- Low-grade fever
- Inspiratory stridor due to subglottic edema
- Hoarse or muffled sounds
- Laryngeal obstruction
- Inflammatory edema or spasms
- Seal-like barking cough due to vocal cords swelling
- Wheezing
- Hoarseness
- Patient prefers to sit upright because of inflammation of the airway

Assessment

- Scene size-up
  - Ensure BSI.
- Initial/primary assessment
  - Assess LOC.
  - Manage ABCs.
  - Treat life-threatening illness/injuries.
  - Transport considerations: Transport in a position of comfort.
- Focused history and physical exam/secondary assessment
  - Obtain SAMPLE history and chief complaint (OPQRST).

Management

- Apply supplemental oxygen.
- Suction, as needed.
- Establish IV access.
- Reassure patient.
- Monitor vital signs.
- Apply cardiac monitor.
- Cool mist oxygen decreases subglottic edema.

Table 17-4 summarizes the treatment of croup.

Table 17-4 Treatment of Croup

Treatment	Purpose	Pediatric Dose	Notes
Albuterol	Bronchodilation	2.5 mg with ipratropium 2.5 mL (first treatment only) < 15 kg (33 lb): 2.5 mg > 15 kg (33 lb): 5.0 mg	Maximum of three treatments

Table 17-4 Treatment of Croup (Continued)

Treatment	Purpose	Pediatric Dose	Notes
Methylprednisolone	Anti-inflammatory	IV: 2 mg/kg	Maximum of 125 mg
Epinephrine (1:1,000)	Stimulates both alpha- and beta-adrenergic receptors	SQ: 0.01 mg/kg	Min: 0.1 mg/kg Max: 0.5 mg
Magnesium sulfate	Smooth muscle relaxant	SIVP: 25-50 mg/kg diluted in 50-100 mL	Administer over 5-10 min
Racemic epinephrine	Relaxes smooth muscle of bronchi	< 15 kg (33 lb): 0.5 mL > 15 kg (33 lb): 1 mL	Mixed with 3 mL of normal saline

IV, intravenous; SQ, subcutaneous; SIVP, slow intravenous push.

Epiglottitis

Pathophysiology

Epiglottitis is a life-threatening condition caused by a bacterial infection in children 3 to 7 years of age. It has a sudden onset and can progress rapidly, completely occluding the airway and resulting in respiratory arrest if the epiglottis swells over the opening of the trachea. The patient will be noticeably drooling and experiencing difficulty swallowing. Avoid upsetting this child if at all possible; agitation may cause increased work of breathing and decompensation.

Signs and Symptoms

- Pain in throat out of proportion to the physical exam appearance of the posterior oropharynx
- Inability to swallow
- Respiratory distress
- High fever
- Patient assumes tripod position
- Drooling
- Patient looks ill
- Mouth open with tongue protruding
- Quiet or muffled voice
- Stridor
- Inspiratory retractions
- Rhonchi

Assessment

- Scene size-up
  - Ensure BSI.
- Initial/primary assessment
  - Assess LOC.
  - Manage ABCs.
  - Treat life-threatening illness/injuries.
  - Do not make an attempt to visualize airway.
  - Keep child calm and comfortable.
  - Transport considerations: Transport in a position of comfort.
- Focused history and physical exam/secondary assessment
  - Obtain SAMPLE history and chief complaint (OPQRST).

Management

- Apply supplemental oxygen.
- Suction, as needed.
- Establish IV access.
- Reassure patient.

- Monitor vital signs.
- Apply cardiac monitor.
- Prepare for management of a complete airway obstruction.

Bacterial Tracheitis

Pathophysiology

Bacterial tracheitis is an uncommon infectious cause of acute upper airway obstruction. Patients may present with crouplike symptoms, such as barking cough, stridor, and fever; however, patients with bacterial tracheitis do not respond to standard therapy and may experience acute respiratory decompensation.

Signs and Symptoms

- Inspiratory stridor (with or without expiratory stridor)
- Barklike or brassy cough
- Hoarseness
- Worsening or abruptly occurring stridor
- Varying degrees of respiratory distress
- Retractions
- Dyspnea
- Nasal flaring
- Cyanosis
- Sore throat
- Fever
- Dysphonia
- No specific position of comfort (the patient may lie supine)

Assessment

- Scene size-up
  - Ensure BSI.
- Initial/primary assessment
  - Assess LOC.
  - Manage ABCs.
  - Treat life-threatening illness/injuries.
  - Do not make an attempt to visualize airway.
  - Keep child calm and comfortable.
  - Transport considerations: Transport in a position of comfort.
- Focused history and physical exam/secondary assessment
  - Obtain SAMPLE history and chief complaint (OPQRST).

Management

- Apply supplemental oxygen.
- Suction, as needed.
- Establish IV access.
- Reassure patient.
- Monitor vital signs.
- Apply cardiac monitor.
- Provide supportive, symptomatic care.

Foreign Body Airway Obstruction

Pathophysiology

An FBAO can result in either a partial or complete blockage of the trachea. Obstruction of the airway can be a result of different causes, including foreign bodies, allergic reactions, infections, anatomic abnormalities, and trauma.

The onset of respiratory distress may be sudden, with a cough. There is often agitation in the early stage of airway obstruction. The signs of respiratory distress include labored, ineffective breathing until the person is no longer breathing (apnea). Loss of consciousness occurs if the obstruction is not relieved.

Signs and Symptoms
- Coughing
- Universal choking sign
- Stridor
- Increased work of breathing
- Cyanosis
- Altered LOC

Assessment
- Scene size-up
  - Ensure BSI.
- Initial/primary assessment
  - Assess LOC.
  - Manage ABCs.
  - Treat life-threatening illness/injuries.
  - Keep child calm and comfortable.
  - Transport considerations: Transport in a position of comfort.
- Focused history and physical exam/secondary assessment
  - Obtain SAMPLE history and chief complaint (OPQRST).

Management
- Apply supplemental oxygen.
- Establish IV access.
- Reassure patient.
- Monitor vital signs.
- Apply cardiac monitor.
- Attempt to relieve obstruction.

For Infants Younger Than 1 Year:
- Five back slaps and five chest thrusts.
- *Never perform a blind finger sweep.*
- Repeat back slaps and chest thrusts until object is expelled or infant becomes unconscious.
- If infant becomes unconscious, start CPR.

For Children Aged 1 Year to Onset of Puberty:
- Heimlich maneuver (abdominal thrusts) (**Figure 17-2**).
- *Never perform a blind finger sweep.*

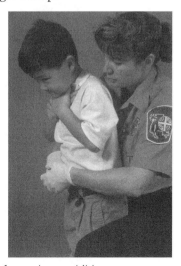

Figure 17-2 Heimlich maneuver performed on a child.

- Repeat the Heimlich maneuver until the object is expelled or the child becomes unconscious.
- If the child becomes unconscious, start CPR.

Lower Airway Emergencies

Lower airway emergencies are usually characterized by wheezing on expiration. Four lower airway conditions that commonly affect children are asthma, status asthmaticus, bronchiolitis, and pneumonia.

Asthma

Pathophysiology

It is estimated that 5% to 10% of children are affected by this disease of the small airways. Asthma rarely occurs before the child's first birthday. It presents in two phases.

- **First phase:** Reaction is characterized by the release of chemical mediators that cause bronchoconstriction and bronchial edema. The treatment goal is to decrease bronchospasms.
- **Second phase:** Inflammation and production of mucus in the bronchioles. The treatment goal is to decrease inflammation and mucus production.

Status asthmaticus is a severe, prolonged asthma attack that does not respond to regular medications (**Table 17-5**). It is considered a life-threatening medical emergency.

Signs and Symptoms
- Tachypnea
- Unproductive cough
- Wheezing

Assessment
- Scene size-up
  - Ensure BSI.
- Initial/primary assessment
  - Assess LOC.
  - Manage ABCs.
  - Treat life-threatening illness/injuries.
  - Keep child calm and comfortable.
  - Transport considerations: Transport in a position of comfort.
- Focused history and physical exam/secondary assessment
  - Obtain SAMPLE history and chief complaint (OPQRST).

Table 17-5 Initial Medications Used to Treat Asthma

Treatment	Used For	Initial Pediatric Dose
Albuterol	Bronchodilation; adrenergic effects	Nebulizer: 0.03 mg/kg
Methylprednisolone	Anti-inflammatory	IV: 1-2 g
Epinephrine	Vasoconstriction of the peripheral and bronchial vessels; increase in contractility, rate, and overall cardiac output; smooth muscle relaxant	SQ: 0.15 mg
Magnesium sulfate	Bronchodilation; anticholinergic effects; decreases histamine release	IV: 25-50 mg/kg
Levalbuterol	Bronchodilation	Nebulizer: 0.625 mg

Management
- Apply supplemental oxygen.
- Establish IV access.
- Reassure patient.
- Monitor vital signs.
- Apply cardiac monitor.

Bronchiolitis
Pathophysiology
Bronchiolitis is a viral infection of the middle airway that primarily affects children in the first year of life. The most common cause is the RSV, which affects the lining of the bronchioles. **Table 17-6** lists initial medications for treating bronchiolitis.

Signs and Symptoms
- Expiratory wheezing
- Fever

Assessment
- Scene size-up
  - Ensure BSI.
- Initial/primary assessment
  - Assess LOC.
  - Manage ABCs.
  - Treat life-threatening illness/injuries.
  - Keep child calm and comfortable.
  - Transport considerations: Transport in a position of comfort.
- Focused history and physical exam/secondary assessment
  - Obtain SAMPLE history and chief complaint (OPQRST).

Management
- Apply humidified supplemental oxygen.
- Establish IV access.
- Reassure patient.
- Monitor vital signs.
- Apply cardiac monitor.

Pneumonia
Pathophysiology
Pneumonia is an infection of the lower airway that may be caused by bacteria, viruses, fungi, or other organisms. In children 1 to 5 years old, the cause is generally viral.

Table 17-6 Initial Medications Used to Treat Bronchiolitis

Treatment	Used For	Initial Pediatric Dose
Albuterol	Bronchodilation; adrenergic effects	Nebulizer: 0.03 mg/kg
Methylprednisolone	Anti-inflammatory	IV: 1-2 g
Epinephrine	Vasoconstriction of the peripheral and bronchial vessels; increase in contractility, rate, and overall cardiac output; smooth muscle relaxant	SQ: 0.15 mg
Magnesium sulfate	Bronchodilation; anticholinergic effects; decreases histamine release	IV: 25-50 mg/kg
Levalbuterol	Bronchodilation	Nebulizer: 0.625 mg

Signs and Symptoms
- History of respiratory infection
- Fever
- Decreased breath sounds
- Crackles, rhonchi, chest pain
- Chest pain (may be **pleuritic**)

Assessment
- Scene size-up
  - Ensure BSI.
- Initial/primary assessment
  - Assess LOC.
  - Manage ABCs.
  - Treat life-threatening illness/injuries.
  - Keep child calm and comfortable.
  - Transport considerations: Transport in a position of comfort.
- Focused history and physical exam/secondary assessment
  - Obtain SAMPLE history and chief complaint (OPQRST).

Management
- Apply humidified supplemental oxygen.
- Establish IV access.
- Reassure patient.
- Monitor vital signs.
- Apply cardiac monitor.
- Provide supportive, symptomatic care.

Hypovolemia

Pathophysiology

Hypovolemia, characterized by internal or external fluid loss or both, is the most common type of shock in pediatric patients.

Signs and Symptoms
- Confusion, anxiety
- Lightheadedness
- Nausea
- Tachycardia
- Weak, thready, narrow pulse
- Tachypnea
- Cold, clammy, pale skin
- Low urine output
- Altered mental status

Assessment
- Scene size-up
  - Ensure BSI.
- Initial/primary assessment
  - Assess LOC.
  - Manage ABCs.
  - Treat life-threatening illness/injuries.
  - Keep child calm and comfortable.
  - Transport considerations: Transport in a position of comfort.

Tip

Children descend very rapidly into irreversible shock. Time is of the essence; diligently monitor their vital signs and appearance. Provide rapid treatment and rapid transport.

- Focused history and physical exam/secondary assessment
  - Obtain SAMPLE history and chief complaint (OPQRST).

Management

- Apply humidified supplemental oxygen.
- Reassure patient.
- Monitor vital signs.
- Apply cardiac monitor.
- Infant: 10 mL/kg of isotonic crystalloid (up to 40–60 mL/kg/h)
- Child: 20 mL/kg of isotonic crystalloid (up to 40–60 mL/kg/h)

Allergic Reaction

Pathophysiology

The pathophysiology of allergic reactions is discussed in Chapter 11. **Table 17-7** summarizes the treatment of pediatric allergic reactions.

Signs and Symptoms

- Urticaria
- Wheezing
- Edema
- Itching
- Dyspnea
- Hypotension
- Agitation, anxiety
- Stridor
- Altered LOC
- Vomiting
- Throat or chest tightness
- Difficulty swallowing
- Diarrhea

Assessment

- Scene size-up
  - Ensure BSI.
- Initial/primary assessment
  - Assess LOC.
  - Manage ABCs.
  - Treat life-threatening illness/injuries.
  - Keep child calm and comfortable.
  - Transport considerations: Transport in a position of comfort.
- Focused history and physical exam/secondary assessment
  - Obtain SAMPLE history and chief complaint (OPQRST).

Management

- Apply supplemental oxygen.
- Reassure patient.
- Monitor vital signs.
- Apply cardiac monitor.
- Infant: 10 mL/kg of isotonic crystalloid (up to 40–60 mL/kg/h)
- Child: 20 mL/kg of isotonic crystalloid (up to 40–60 mL/kg/h)

Table 17-7 Treatment of Pediatric Allergic Reaction

Treatment	Purpose	Pediatric Dose	Notes
0.9% normal saline	Perfusion; increase or maintain blood pressure	IV: 20 mL/kg	Up to 40-60 mL/kg/h
Albuterol	Bronchodilation; adrenergic effects	Nebulizer: 0.03 mg/kg	Maximum of three doses
Diphenhydramine	Anticholinergic; blocks histamines	IV/IM: 1-2 mg/kg	N/A
Epinephrine	Vasoconstriction of the peripheral and bronchial vessels; increases contractility, rate, and overall cardiac output; smooth muscle relaxant	SQ: 0.15 mg IV: 0.15-0.03 mg	Maximum dose 0.3 mg
Levalbuterol	Bronchodilation	Nebulizer: 0.625 mg	No maximum dose
Methylprednisolone	Anti-inflammatory	IV: 1-2 g/kg	Maximum dose: 125 mg
Oxygen	Increase cellular perfusion	12-15 L/min via nonrebreathing mask	N/A
IM, intramuscular.			

Seizures

For an in-depth discussion of seizures, see Chapter 11. Seizures in children may be characterized by a wide variety of presentations. Common presentations follow.

- **Subtle:** Chewing motions, excessive salivation, blinking, sucking, swimming motions (arms), pedaling motion (legs), apnea, color change
- **Tonic:** Rigid posturing of extremities and trunk; fixed eyes; common in premature infants
- **Clonic:** Jerking
- **Focal clonic:** Rhythmic twitching of muscle groups in extremities and face; jerking
- **Multifocal:** Brief focal or generalized jerks of the extremities or parts of distal muscle groups

Febrile Seizures
Pathophysiology
Febrile seizures affect about 1 in 25 children between the ages of 6 months and 6 years. They are caused by the body's rapid change in temperature, not the temperature itself. Simple febrile seizures are not dangerous, but complicated febrile seizures may indicate serious disease. Characteristics of complicated febrile seizures include long seizure activity and failure to return quickly to preictal mental status. Often there is a family history of febrile seizures.

Signs and Symptoms
- High fever

Assessment
- Scene size-up
  - Ensure BSI.

– Protect the patient from further harm; clear the immediate area of potential hazards.
- Initial/primary assessment
  – Assess LOC.
  – Manage ABCs.
  – Treat life-threatening illness/injuries.
  – Keep child calm and comfortable.
  – Transport considerations: Transport in a position of comfort.
- Focused history and physical exam/secondary assessment
  – Obtain SAMPLE history and chief complaint (OPQRST).
  – The family or bystanders can provide helpful information regarding the history of the seizure, preceding events, and other possible illnesses or causes.

Management
- See Chapter 11 for the management and treatment of seizures.

Meningitis

Pathophysiology

An in-depth discussion of meningitis can be found in Chapter 11. **Table 17-8** summarizes the treatment of meningitis.

Signs and Symptoms

- Fever
- Altered LOC
- Irritability
- Headache
- Photophobia (eye sensitivity to light)
- Stiff neck
- Skin rashes
- Seizures

Assessment

- Scene size-up
  – Ensure BSI.
- Initial/primary assessment
  – Assess LOC.
  – Manage ABCs.
  – Treat life-threatening illness/injuries.
  – Keep child calm and comfortable.
  – Transport considerations: Transport in a position of comfort.
- Focused history and physical exam/secondary assessment
  – Obtain SAMPLE history and chief complaint (OPQRST).

Management

- Apply supplemental oxygen.
- Reassure patient.
- Monitor vital signs.
- Apply cardiac monitor.
- Establish IV access.
- Provide supportive, symptomatic care.

> **Tip**
>
> Thirty percent of children with meningitis develop permanent complications; 5% to 15% of children with bacterial meningitis die. Always assume meningitis in a pediatric patient with a fever unless otherwise ruled out! Take appropriate universal precautions to protect you and your coworkers.

Table 17-8 Treatment of Meningitis

Treatment	Purpose	Pediatric Dose
Acetaminophen or ibuprofen	Relieve headache and fever	PR/PO: 15 mg/kg
PR, rectal administration; PO, by mouth.		

Diabetic Ketoacidosis

For an in-depth discussion of the pathophysiology and signs and symptoms of diabetic ketoacidosis, see Chapter 10. **Table 17-9** summarizes the treatment of pediatric diabetic ketoacidosis.

Assessment

- Scene size-up
  - Ensure BSI.
- Initial/primary assessment
  - Assess LOC.
  - Manage ABCs.
  - Treat life-threatening illness/injuries.
  - Keep child calm and comfortable.
  - Transport considerations: Transport in a position of comfort.
- Focused history and physical exam/secondary assessment
  - Obtain SAMPLE history and chief complaint (OPQRST).

Management

- Apply supplemental oxygen.
- Reassure patient.
- Monitor vital signs.
- Monitor blood glucose levels.
- Apply cardiac monitor.
- Establish IV access.

Table 17-9 Treatment of Diabetic Ketoacidosis

Treatment	Purpose	Pediatric Dose
0.9% normal saline	Perfusion; increase or maintain radial pulses; attempt to "dilute" circulating glucose	IV: 20 mL/kg

Hypoglycemia

See Chapter 10 for a full discussion of the pathophysiology and signs and symptoms of hypoglycemia. **Table 17-10** summarizes the treatment of hypoglycemia.

Assessment

- Scene size-up
  - Ensure BSI.
- Initial/primary assessment
  - Assess LOC.
  - Manage ABCs.
  - Treat life-threatening illness/injuries.
  - Keep child calm and comfortable.
  - Transport considerations: Transport in a position of comfort.
- Focused history and physical exam/secondary assessment
  - Obtain SAMPLE history and chief complaint (OPQRST).

Management

- Apply supplemental oxygen.
- Reassure patient.
- Monitor vital signs.
- Monitor blood glucose levels.
- Apply cardiac monitor.
- Establish IV access.
- For responsive patients with an intact gag reflex, administer oral glucose.
- For unresponsive patients without an intact gag reflex, administer D_{25} if the blood glucose level falls below 60 mg/dL.

Table 17-10 Treatment of Hypoglycemia

Treatment	Purpose	Pediatric Dose	Notes
Dextrose 25%	Increase glucose levels	2 mg/kg	Do not allow infusion into skin from nonpatent IV. Infiltration of an IV with dextrose solution will lead to necrosis of the tissue.

Pediatric Arrhythmias

Ventricular Fibrillation

Ventricular fibrillation (v-fib) (**Figure 17-3**) is caused by erratic firing from multiple sites in the ventricle. It is rare in pediatric prehospital cardiac arrest. **Table 17-11** summarizes treatment of v-fib.

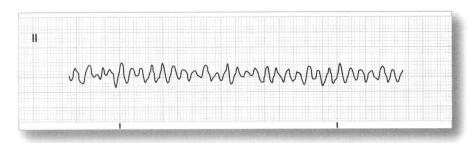

Figure 17-3 Ventricular fibrillation.

Table 17-11 Treatment of Ventricular Fibrillation

Treatment	Purpose	Pediatric Dose
Defibrillation	Cardiac reset	2 J/kg, 4 J/kg
Epinephrine	Stimulates both alpha- and beta-adrenergic receptors	IV: 0.01 mg/kg ETT: 0.1 mg/kg
Lidocaine *or* Amiodarone (preferred)	Suppresses automaticity and spontaneous depolarization of ventricles Prolongs action potential and refractory period; slows sinus rate; PR and QT intervals; vasodilation	IV: 1 mg/kg ETT: 1.5 mg/kg IV: 5 mg/kg
Magnesium sulfate	Important for muscle contraction and nerve transmission	IV: 50 mg/kg

Asystole ("Flat Line")

Asystole is an absence of cardiac activity (**Figure 17-4**), electrical or mechanical. Mechanical equipment difficulty can mimic asystole. Be sure to confirm in two or more leads if this rhythm is present.

Table 17-12 summarizes treatment of asystole.

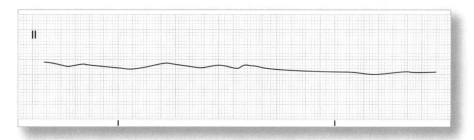

Figure 17-4 Asystole.

Table 17-12 Treatment of Asystole

Treatment	Purpose	Pediatric Dose
Epinephrine	Stimulates both alpha- and beta-adrenergic receptors; positive inotrope (increases strength of cardiac contractions) and increases heart rate	IV/IO (1:10,000): 0.1 mL/kg IV/IO (1:1,000): 0.1 mL/kg
Atropine	Increases heart rate; blocks parasympathetic nervous system	IV/IO: 0.02 mg/kg
IO, intraosseus.		

If the child has bradycardia and an initial assessment demonstrates oxygenation, ventilation, or perfusion abnormalities, provide 100% oxygen and transport. If the child does not respond to oxygen, begin assisted bag-mask ventilation. In rare cases, chest compressions for bradycardia are necessary.

If the heart rate does not rise in response to assisted ventilations, in most cases you should administer epinephrine as the first-line drug at 1:10,000, 0.01 mg/kg IV or IO, or 0.1 mL kg, every 3 to 5 min. Also administer atropine, 0.02 mg/kg IV or IO (minimum dose 0.1 mg) after epinephrine.

Pediatric Interventions

Fluid Replacement

- Child: 20 mL/kg normal saline or lactated Ringer's solution over 20 minutes.
- Infant: 10 mL/kg normal saline or lactated Ringer's solution over 5 to 10 minutes.
- Normal saline and lactated Ringer's solution stay in vascular spaces longer than dextrose.
- Rapid fluid bolus is acceptable in pediatric patients because they are less likely to develop pulmonary edema.
- Repeat if
  - Good response but circulation is inadequate
  - No response

- In childhood diabetic ketoacidosis, hypotonic fluids can increase cerebral edema and increase intracranial pressure.

Pediatric Infusions

Intraosseous Infusion Procedure
- Find the anterior medial flat surface of the tibia.
- Go 2 cm below the growth plate (tibial tuberosity).
- Clean site with alcohol.
- Place needle in the leg in a twisting motion; if you are using an IO device other than manual, activate trigger. You will hear and feel a popping sensation when you enter the bone marrow space.
- Aspirate for bone marrow. It should be noted that even if you have correct placement, you may not be able to aspirate marrow.
- Infuse fluids as you would an IV site.
- Secure the needle and site.

Administering Pediatric Drugs

Table 17-13 summarizes pediatric drug information.

Table 17-13 Pediatric Drug Information

Drug *Type (Concentration)*	Uses	Dose	Notes
Acetaminophen Analgesic	Fever	PO: 15 mg/kg	Every 4 hours
Adenosine Antiarrhythmic	Supraventricular tachycardia (SVT)/ paroxysmal supraventricular tachycardia (PSVT)	IV/IO: 0.1 mg/kg; repeat at 0.2 mg/kg	Follow with rapid flush of normal saline, max 6 mg
Albuterol Bronchodilator	Respiratory distress	Nebulizer: 0.03 mL/kg	Repeat as needed
Amiodarone Antiarrhythmic	Ventricular fibrillation (v-fib) Pulseless ventricular tachycardia (v-tach) Stable wide complex tachycardia	IV/IO: 5 mg/kg	Rapid IV push in cardiac arrest Over 10 minutes in perfusing rhythms
Atropine Anticholinergic	Symptomatic bradycardia refractory to epinephrine	IV/IO/ETT: 0.02 mg/kg	Min single dose = 0.1 mg Max child dose = 0.5 mg Max adolescent dose = 1 mg
Dextrose	Hypoglycemia	IV/IO: 0.5 g/kg $D_{25}W$: 2–4 mL/kg $D_{10}W$: 5–10 mL/kg	Slow IV push (SIVP), ensuring a patent site
Diphenhydramine Antihistamine	Allergic reaction	IV/IO/IM: 1–2 mg/kg	Max: 50 mg
Dopamine infusion	Hypotension	10 µg/kg/min	Titrate to adequate blood pressure

Continues

Table 17-13 Pediatric Drug Information (Continued)

Drug Type (Concentration)	Uses	Dose	Notes
Epinephrine Sympathomimetic (1:10,000) (1:1,000)	Anaphylaxis (1:1,000) V-fib Pulseless v-tach Asystole Pulseless electrical activity Severe respiratory distress	IV/SQ/ETT: 0.01 mg/kg IV: (1:10,000) 0.01 mg/kg ETT: (1:1,000) 0.1 mg/kg SQ: (1:1,000) 0.01 mg/kg	Max: 0.3-0.5 mg Max: 10-50 µg/kg Drip: 1 µg/mg/min Max: 0.3 mg
Epinephrine infusion	Hypotension	0.1 µg/kg/min	Titrate to adequate blood pressure
Flumazenil Benzodiazepine antagonist	Benzodiazepine overdose	IV/IO: 0.01 mg/kg	Max: single dose 0.2 mg Max overall dosage: 1 mg
Glucagon	Hypoglycemia	IV/IM/SQ/IN, < 20 kg: 0.5 mg IV/IM/SQ/IN, > 20 kg: 1.0 mg	If unable to establish vascular access
Lidocaine Antiarrhythmic	Wide complex tachycardia V-fib Pulseless v-tach	IV/IO/ETT: 1.0-1.5 mg/kg	Maximum dose of 3 mg/kg
Lidocaine infusion	Ventricular irritability	20-50 µg/kg/min	Titrate to continued suppression of arrhythmia
Lorazepam Anticonvulsant	Status epilepticus (seizure activity)	IV/IO/IM: 0.05-0.2 mg/kg	Max: 4 mg
Magnesium sulfate Electrolyte	Torsades Refractory v-fib/ pulseless v-tach Asthma	IV/IO: 25-50 mg/kg every 10-20 min	Max: 2 g
Methylprednisolone Anti-inflammatory	Inflammation	IV: 2-4 mg/kg	Max: 125 mg
Naloxone Opioid antagonists	Narcotic overdose	IV/IO/ETT/IN: 0.1 mg/kg	Max: 2 mg
Terbutaline Bronchodilator	Respiratory distress	IV/SQ: 0.01 mg/kg	Max: 0.4 mg

Table 17-14 outlines pediatric drug dosages for rapid-sequence intubation (RSI).

Table 17-14 Pediatric Rapid-Sequence Intubation Drug Dosages

Drug	Name	Dosage	Notes
Sedatives: Presentation for RSI			
Diazepam	Valium	IV/IO: 0.25 mg/kg	Hypotension/respiratory depression
Midazolam	Versed	IV: 2.5 mg IM: 5 mg	Hypotension May repeat in 5 min at 1.0-1.5 mg
Etomidate	Amidate	IV/IO: 0.2-0.6 mg/kg	Do not use for head injury

Table 17-14 Pediatric Rapid-Sequence Intubation Drug Dosages (Continued)

Drug	Name	Dosage	Notes
Sublimaze	Fentanyl	IV/IO: 3 μg/kg	Can cause muscle rigidity in chest wall if administered quickly and/or in high (> 5 μg/kg) doses
Neuromuscular Blocking Agents			
Depolarizing (binds to the acetylcholine receptors at the neuromuscular junction)			
Succinylcholine*	Anectine	IV/IO: 2 mg/kg (infant) IV/IO: 1.0 mg/kg (peds)	Facilitate intubation of the conscious patient
Nondepolarizing (binds to the same receptors and blocks acetylcholine at the junction)			
Pancuronium	Pavulon	IV/IO: 0.06–0.1 mg/kg in children > 1 month	Facilitate intubation of the conscious patient
Vecuronium	Norcuron	IV/IO: 0.1 mg/kg in children > 10 years	Facilitate intubation of the conscious patient
Adjunctive RSI Agents			
Atropine sulfate	Atropine	IV/IO: 0.02 mg/kg	Pediatric patients are premedicated with atropine prior to intubation to prevent bradycardia.
Lidocaine hydrochloride	Xylocaine	IV/IO: 1.5 mg/kg	Decrease intracranial pressure in head injury Decrease gag reflex/laryngospasm

* Causes muscle fasciculations (twitching).

Vital Vocabulary

Apgar score A scoring system for assessing the status of a newborn that assigns a number value to each of five areas of assessment.

bronchiolitis A condition seen in children younger than 2 years, characterized by dyspnea and wheezing.

croup A childhood viral disease characterized by edema of the upper airways with barking cough, difficulty breathing, and stridor.

epiglottitis Inflammation of the epiglottis.

Glasgow Coma Scale An evaluation tool used to determine a patient's neurologic status, which evaluates three categories: eye opening, verbal response, and motor response; effective in helping to determine the extent of neurologic injury.

pleuritic Inflammation of the pleura (the membrane around the lungs).

pneumonia An inflammation of the lungs caused by bacteria, viruses, fungi, or other organisms.

status asthmaticus A severe, prolonged asthma attack that cannot be broken with epinephrine.

Geriatric Considerations

Geriatric patients are defined as people aged 65 years or older. In the year 2000, the number of Americans over age 65 increased to 13% of the population. Estimates are that by the year 2030, over 20% of the population will be older than 65 years. Because of this increasing geriatric population, and the independence of geriatric individuals, more and more prehospital providers are being called on to care for and transport these patients.

Geriatric Patients

Because of the physiologic changes that characterize the aging process, treatment of geriatric patients is different in many respects from treatment of young to middle-aged adults and requires a greater understanding of the changes seen with age. **Table 18-1** lists a few of the more prominent systemic changes in the geriatric patient.

Geriatric Assessment

The GEMS Diamond

The GEMS diamond (**Table 18-2**) was created to help providers recall key themes when dealing with geriatric patients. It was designed to assist the prehospital professional in the assessment and treatment of elderly patients. The GEMS diamond provides a concise way to remember the important issues for older patients.

"G" stands for *geriatric patient*. The provider's thought process needs to be geared to the possible problems of an aging patient. Remember that older patients are different from younger patients and may present atypically.

"E" stands for an *environmental assessment*. Assessment of the environment can help give clues to the patient's condition or the cause of the emergency.

"M" stands for *medical assessment*. Older patients tend to have a variety of medical problems and may be taking numerous prescription, over-the-counter, and herbal medications. Obtaining a thorough history is very important in older patients.

"S" stands for *social assessment*. Older people may have less of a social network, because of the death of a spouse, family members, or friends. Older people may also need assistance with activities of daily living, such as dressing and eating. There are numerous social agencies that are readily available to help geriatric patients.

Factors Complicating Assessment

- Variability: Older people differ tremendously from one another both physically and mentally.
- Physiologic age is more important than chronologic age.
- Response to illness differs.
- Patients seek help for only a small part of their symptoms.
- Patients perceive symptoms as "just getting old."
- Patients delay seeking treatment.

Table 18-1 Physiologic Changes in Geriatric Patients

System	Increased Due to Aging	Decreased Due to Aging	Pathophysiologic Results
Cardiovascular	Systolic blood pressure (BP), peripheral resistance, left ventricular stiffness, ventricular filling due to atrial contraction (late diastolic phase), arrhythmias Other: **Atherosclerosis** increases vessel stiffness	Cardiac output, vasoconstriction, response time (to catecholamines), force, compliance, response in heart rate, pacemaker cells	Higher BP, hypertrophy of left ventricle, prolonged contraction, reduction in cardiac output, increased susceptibility to diastolic heart failure, S_4 heart tone, reduced response in heart rate to exercise, reduced blood supply to organs, resting bradycardia
Respiratory	Increased size of individual alveoli (however, they decrease in total number)	Elastic recoil, smooth muscle strength, alveolar surface, lung defenses, lining of the airway (cilia)	Greater susceptibility to aspiration and respiratory infections; decreased cough reflex, carbon dioxide diffusion, Pao_2; strength of smooth muscles can cause the airway to swell or collapse with the positive and negative pressures of ventilation
Renal		Loss of functioning nephrons; decrease in overall mass of kidneys, renal artery size, renal blood flow	Medication dosage changes may be required due to the inability of the renal system to process the medications; increase in urinary frequency and incontinence
Musculoskeletal		Muscle mass, lean body mass, progressive loss of bone mineral density (**osteoporosis**), atrophy, loss of elasticity	Impaired mobility; susceptibility to trauma, postural changes, arthritis
Glucose regulation		Insulin sensitivity	Glucose regulation issues such as hypoglycemia and hyperglycemia
Sexual function		Declines	Patients may require medication to restore sexual function.
Gastrointestinal		Diminished sense of taste and smell; less saliva and dental loss; reduced gastric secretions and slower gastric emptying; loss of anal sphincter elasticity	More gastric acid produced, acid reflux, lactose intolerance, constipation, fecal incontinence

Table 18-1 Physiologic Changes in Geriatric Patients (Continued)

System	Increased Due to Aging	Decreased Due to Aging	Pathophysiologic Results
Nervous		Decreased brain weight and cerebral blood flow; peripheral nervous system slowing; fewer pain receptors and nerve cells (causing an increase in length and dendritic connections of remaining nerve cells)	Acute or chronic behavior and cognitive changes; potential for increased subdural hematomas due to brain shrinkage; increased neuron travel time, causing a delay in processing information; decreased sensation and slowed reflexes; altered or absent pain response
Immune	Increased levels of IgG and IgA	Decreased cell-mediated immunity, basal and stimulated interleukin levels, response of lymphocytes to antigens, IgM, response to antigens, number and effectiveness of killer T cells	Pneumonia and urinary tract infection prevalent; greater susceptibility to cancer
Integumentary		Decreased sweat glands activity, resiliency of the skin, elasticity, size of subcutaneous fatty layer	Decreased elastin and collagen causes decrease in strength and pliability; dermis becomes drier, allowing for easier lacerations and increasing risk of trauma due to thinning of the subcutaneous tissue and decreasing shock-absorbing capabilities

- Patients trivialize chief complaints.
- Presence of multiple pathologies: 85% have one chronic disease; 30% have three or more
- Acute illness in one system stresses the reserve capacity of other systems.
- Symptoms or treatment of one disease may mask another disease.
- Altered presentation
- Diminished or absent pain
- Depressed temperature regulation
- Depressed thirst mechanisms
- Confusion, restlessness, hallucinations
- Generalized deterioration
- Vague, poorly defined complaints
- Communication problems
- Diminished cognitive function
- Depression
- Poor cooperation
- Limited mobility
- Polypharmacy

Table 18-2 The GEMS Diamond

G—Geriatric Patients	E—Environmental Assessment
• Present atypically • Deserve respect • Experience normal changes with age	• Check the physical condition of the patient's home: Is the exterior of the home in need of repair? Is the home secure? • Check for hazardous conditions that may be present (eg, poor wiring, rotted floors, unventilated gas heaters, broken window glass, clutter that prevents adequate egress) • Are smoke detectors present and working? • Is the home too hot or too cold? • Is there an odor of feces or urine in the home? Is bedding soiled or urine-soaked? • Is food present in the home? Is it adequate and unspoiled? • Are liquor bottles present? If so, are they lying empty? • If the patient has a disability, are appropriate assistive devices (eg, a wheelchair or walker) present? • Does the patient have access to a telephone? • Are medications outdated or unmarked, or are prescriptions for the same or similar medications from many physicians? • If living with others, is the patient confined to one part of the home? • If the patient is residing in a nursing facility, does the care appear to be adequate to meet the patient's needs?
M—Medical Assessment	**S—Social Assessment**
• Older patients tend to have a variety of medical problems, making assessment more complex. Keep this in mind in all cases—both trauma and medical. A trauma patient may have an underlying medical condition that could have caused or may be exacerbated by the injury • Obtaining a medical history is important in older patients, regardless of the chief complaint • Initial assessment • Ongoing assessment	• Assess activities of daily living (eating, dressing, bathing, toileting) • Are these activities being provided for the patient? If so, by whom? • Are there delays in obtaining food, medication, or other necessary items? The patient may complain of this, or the environment may suggest this • If in an institutional setting, is the patient able to feed himself or herself? If not, is food still sitting on the food tray? Has the patient been lying in his or her own urine or feces for prolonged periods? • Does the patient have a social network? Does the patient have a mechanism to interact socially with others on a daily basis?

History Taking

- Probe for significant, life-threatening complaints.
- Chief complaint may seem trivial and unrelated to the acute problem. The chief complaint may be vague and nonspecific.

- Patient may not volunteer information.
- Dealing with communication difficulties:
  - Talk to the patient first.
  - If possible, talk to the patient alone, in a quiet, nondistracting location.
  - Use a formal, respectful approach.
  - Position yourself near the middle of the patient's visual field, at eye level.
  - Do not assume deafness and shout.
  - Speak slowly and enunciate clearly.
  - Do *not* assume that a confused or disoriented patient is "just senile."
  - Obtain a thorough medication history regarding:
    - More than one doctor
    - More than one pharmacy
    - Old versus current medications
    - Shared medications
    - Over-the-counter medications
    - Medication compliance

Physical Examination

- Examine the patient in a warm, well-lit area.
- The patient may fatigue easily.
- The patient may have difficulty with positioning. Older patients may require more time than younger patients because of decreased agility.
- Consider the patient's modesty.
- Decreased pain sensation requires a thorough examination.
- If the patient says it hurts, it probably *really* hurts!
- Examine patient carefully.
- Findings may be misleading; for example, bradycardia may be due to unintentional beta-blocker overdose and not due to a heart block or failing pacemaker, and inelastic skin may mimic decreased turgor.
- Mouth breathing may give the impression of dyspnea.
- Inactivity or the dependent position of the feet may cause peripheral edema.
- Crackles or rales in lung bases may be **nonpathologic**.
- Peripheral pulses may be difficult to feel.

Elder Abuse

Reports of physical, emotional, and financial elder abuse have risen dramatically, increasing 150% nationwide since 1986. The role of prehospital providers is not to prove that it has occurred, but to recognize and report your suspicions.

Effective Communication Techniques

- Spend adequate time with the patient.
- Use a private, quiet location.
- Use appropriate nonverbal communication, such as eye contact, hand gestures, facial expressions, and touch.
- Be seated, if possible.
- Establish and maintain eye contact.
- Demonstrate empathy.
- Be respectful.
- Address the patient and loved ones by their given name (ie, Mr. Jones, Mrs. Smith) until directed otherwise.

Mnemonic for Identifying and Treating Elder Abuse

Identification		Treatment	
S	Screen	S	Safety
C	Central injuries	C	Crime
R	Repetitive injuries	R	Referral
A	Abuse (physical + psychological)	A	Acknowledge abuse
P	Possessive caregiver	P	Protocols
E	Explanation inconsistent	E	Evidence collection
D	Direct questions	D	Documentation

- Use understandable language (avoid medical jargon).
- Ask open-ended questions.
- Employ active listening techniques.
- Use reassurance to resolve feelings of guilt or blame.
- Accept the emotions of patients and loved ones.
- Avoid condescending speech or behavior.
- Use additional resources (nursing, psychiatry, pastoral care, social service, etc.).

Pharmacology and the Geriatric Patient

When attending to geriatric patients, remember that many of them are on multiple medications, prescribed and unprescribed (including over-the-counter medications and herbal remedies), by many different physicians. This can lead to several complications such as adverse drug reactions and drug-to-drug interactions. In fact, each additional drug prescribed or taken increases the risk for an **adverse drug-related event** exponentially. In the elderly, pharmacodynamics and pharmacokinetics are altered by metabolic changes, renal decline, and decreased liver function. **Table 18-3** lists medications that pose potential risks to older adults.

Table 18-3 Potentially Inappropriate Medications for the Elderly

A
Alprazolam (Xanax)
Amiodarone (Cordarone)
Amitriptyline (Elavil)
Amphetamines
Anorexic agents

B
Barbiturates
Belladonna alkaloids (Donnatal)
Bisacodyl (Dulcolax)

C
Carisoprodol (Soma)
Cascara sagrada
Chlordiazepoxide (Librium, Mitran)
Chlordiazepoxide-amitriptyline (Limbitrol)
Chlorpheniramine (Chlor-Trimeton)
Chlorpropamide (Diabinese)
Chlorzoxazone (Paraflex)
Cimetidine (Tagamet)
Clidinium-chlordiazepoxide (Librax)
Clonidine (Catapres)
Clorazepate (Tranxene)
Cyclandelate (Cyclospasmol)
Cyclobenzaprine (Flexeril)
Cyproheptadine (Periactin)

D
Desiccated thyroid
Dexchlorpheniramine (Polaramine)
Diazepam (Valium)
Dicyclomine (Bentyl)
Digoxin (Lanoxin)
Diphenhydramine (Benadryl)
Dipyridamole (Persantine)
Disopyramide (Norpace, Norpace CR)
Doxazosin (Cardura)
Doxepin (Sinequan)

Table 18-3 Potentially Inappropriate Medications for the Elderly (Continued)

E
Ergoloid mesylates (Hydergine) Estrogens Ethacrynic acid (Edecrin)
F
Ferrous sulfate (iron) Fluoxetine (Prozac) Flurazepam (Dalmane)
G
Guanadrel (Hylorel) Guanethidine (Ismelin)
H
Halazepam (Paxipam) Hydroxyzine (Vistaril, Atarax)
I
Indomethacin (Indocin, Indocin SR) Isoxsuprine (Vasodilan)
K
Ketorolac (Toradol)
L
Lorazepam (Ativan)
M
Meperidine (Demerol) Meprobamate (Miltown, Equanil) Mesoridazine (Serentil) Metaxalone (Skelaxin) Methocarbamol (Robaxin) Methyldopa (Aldomet) Methyldopa-hydrochlorothiazide (Aldoril) Methyltestosterone (Android, Virilon, Testred) Mineral oil
N
Naproxen (Naprosyn, Anaprox, Aleve) Neoloid Nifedipine (Procardia, Adalat) Nitrofurantoin (Macrodantin)
O
Orphenadrine (Norflex) Oxaprozin (Daypro) Oxazepam (Serax) Oxybutynin (Ditropan)
P
Pentazocine (Talwin) Perphenazine-amitriptyline (Triavil) Piroxicam (Feldene) Promethazine (Phenergan) Propantheline (Pro-Banthine) Propoxyphene (Darvon) and combination products

Continues

Table 18-3 Potentially Inappropriate Medications for the Elderly (Continued)

Q
Quazepam (Doral)
R
Reserpine (Serpalan, Serpasil)
T
Temazepam (Restoril) Thioridazine (Mellaril) Ticlopidine (Ticlid) Triazolam (Halcion) Trimethobenzamide (Tigan) Tripelennamine (Pyribenzamine)
Fick DM, Cooper JW, Wade WE, Waller JL, MacLean R, Beers MH: Updating the Beers criteria for potentially inappropriate medication use in older adults. *Arch Intern Med* 2003; 163: 2716–2724.

Common Geriatric Conditions

Cardiovascular Disorders
- Angina pectoris
- Dysrhythmias
- Aortic dissection/aneurysm
- Hypertension
- Syncope
- Acute myocardial infarction ("silent MI")
- Congestive heart failure

Respiratory Disorders
- Pneumonia
- Chronic obstructive pulmonary disease
- Pulmonary embolism
- Pulmonary edema
- Lung cancer

Neurologic Disorders
- Cerebrovascular disease (stroke)
- Seizures
- Dizziness/vertigo
- Parkinson's disease
- Alzheimer's disease
- Dementia versus delirium
- Neuropsychiatric disease
- Altered mental status

Table 18-4 describes the possible causes of altered mental status in geriatric patients, and **Table 18-5** lists possible causes of delirium.

Musculoskeletal Disorders
- Osteoarthritis
- Osteoporosis

Endocrine Disorders
- Diabetes mellitus
- Thyroid disorders

> **Tip**
>
> **Hint:** Remember that delirium is an acute cognitive change, whereas dementia is more of a chronic cognitive change.

Table 18-4 Possible Causes of Altered Mental Status in Geriatric Patients: VITAMINS-CD

V	Vascular
I	Inflammation
T	Toxins, trauma, tumors
A	Autoimmune
M	Metabolic
I	Infection
N	Narcotics
S	Systemic
C	Congenital
D	Degenerative

Table 18-5 Possible Causes of Delirium: DELIRIUMS

D	Drugs and toxins
E	Emotional
L	Low partial pressure of oxygen
I	Infection
R	Retention
I	Ictal state
U	Undernutrition/dehydration
M	Metabolism
S	Subdural hematoma

Gastrointestinal Disorders
- Gastrointestinal (GI) hemorrhage
- Upper GI bleed
- Lower GI bleed
- Bowel obstruction

Renal Disorders
- **Glomerulonephritis**
- Urinary disorders
- Urinary tract infections

Congestive Heart Failure
Signs and Symptoms
- Fatigue, in left-sided heart failure.
- Dependent edema may signal right-sided failure.
- Shortness of breath, or dyspnea, on exertion.
- Patients may experience orthopnea, or difficulty breathing while lying down. The number of pillows a patient needs to lie on to relieve the discomfort is an indication of the severity of the condition.
- Nocturnal confusion.

- Large, fluid-filled blisters may develop on the legs, especially if the patient sleeps sitting up. Bedridden patients may have fluid over sacral areas rather than the feet or legs.
- A dry, hacking cough that progresses to a productive cough may indicate heart failure.
- **Nocturia.**
- **Anorexia.**
- **Hepatomegaly.**

Assessment
- Scene size-up
  - Ensure body substance isolation (BSI).
- Initial/primary assessment
  - Assess level of consciousness (LOC).
  - Manage ABCs (airway, breathing, circulation).
  - Treat life-threatening illness/injury.
- Focused history and physical exam/secondary assessment
  - Obtain SAMPLE history and chief complaint (OPQRST).
  - Assess vital signs.

Management
- Establish patent airway; if patient has vomited, immediately suction airway to prevent aspiration.
- Administer 100% oxygen.
  - Via nonrebreathing mask if patient is breathing adequately.
  - Via bag-mask ventilation if breathing is inadequate.
- Establish intravenous (IV) access.
- Attach cardiac monitor; evaluate for any arrhythmias.
- If pulmonary edema is present, with an increased work of breathing, apply continuous positive airway pressure at 5 cm H_2O, titrating upward to patient's response.
- Consider vasodilators if the patient is not hypotensive. Vasodilation increases venous capacitance to decrease pulmonary congestion and also decreases after load, thereby increasing cardiac output.

Acute Myocardial Infarction

Signs and Symptoms
- Chest pain is less common in the elderly. In fact, there is a much greater incidence of silent MI in the elderly.
- Dyspnea, or shortness of breath, is the most common sign in patients older than 85 years.
- Any nonspecific complaint of upper trunk discomfort should be considered a possible symptom of MI.
- Vague symptoms, such as weakness, fatigue, syncope, incontinence, or confusion, are possible.

Assessment
- Scene size-up
  - Ensure BSI.
- Initial/primary assessment
  - Assess LOC.
  - Manage ABCs.
  - Treat life-threatening illness/injury.

- Focused history and physical exam/secondary assessment
  - Obtain SAMPLE history and chief complaint (OPQRST).
  - Assess vital signs.

Management

- Establish patent airway; if patient has vomited, immediately suction airway to prevent aspiration.
- Administer 100% oxygen.
  - Via nonrebreathing mask if patient is breathing adequately.
  - Via bag-mask ventilation if breathing is inadequate.
- Establish intravenous IV access.
- Attach cardiac monitor; evaluate for any arrhythmias.
- Administer medications for acute MI (aspirin, nitroglycerin, and morphine), per local protocols.

Vital Vocabulary

adverse drug-related event When a person experiences unwanted, negative effects associated with the use of given medications.

anorexia Inadequate consumption of food. May be due to poor appetite, inadequate strength or energy to eat, or a psychological eating disorder.

atherosclerosis A disorder in which cholesterol and calcium build up inside the walls of the blood vessels, forming plaque, which eventually leads to partial or complete blockage of blood flow.

glomerulonephritis A dry, hacking cough that may progress to a cough that produces pink frothy sputum (as opposed to a mucus or purulent cough in infections).

hepatomegaly Enlargement of the liver, often the result of congestive heart failure or liver disease.

nocturia When a person's need to urinate at night interrupts his or her sleep cycle.

nonpathologic Not resulting from a disease or physical condition.

osteoporosis A condition characterized by decreased bone mass and density and increased susceptibility to fractures.

References

Aehlert B: *Comprehensive Pediatric Emergency Care*, rev ed. St. Louis, MO, Mosby, 2007.

American Academy of Pediatrics: *Pediatric Education for Prehospital Professionals*, rev ed 2. Sudbury, MA, Jones and Bartlett Publishers, 2006.

Beck RK: *Pharmacology for the EMS Provider*, ed 3. Albany, NY, Delmar Thompson Learning, 2002.

Caroline NL: *Emergency Care in the Streets*, ed 6. Sudbury, MA, Jones and Bartlett Publishers, 2007.

Chiras DD: *Human Biology*, ed 6. Sudbury, MA, Jones and Bartlett Publishers, 2008.

Dalton AL, Limmer D, Mistovich JJ, Werman H: *Advanced Medical Life Support*, ed 3. Upper Saddle River, NJ, Pearson Prentice Hall, 2006.

Deglin JH, Vallerand AH: *Davis's Drug Guide for Nurses, Your Best Resources for Drugs*, ed 11. Philadelphia, PA, FA Davis, 2008.

Elson RC, Johnson WD: *Essentials of Biostatistics*, ed 2. Philadelphia, PA, FA Davis, 1994.

Garcia T, Miller G: *Arrhythmias: The Art of Interpretation*. Sudbury, MA, Jones and Bartlett Publishers, 2004.

Holleran R: *Air and Surface Patient Transport: Principles and Practice*, ed 3. St. Louis, MO: Mosby, 2002.

Hung O, Murphy M: *Management of the Difficult and Failed Airway*. New York, NY, McGraw-Hill Professional. 2007.

National Association of Emergency Medical Technicians: *Prehospital Trauma Life Support*. St. Louis, MO: Mosby, 2007.

Quinn E: High altitude illness and acute mountain sickness. http://sportsmedicine.about.com/od/enviromentalissues/a/AltitudeIllness.htm.

Ritchison G: Human physiology: Cell structure and function. http://www.people.eku.edu/ritchisong/RITCHISO/301notes1.htm.

Snyder DR, Christmas C (eds): *Geriatric Education for Emergency Medical Services*. Sudbury, MA, Jones and Bartlett Publishers, 2003.

Walls RM, Murphy MF, Luten RC (eds): *Manual of Emergency Airway Management*, ed 3. Philadelphia, PA, Lippincott Williams & Wilkins, 2008.

Glossary

abandonment Unilateral termination of care by a prehospital provider without the patient's consent and without making provisions for transferring care to another medical professional with skills at the same level or higher.

abdominal aortic aneurysm A saclike widening in the abdominal aorta that is present in 2% to 4% of the population. Rupture results in a 35% mortality rate.

abruptio placentae A premature separation of the placenta from the wall of the uterus.

absorption The process by which a substance's molecules are moved from the site of entry or administration into the body and into systemic circulation.

acidosis A blood pH of less than 7.35—a pathologic condition resulting from the accumulation of acids in the body.

active transport The movement of molecules across a cell membrane from an area of low concentration to an area of higher concentration, using a helper protein and ATP to move the substance against a concentration gradient.

acute mountain sickness (AMS) An altitude illness characterized by headache, dizziness, irritability, breathlessness, and euphoria.

adenoids Lymphatic tissues located on the posterior nasopharyngeal wall that filter bacteria.

adenosine triphosphate (ATP) An organic compound that is the energy source in cells.

adrenal cortex The outer part of the adrenal glands that produces corticosteroids.

adrenal medulla The inner portion of the adrenal glands that synthesizes, stores, and eventually releases epinephrine and norepinephrine.

adrenergic drugs Drugs that affect the sympathetic nervous system (sympathomimetics), which act by directly stimulating the adrenal medulla.

advance directive A written document that expresses the wants, needs, and desires of a patient in reference to future medical care; examples include living wills, do not resuscitate (DNR) orders, and organ donation cards.

adverse drug-related event When a person experiences unwanted, negative effects associated with the use of given medications.

agonists Substances that mimic the actions of a specific neurotransmitter or hormone by binding to the specific receptor of the naturally occurring substance.

alkalosis A blood pH of greater than 7.45—a pathologic condition resulting from the accumulation of bases in the body.

allergens Substances that cause a hypersensitivity reaction.

allergic reaction An abnormal immune response the body develops when reexposed to a substance or allergen.

altered mental status A decrease from the baseline mental status, from conscious and alert, progressing to complete unresponsiveness.

anaphylactic shock A severe hypersensitivity reaction that involves bronchoconstriction and cardiovascular collapse.

anaphylaxis An extreme systemic form of an allergic reaction involving two or more body systems.

androgens Hormones that are involved in the development of male sexual characteristics but are also present in females.

anisocoria A condition in which the pupils are not of equal size.

anorexia Inadequate consumption of food. May be due to poor appetite, inadequate strength or energy to eat, or a psychological eating disorder.

antagonists Molecules that block the ability of a given chemical to bind to its receptor, preventing a biologic response.

anterior cord syndrome A condition that occurs with flexion injuries or fractures resulting in the displacement of bony fragments into the anterior portion of the spinal cord; findings include paralysis below the level of the insult and loss of pain, temperature, and touch sensation.

antiarrhythmics The medications used to treat and prevent cardiac rhythm disorders.

antibodies Proteins secreted by certain immune cells that bind antigens to make them more visible to the immune system.

antiemetic Medication that relieves nausea, to prevent vomiting.

antigens Agents that, when taken into the body, stimulate the formation of specific protective proteins called antibodies.

aortic valve The valve between the left ventricle and the aorta.

Apgar score A scoring system for assessing the status of a newborn that assigns a number value to each of five areas of assessment.

apneustic center Portion of the brainstem that influences the respiratory rate by increasing the number of inspirations per minute.

arrhythmias Disturbances in cardiac rhythm. Also called *dysrhythmias*.

arteries The blood vessels that carry oxygenated blood away from the heart.

arterioles A small-diameter blood vessel that extends and branches out from an artery and leads to capillaries.

ascites Abnormal accumulation of fluid in the peritoneal cavity.

assault To create in another person a fear of immediate bodily harm or invasion of bodily security.

asystole A state of no cardiac electrical activity.

atherosclerosis A disorder in which cholesterol and calcium build up inside the walls of the blood vessels, forming plaque, which eventually leads to partial or complete blockage of blood flow.

atrial fibrillation A rhythm in which the atria no longer contract but fibrillate or quiver without any organized contraction.

atrial tachycardia Any rapid heart rhythm originating in the atria, such as atrial fibrillation and atrial flutter.

atrioventricular (AV) node A specialized structure located in the AV junction that slows conduction through the AV junction.

atrium Upper chamber of the heart.

aura Sensations experienced by a patient before an attack occurs. Common in seizures and migraine headaches.

autoimmunity The production of antibodies or T cells that work against the tissues of a person's own body, producing autoimmune disease.

automaticity Spontaneous initiation of depolarizing electric impulses by pacemaker sites within the electric conduction system of the heart.

autonomic nervous system A subdivision of the nervous system that controls primarily involuntary body functions. It comprises the sympathetic and parasympathetic nervous systems.

autorhythmic cells Cells distributed in an orderly fashion through the heart. They make up the heart's conduction system and are concentrated in the sinoatrial (SA) node, atrioventricular (AV) node, atrioventricular (AV) bundle (bundle of His), and Purkinje fibers.

AVPU A method of assessing mental status by determining whether a patient is awake and alert, responsive to verbal stimuli, responsive to pain, or unresponsive.

bacteria Small organisms that can grow and reproduce outside the human cell in the presence of the proper temperature and nutrients, and that cause disease by invading and multiplying in the tissues of the host.

basophils White blood cells that work to produce chemical mediators during an immune response.

battery Unlawfully touching a person; this includes providing emergency care without consent.

beta-adrenergic blockers Medical treatments that block the inhibitory effects of sympathetic nervous system agents, such as epinephrine.

bicuspid (or mitral) valve The valve located between the left atrium and the left ventricle of the heart.

bipolar Monitor leads that contain two electrodes (positive and negative). Applied to the arms and legs. Found in leads I, II, and III.

Boyle's law At a constant temperature, the volume of gas is inversely proportional to its pressure (if you double the pressure on a gas, you halve its volume); written as $PV = K$, where P = pressure, V = volume, and K = a constant.

brainstem The area of the brain between the spinal cord and cerebrum, surrounded by the cerebellum; controls functions that are necessary for life, such as respiration.

breech presentation A delivery in which the buttocks come out first.

bronchiolitis A condition seen in children younger than 2 years, characterized by dyspnea and wheezing.

buffers Molecules that modulate changes in pH to keep it in the physiologic range.

bundle branch blocks Disturbances in electric conduction through the right or left bundle branch from the bundle of His.

bundle of His The portion of the electric conduction system in the interventricular septum that conducts the depolarizing impulse from the atrioventricular junction to the right and left bundle branches.

burn shock Hypovolemic shock resulting from burns, caused by fluid loss across burned skin and volume shifts in the body.

calcitonin Hormone secreted by the thyroid gland; helps maintain normal calcium levels in the blood.

cancellous bone Trabecular or spongy bone.

capillaries Extremely narrow blood vessels composed of a single layer of cells through which oxygen and nutrients pass to the tissues. Capillaries form a network between arterioles and venules.

carbon monoxide A chemical asphyxiant that results in cellular respiratory failure; this gas binds to hemoglobin to the extent that oxygen in the blood becomes inaccessible to the cells.

cardiac cycle The period from one cardiac contraction to the next. Each cardiac cycle consists of ventricular contraction (systole) and relaxation (diastole).

cardiac output (CO) Amount of blood pumped by the heart per minute, calculated by multiplying the stroke volume by the heart rate per minute.

cardiogenic shock A condition caused by loss of 40% or more of the functioning myocardium; the heart is no longer able to circulate sufficient blood to maintain adequate oxygen delivery.

carina Point at which the trachea divides into the left and right mainstem bronchi.

catecholamines Hormones produced by the adrenal medulla (epinephrine and norepinephrine) that assist the body in coping with physical and emotional stress by increasing the heart and respiratory rates and the blood pressure.

cell-mediated immunity Immune process by which T-cell lymphocytes recognize antigens and then secrete cytokines (specifically, lymphokines) that attract other cells or stimulate the production of cytotoxic cells that kill the infected cells.

cephalic delivery Fetus delivers head first.

chemotaxins Components of the activated complement system that attract leukocytes from circulation to help fight infections.

chronic bronchitis Chronic inflammatory condition affecting the bronchi that is associated with excess mucus production that results from overgrowth of the mucous glands in the airways.

circumferential burns Burns on the neck or chest that may compress the airway or on an extremity that might act like a tourniquet.

coagulation cascade A series of biochemical activities involving clotting factors that result in the formation of the fibrin clot.

compensated shock The early stage of shock, in which the body can still compensate for blood loss.

complement system A group of plasma proteins whose function is to do one of three things: attract leukocytes to sites of inflammation, activate leukocytes, and directly destroy cells.

concentration The total weight of a drug contained in a specific volume of liquid.

conduction Transfer of heat to a solid object or a liquid by direct contact.

conductivity The ability to transmit an electrical impulse from one cell to the next.

contractile cells Cells that make up the muscle walls of the atria and ventricles. They give the heart its ability to pump blood through the body.

contractility The strength of heart muscle contractions.

contralateral The opposite side.

convection Mechanism by which body heat is picked up and carried away by moving air currents.

convulsions Involuntary contraction of the voluntary muscles.

corticosteroids Hormones that regulate the body's metabolism, the balance of salt and water in the body, the immune system, and sexual function.

coup-contrecoup Dual impacting of the brain into the skull.

cricothyroid membrane A thin, superficial membrane located between the thyroid and cricoid cartilages that is relatively avascular and contains few nerves; the site for emergency surgical and nonsurgical access to the airway.

croup A childhood viral disease characterized by edema of the upper airways with barking cough, difficulty breathing, and stridor.

crowning The appearance of the infant's head at the vaginal opening during labor.

Cullen sign Ecchymotic discoloration of the umbilicus—a sign of intraperitoneal hemorrhage.

cytoplasm The protoplasm surrounding the nucleus, which plays a part in cell division and forms the larger part of the human cell.

Dalton's law Each gas in mixture exerts the same partial pressure that it would exert if it were alone in the same volume, and the total pressure of a mixture of gases is the sum of the partial pressures of all the gases in the mixture.

decompensated shock The late stage of shock, when blood pressure is falling.

dehydration Depletion of the body systemic fluid volume.

delirium tremens A severe withdrawal syndrome seen in people with alcoholism who are deprived of ethyl alcohol; characterized by restlessness, fever, sweating, disorientation, agitation, and seizures.

depolarization The process of discharging resting cardiac muscle fibers by an electric impulse that causes them to contract.

depression fracture A fracture in which the broken region of the bone is pushed deeper into the body than the remaining intact bone.

diaphoresis Extreme sweating.

diastasis An increase in the distance between the two sides of a joint.

diastole The period of ventricular relaxation during which the ventricles passively fill with blood.

diencephalon The part of the brain between the brainstem and the cerebrum that includes the thalamus, the subthalamus, hypothalamus, and epithalamus.

diffusion A process in which molecules move from an area of high concentration to an area of lower concentration.

distraction injury An injury that results from a force that tries to increase the length of a body part or separate one body part from another.

distributive shock A condition that occurs when there is widespread dilation of the resistance vessels (small arterioles), the capacitance vessels (small venules), or both.

diverticulosis Irritation or bleeding of the diverticula of the large intestine, thought to be caused by increased pressure within the colon.

dose on hand (DOH) Dose of medication available to the caregiver.

drowning The process of experiencing respiratory impairment from submersion or immersion in liquid.

eclampsia The most severe form of pregnancy-induced hypertension, characterized by seizures.

ectopic beat Any cardiac impulse originating outside the SA node; considered abnormal.

ectopic pregnancy A pregnancy in which the ovum implants somewhere other than the uterine endometrium.

edema A condition in which excess fluid accumulates in tissues, manifested by swelling.

emancipated minors Persons who are under the legal age of consent in a given state but, because of other circumstances, have been legally declared adults by the courts.

endocardium The thin membrane lining the inside of the heart.

endometriosis A condition in which endometrial tissue grows outside the uterus.

endometritis An inflammation of the endometrium that often is associated with a bacterial infection.

eosinophils Cells that make up approximately 1% to 3% of the leukocytes; they play a major role in allergic reactions and bronchoconstriction in an asthma attack.

epicardium The thin membrane lining the outside of the heart.

epiglottitis Inflammation of the epiglottis.

erythrocytes Red blood cells.

erythropoiesis The formation of erythrocytes, taking place mainly in the marrow of the sternum, ribs, vertebral processes, and skull bones in adults.

eschar The damaged tissue that forms on the skin over a burn injury.

estrogen One of the major female hormones. At puberty, estrogen brings about the secondary sex characteristics.

evaporation The conversion of a liquid to a gas.

excitability The ability to respond to an electrical impulse.

expressed consent A type of informed consent that occurs when the patient does something, either through words or action, that demonstrates permission to provide care.

extensibility The ability to stretch.

extracellular fluid The water outside the cells; accounts for approximately 20% of body weight.

facilitated diffusion The movement of a specific molecule across a cell membrane from an area of high concentration to an area of low concentration using a helper protein.

first-degree AV block A partial disruption of the conduction of the depolarizing impulse from the atria to the ventricles, causing prolongation of the PR interval.

flail chest An injury that involves two or more adjacent ribs fractured in two or more places, allowing the segment between the fractures to move independently of the rest of the thoracic cage.

Frank-Starling mechanism The increase in strength of contraction due to increased end diastolic volume (the volume of blood in the heart just before the ventricles begin to contract).

full-thickness burn A burn that extends through the epidermis and dermis into the subcutaneous tissues beneath; previously called a third-degree burn.

ganglion Groupings of nerve cell bodies located in the peripheral nervous system.

gastroesophageal reflux disease (GERD) Also known as acid-reflux disease. Abnormal reflux in the esophagus, which results in persistent symptoms and may ultimately cause damage to the esophageal lining.

gestation Period of time from conception to birth. For humans, the full period is normally 9 months.

Glasgow Coma Scale An evaluation tool used to determine a patient's neurologic status, which evaluates three categories: eye opening, verbal response, and motor response; effective in helping to determine the extent of neurologic injury.

glomerulonephritis A dry, hacking cough that may progress to a cough that produces pink frothy sputum (as opposed to a mucus or purulent cough in infections).

glottis The space in between the vocal chords that is the narrowest portion of the adult's airway; also called the glottic opening.

glucagon Hormone produced by the pancreas that is vital to the control of the body's metabolism and blood glucose level. Glucagon stimulates the breakdown of glycogen to glucose.

glucose The main "food" used by cells for energy.

glycogen The storage form of glucose occurring mainly in the liver and muscles.

Grey Turner sign Ecchymosis of the flanks.

guarding Muscles of the abdomen wall contract and remain tense, to protect inflamed internal organs from external pressure.

gynecology The branch of medicine that deals with the health maintenance and diseases of women, primarily of the reproductive system.

heart rate (HR) The number of cardiac contractions (heartbeats) per minute—in other words, the pulse rate.

hematemesis Vomit with blood. Can either be like coffee grounds in appearance, indicating partially digested blood, or contain bright red blood, indicating current active bleeding.

hematochezia The passage of stools containing blood.

hemoglobin An iron-containing protein within red blood cells that has the ability to combine with oxygen.

hemophilia A bleeding disorder that is primarily hereditary, in which clotting does not occur or occurs insufficiently.

hemopneumothorax A collection of blood and air in the pleural cavity.

hemostasis The stoppage of bleeding.

hemothorax The collection of blood within the normally closed pleural space.

Henry's law The amount of gas dissolved in a liquid is directly proportional to the partial pressure of the gas above the liquid.

hepatomegaly Enlargement of the liver, often the result of congestive heart failure or liver disease.

high-altitude cerebral edema (HACE) An altitude illness in which there is a change in mental status and/or ataxia.

high-altitude pulmonary edema (HAPE) An altitude illness characterized by dyspnea at rest, cough, severe weakness, and drowsiness that may eventually lead to central cyanosis, audible rales or wheezing, tachypnea, and tachycardia.

hilum Point of entry of all of the blood vessels and the bronchi into each lung.

humoral immunity The use of antibodies dissolved in the plasma and lymph to destroy foreign substances.

hyperkalemia An increased level of potassium in the blood.

hypermotility Overactivity of the gastrointestinal tract.

hypernatremic dehydration Occurs when the body loses more water than sodium; causes include excess use of diuretics, increased intake of sodium and decreased intake of water, excessive sodium loss, and diarrhea.

hypertension High blood pressure, usually a diastolic pressure of greater than 90 mm Hg.

hypertonic A solution that has a greater concentration of sodium than does the cell; the increased osmotic pressure can draw water out of the cell and cause it to collapse.

hyphema Bleeding into the anterior chamber of the eye; results from direct ocular trauma.

hypocapnia Decreased carbon dioxide content in arterial blood.

hypokalemia A low blood serum potassium level.

hyponatremic dehydration Occurs when the body loses more sodium than water; causes include increased water intake, diuretics, and sodium loss from renal disorder.

hypoperistalsis Decreased bowel movement.

hypotonic A solution that has a lower concentration of sodium than does the cell; the increased osmotic pressure lets water flow into the cell, causing it to swell and possibly burst.

hypovolemic shock Hypovolemic shock is an emergency condition in which severe blood and fluid loss makes the heart unable to pump enough blood to the rest of the body.

immune system The body system that includes all of the structures and processes designed to mount a defense against foreign substances and disease-causing agents.

immunity The body's ability to protect itself from acquiring a disease.

implied consent Assumption, on behalf of a person unable to give consent, that he or she would want life-saving treatment initiated.

inflammation A reaction by tissues of the body to irritation or injury, characterized by pain, swelling, redness, and heat.

informed consent A patient's voluntary agreement to be treated after being told about the nature of the disease, the risks and benefits of the proposed treatment, alternative treatments, and the choice of no treatment at all.

ingestion Eating or drinking materials for absorption through the gastrointestinal tract.

inhalation injury Injury to the airway or lungs that results from inhaling toxic or superheated gases.

inhalation The process by which a substance enters the body through the nose or mouth, moving into the lungs.

injection When the skin is pierced, and foreign material is deposited into the skin.

insulin Hormone produced by the pancreas that is vital to the control of the body's metabolism and blood glucose level. Insulin causes sugar, fatty acids, and amino acids to be taken up and metabolized by cells.

interferon Protein produced by cells in response to viral invasion. Interferon is released into the bloodstream or intercellular fluid to induce healthy cells to manufacture an enzyme that counters the infection.

interstitial fluid The water bathing the cells; accounts for about 10% of body weight; includes special fluid collections, such as cerebrospinal fluid and intraocular fluid.

interstitium An area of tissue between the alveoli and capillaries that allows for exchange of oxygen, nutrients, and waste to occur. During inspiration, the alveoli expand with air, and the interstitium stretches into a very thin layer, allowing for diffusion.

intracellular fluid The water contained inside the cells; normally accounts for 40% of body weight.

irreversible shock The final stage of shock, resulting in death.

ischemia Tissue anoxia from diminished blood flow to tissue, usually caused by narrowing or occlusion of the artery.

isotonic A solution that has the same concentration of sodium as does the cell. In this case, water does not shift, and no change in cell shape occurs.

isotonic dehydration The excessive loss of equal amounts of sodium and water. It results from severe or excessive vomiting or diarrhea.

junctional rhythms Arrhythmias arising from ectopic foci in the area of the atrioventricular junction; often show an absence of the P wave, a short PR interval, or a P wave appearing after the QRS complex.

junctional tachycardia Occurs when impulses originate in the atrioventricular junctional pacemaker at a rate of anywhere between 100 and 220 beats/min and are conducted retrograde to the atria and antegrade to the ventricles.

Kehr's sign Left shoulder pain that may indicate a ruptured spleen.

Kernig sign Considered positive when the leg is fully bent at the hip and knee, and subsequent extension of the knee is painful. Often an indicator of meningitis.

kidnapping Moving a patient from one place to another without the patient's consent, or restraining a person without proper justification; both may result in civil or criminal liability.

kinins A group of polypeptides that mediate inflammatory responses by stimulating visceral smooth muscle and relaxing vascular smooth muscle to produce vasodilation.

larynx A complex structure formed by many independent cartilaginous structures that all work together; where the upper airway ends and the lower airway begins.

leukocytes White blood cells.

Lund and Browder chart A detailed version of the rule of nines chart that takes into consideration the changes in body surface area brought on by growth.

lymphocytes The white blood cells responsible for a large part of the body's immune protection.

Mallory-Weiss syndrome A tear at the junction between the esophagus and the stomach, usually caused by severe retching, vomiting, or coughing. Additional causes include chronic alcoholism as well as eating disorders.

medulla Continuous inferiorly with the spinal cord; serves as a conduction pathway for ascending and descending nerve tracts; coordinates heart rate, blood vessel diameter, breathing, swallowing, vomiting, coughing, and sneezing. Also refers to part of the internal anatomy of the kidney, namely, the middle layer.

medulla oblongata The inferior portion of the midbrain, which serves as a conduction pathway for both ascending and descending nerve tracts.

meningitis An inflammation of the meningeal coverings of the brain and spinal cord, usually caused by a virus or bacterium.

metabolites Smaller chemical compounds that are produced as a result of metabolism (eg, of a drug).

midbrain The part of the brain that is responsible for helping to regulate level of consciousness.

minors Persons who are not yet legally considered adults. Patients who are minors cannot consent to or refuse medical care; consent must be obtained from a parent or legal guardian of the patient; in the case of life-threatening emergencies, consent may be implied.

monocytes Mononuclear phagocytic white blood cells derived from myeloid stem cells. They circulate in the bloodstream for about 24 hours and then move into tissues to mature into macrophages.

myasthenia gravis An abnormal condition characterized by the chronic fatigability and weakness of muscles, especially in the face and throat. It is the result of a defect in the conduction of nerve impulses at the nerve junction. This deficit is caused by a lack of acetylcholine.

myocardial infarction (MI) Occurs when the heart muscle does not get adequate oxygen because of decreased blood supply, an increased need for oxygen, or both. The main site of infarct (tissue death) is the left ventricle.

myocardium The cardiac muscle.

myxedema coma Decompensated hypothyroidism. Usually precipitated by a stressful event.

natural killer cells A distinct group of lymphocytes with no immunologic memory. Their specific function is to kill infected and cancerous cells by lysing their membranes on first exposure.

negligence Professional action or inaction on the part of the prehospital care provider that does not meet the standard of ordinary care expected of similarly trained and prudent prehospital care providers or that results in injury to the patient.

neurogenic shock Circulatory failure caused by paralysis of the nerves that control the size of the blood vessels, leading to widespread dilation; seen in spinal cord injuries.

neutrophils Cells that make up approximately 55% to 70% of the leukocytes responsible in large part for the body's protection against infection. They are readily attracted by foreign antigens and destroy them by phagocytosis.

nocturia When a person's need to urinate at night interrupts his or her sleep cycle.

nondisplaced fracture A break in which the bone remains aligned in its normal position.

nonpathologic Not resulting from a disease or physical condition.

NSTEMI Non-ST-segment-elevation myocardial infarction. Characterized as a myocardial infarction without ST-segment elevation.

nuchal rigidity Inability to flex the head forward and touch the chin to the chest as a result of rigidity of the neck muscles.

nucleus A cellular organelle that contains the genetic information. The nucleus controls the function and structure of the cell.

obstetrics The branch of medicine that deals specifically with the care of women throughout pregnancy.

obstructive shock Shock that occurs when blood flow in the heart or great vessels becomes blocked.

open pneumothorax The result of a defect in the chest wall that allows air to enter the thoracic space.

OPQRST A mode of patient questioning used to evaluate the specific details of the medical emergency and determine the chief complaint.

opsonins Antibodies that cause bacteria and other foreign cells to become more susceptible to phagocytosis.

organelles Internal cellular structures that carry out specific functions for the cell.

osmosis The movement of water across a semipermeable membrane (for example, the cell wall) from an area of lower to higher concentration of solute molecules.

osteoporosis A condition characterized by decreased bone mass and density and increased susceptibility to fractures.

ovarian cysts Fluid-filled pockets that form on or in an ovary.

ovaries Female gonads; ovaries release eggs and secrete the female hormones.

overriding The overlap of a bone that occurs from the muscle spasm that follows a fracture, leading to a decrease in the length of the bone.

pancreatitis Inflammation of the pancreas, which may be acute or chronic. Acute pancreatitis is a condition associated with tissue damage as a result of the inappropriate activation of enzymes.

parathyroid hormone (PTH) A hormone secreted by the parathyroids that acts as an antagonist to calcitonin. PTH is secreted when calcium blood levels are low.

parietal peritoneum The membrane that lines the abdominal wall and the pelvic cavity.

Parkland formula A formula that recommends giving 4 mL of normal saline for each kilogram of body weight, multiplied by the percentage of total body surface area burned; sometimes used to calculate fluid needs during lengthy transport times.

paroxysmal SVT (PVST) A tachycardia that originates in tissue above the ventricles and begins and ends suddenly.

partial-thickness burn A burn that involves the epidermis and part of the dermis, characterized by pain and blistering; previously called a second-degree burn.

passive transport The process by which water and dissolved particles move across the cell membrane, requiring no expenditure of energy by the cells; consists of two movements, osmosis and diffusion.

pelvic inflammatory disease An infection of the female upper organs of reproduction, specifically the uterus, ovaries, and fallopian tubes.

peptic ulcer disease Abrasion of the stomach or small intestine.

perfusion The circulation of blood within an organ or tissue in adequate amounts to meet the cells' needs.

pericardial tamponade Impairment of diastolic filling of the right ventricle as the result of significant amounts of fluid in the pericardial sac surrounding the heart, leading to a decrease in the cardiac output.

pericardiocentesis A procedure in which fluid is aspirated from the pericardial sac.

pericardium The double-layered sac containing the heart and the origins of the superior vena cava, inferior vena cava, and pulmonary artery.

peripheral neuropathy A group of conditions in which the nerves leaving the spinal cord become damaged.

periumbilical Around the navel.

pH The measurement of hydrogen ion concentration of a solution.

phagocytosis Process in which one cell eats or engulfs a foreign substance to destroy it.

placenta previa A condition in which the placenta develops over and covers the cervix.

pleuritic Inflammation of the pleura (the membrane around the lungs).

plexus A cluster of nerve roots that permits peripheral nerve roots to rejoin and functions as a group.

pneumonia An inflammation of the lungs caused by bacteria, viruses, fungi, or other organisms.

pneumotaxic center Area of the brainstem that has an inhibitory influence on inspiration.

poison A substance whose chemical action could damage structures or impair function when introduced into the body.

pons The portion of the brainstem that lies below the midbrain and contains nerve fibers that affect sleep and respiration.

postganglia Occurring after the ganglia.

postictal The period of time after a seizure during which the brain is reorganizing activity.

precordial Leads that are applied to the chest, allowing for a horizontal view of the heart. Found in leads V_1, V_2, V_3, V_4, V_5, and V_6.

preeclampsia A condition of late pregnancy that involves the gradual onset of hypertension, headache, visual changes, and swelling of the hands and feet, also called pregnancy-induced hypertension or toxemia of pregnancy.

preganglia Occurring before the ganglia.

preload The pressure under which a ventricle fills; it is influenced by the volume of blood returned by the veins to the heart.

premature atrial complex (PAC) Heartbeats originating from the atrium and occurring before the beat coming from the sinoatrial node.

premature junctional complex (PJC) Caused by premature electrical impulses that occur in the atrioventricular junction.

premature ventricular complex (PVC) An extra heartbeat originating in the ventricles and a wide QRS complex without a P wave. It is usually followed by a pause called the compensatory pause.

primary response The first encounter with the foreign substance to begin the immune response.

prodrome Signs or symptoms that precede a disease or condition.

progesterone One of the major female hormones.

prolapsed umbilical cord When the umbilical cord presents itself outside the uterus while the fetus is still inside; an obstetric emergency during pregnancy or labor that acutely endangers the life of the baby; can happen when the water breaks and the cord comes along with the gush of water.

proprioception The ability to perceive the position and movement of one's body or limbs.

prostaglandins A group of lipids that act as chemical messengers.

protoplasm A fluid made up of many compounds, such as water, proteins, lipids, ions, and amino acids, that composes the basic units of life.

pulmonary edema Congestion of the pulmonary air spaces with exudate and foam, often secondary to left-sided heart failure.

pulmonic valve The valve between the right ventricle and the pulmonary artery.

pulseless electrical activity (PEA) An electrical rhythm is present but there is no ventricular response and therefore no pulse.

pulsus paradoxus A drop in the systolic blood pressure of 10 mm Hg or more; commonly seen in patients with pericardial tamponade or severe asthma.

Purkinje fibers A system of fibers in the ventricles that conducts the excitation impulse from the bundle branches to the myocardium.

radiation Emission of heat from an object into surrounding, colder air.

rate The number of drops per minute (gtt/min) to which an IV administration must be established to administer the desired dose.

repolarization The return of ions to their previous resting state, which corresponds with the relaxation of the myocardial muscle. It results from the outward diffusion of potassium.

respiration The exchange of gases between a living organism and its environment.

respiratory acidosis A condition that occurs when exhalation of carbon dioxide is inhibited as a result of hypoventilation due to central nervous system depression or obstructive lung disease. Carbon dioxide retention leads to an increase in hydrogen ion levels and $Paco_2$ (> 45 mm Hg). The results are lowered pH and an increase in carbonic acid.

respiratory alkalosis A condition in which the amount of carbon dioxide found in the blood drops to a level below normal range. This condition produces a shift in the body's pH balance and causes the body's system to become more alkaline (basic). This condition is brought on by rapid, deep breathing called hyperventilation.

retinal detachment Separation of the inner layers of the retina from the underlying choroid, the vascular membrane that nourishes the retina.

rhabdomyolysis Caused by injury to skeletal muscle; myoglobin (a toxin) is released into plasma, often resulting in damage to the kidneys as they attempt to filter the myoglobin out of the bloodstream.

rhythmicity area Portion of the medulla oblongata that controls inspiratory and expiratory phases.

rule of nines A system that assigns percentages to sections of the body, allowing calculation of the amount of skin surface involved in the burn area.

rule of palms A system that estimates total body surface area burned by comparing the affected area with the size of the patient's palm, which is roughly equal to 1% of the patient's total body surface area.

SAMPLE history A mode of patient questioning used to determine the history of the present illness; links the current medical emergency with the patient's preexisting medical conditions.

scaphoid A concave shape of the abdomen. This can be caused by evisceration.

secondary response The body's reaction when it is exposed to an antigen for which it already has antibodies, in which it responds by killing the invading substance.

second-degree AV block, Mobitz type I A progressive prolongation of the PR interval on consecutive beats, followed by a "dropped" QRS complex.

second-degree AV block, Mobitz type II Electrical impulses are delayed in an irregular fashion in the heart, such that beats are occasionally skipped. Less common yet more severe than type I, because it is more likely to progress to complete heart block (third-degree AV block).

seizures Paroxysmal alterations in neurologic function (ie, behavioral and/or autonomic function).

septic shock Shock that occurs as a result of widespread infection, usually bacterial. Untreated, the result is multiple organ dysfunction syndrome (MODS) and often death.

sick sinus syndrome (SSS) The result of long-term damage to the sinoatrial node, which impairs its ability to effectively conduct electrical impulses through the heart.

simple pneumothorax The collection of air within the normally closed pleural space.

sinoatrial (SA) node or **sinus node** The dominant pacemaker of the heart, located at the junction of the superior vena cava and the right atrium.

sinus bradycardia A sinus rhythm with a heart rate of less than 60 beats/min.

sinus tachycardia A sinus rhythm with a heart rate of greater than 100 beats/min.

spontaneous abortion Expulsion of the fetus that occurs naturally; also called miscarriage.

status asthmaticus A severe, prolonged asthma attack that cannot be broken with epinephrine.

status epilepticus A seizure that lasts for longer than 4 to 5 minutes or two or more consecutive seizures that occur without a return to consciousness between seizure episodes.

STEMI ST-segment-elevation myocardial infarction. Characterized as a myocardial infarction with ST segment elevation.

stridor A harsh, high-pitched, crowing inspiratory sound, such as the sound often heard in acute laryngeal obstruction.

stroke volume The amount of blood pumped out by either ventricle in a single contraction (heartbeat).

subglottic Vocal cords and laryngeal portions of the airway structure.

subluxation A partial or incomplete dislocation.

superficial burn A burn involving only the epidermis, producing very red, painful skin; previously called a first-degree burn.

supine hypotensive syndrome Low blood pressure resulting from compression of the inferior vena cava by the weight of the pregnant uterus when the mother is supine.

supraventricular tachycardia (SVT) An abnormal heart rhythm with a rapid, narrow QRS complex.

surfactant A liquid protein substance that coats the alveoli in the lungs, decreases alveolar surface tension, and keeps the alveoli expanded.

syncope Fainting; brief loss of consciousness caused by transient and inadequate blood flow to the brain.

systole The period during which the ventricles contract.

tension pneumothorax A life-threatening collection of air within the pleural space; the volume and pressure have both collapsed the involved lung and caused a shift of the mediastinal structures to the opposite side.

testes Male gonads located in the scrotum that produce hormones called androgens.

testosterone The most important androgen in men.

thermogenesis The production of heat in the body.

third-degree (complete) AV block When the heart's electrical signals do not pass from the upper to the lower chambers, and instead operate independently of each other. When this occurs, the ventricular pacemaker takes over. The ventricles contract and pump blood at a slower rate than the atrial pacemaker.

thrombocytes Platelets.

thrombocytopenia Reduction in the number of platelets.

thyrotoxicosis Excessive levels of circulating thyroid hormone.

thyroxine The body's major metabolic hormone. Thyroxine stimulates energy production in cells, which increases the rate at which the cells consume oxygen and use carbohydrates, fats, and proteins.

tricuspid valve The valve between the right atrium and right ventricle of the heart.

tripoding An abnormal position to keep the airway open; involves leaning forward with the hands on the knees with elbows facing outward.

tumor An abnormal anatomic mass or growth, resulting from uncontrolled cell division.

turbinates Three bony shelves that protrude from the lateral walls of the nasal cavity and extend into the nasal passageway, parallel to the nasal floor; serve to increase the surface area of the nasal mucosa, thereby improving the processes of warming, filtering, and humidifying inhaled air.

type 1 diabetes The type of diabetic disease that usually starts in childhood and requires daily injections of supplemental synthetic insulin to control blood glucose levels. Formerly known as juvenile or juvenile onset diabetes.

type 2 diabetes The type of diabetic disease that usually starts later in life and often can be controlled through diet and oral medications. Formerly known as adult-onset diabetes.

uvula A soft-tissue structure located in the posterior aspect of the oral cavity.

vallecula An anatomic space or "pocket" located between the base of the tongue and the epiglottis; an important anatomic landmark for endotracheal intubation.

vascular bed Describes the blood vessels of a particular organ.

vasopressor A drug that causes the muscles of the arteries and capillaries to contract. Administered during cardiac arrest when an IV/IO is in place, after the first or second shock.

veins The blood vessels that carry deoxygenated blood to the heart.

ventricle Lower chamber of the heart.

ventricular fibrillation Heart condition characterized by erratic firing from multiple sites in the ventricle; the most common cause of prehospital cardiac arrest.

ventricular tachycardia Heart condition characterized by three or more PVCs in a row (typically six to ten PVC runs), without P waves, and with a wide QRS complex; ventricular rate is 150–220 beats/min. T wave may not be present.

viruses Small organisms that can only multiply inside a host, such as a human, and cause disease.

visceral peritoneum The portion of the peritoneum that covers the internal organs and forms the outer layer of most of the intestinal tract.

Wernicke encephalopathy An acute disease of the brain caused by thiamine deficiency.

Index

Endocrine system
    emergencies, 199–213
        Addison's disease, 211–212
        Cushing syndrome, 211
        diabetes mellitus, 200–202
        diabetic ketoacidosis, 203–205, 205t
        in geriatric patients, 330
        hyperglycemia, 203–205, 204t
        hyperosmolar hyperglycemic nonketotic
            syndrome, 205–206, 207t
        hyperthyroidism, 209
        hypoglycemia, 202–203, 203t, 205t
        hypothyroidism, 210
        metabolic acidosis, 208, 209t
        metabolic alkalosis, 207
    function of, 201f
Endometriosis, 299, 300
Endometritis, 298–299, 300
Endoplasmic reticulum (ER), 2, 3f
Endotracheal tube
    cuffed vs. uncuffed, 103
    intubation procedure, 104–106
    placement confirmation, 107
    sizes, 103t–104t
Energy metabolism, cellular, 6–7
Enteral route, 25
Environmental emergencies, 267–281
    bites and stings, 273–274
    diving-associated, 276–279
    drowning, 274–276, 281
    heat-related illness, 270–273
    local cold injuries, 268–270
    predisposing factors, 267
Eosinophils, 253, 265
Epicardium, 124, 178
Epidural hematomas, 52
Epiglottis, 98, 99f, 307–308, 322
Epinephrine
    for allergic reactions/anaphylaxis, 217t
    for anaphylactic shock, 83t
    for anaphylaxis, 36t
    for ARDS, 117t
    for asthma, 115t, 310t
    for asystole, 36t, 165t, 318t
    for bradycardias, 36t
    for bronchiolitis, 311t
    for cardiogenic shock, 77t
    for congestive heart failure, 133t
    for COPD, 112t
    for croup, 307t
    for emphysema, 114t
    hyperventilation and, 118
    pediatric administration, 320t
    for pediatric allergic reactions, 314t
    pharmacology, 120t
    for pulseless electrical activity, 36t
    for pulseless ventricular tachycardia, 39t
    for respiratory distress, 38t
    for ventricular fibrillation, 39t, 162t, 317t
Epiphyseal fracture, 64
Epistaxis (nosebleed), 68

ER (endoplasmic reticulum), 2, 3f
Erosive gastroenteritis, 231t
Erythrocytes, 252, 265
Erythropoiesis, 252, 265
Escape beats, 131
Escape rhythm, 131
Escape rhythms. See Junctional escape rhythms
Eschar, 90, 96
Esophageal varices, 231t, 233t, 235
Esophagitis, 235
Esophagus, bleeding from, 232t
Estrogen, 199, 213
Ethanol poisoning, 248–249, 250t
Ethical issues, for EMS provider, 16–17
Etomidate, for rapid-sequence intubation, 106t, 320t
Eupnea, 102t
Evaporation, 268, 281
Eviscerations, 68
Excitability, 128, 178
Exocrine glands, 199
Expressed consent, 17, 19
Expressive aphasia, 188
Extensibility, 128, 178
External bleeding, management, 72–73
Extracellular fluid, 5,10
Extremities, physical exam, 48
Extrinsic asthma, 114
Extrinsic control, of arterioles, 125
Eyelid
    evaluation, 62
    injuries, 62
Eyes
    injuries of, 61–62
    irrigation of, 62, 63f
    movement of, 62
    orbital fractures, 60
    rapid trauma assessment, 50

F

Facial droop, 189f
Facial injuries, 60–64
    assessment, 60–61
    ear, 62–63
    of eye, 61–62
    management, 61
    oral and dental, 63–64
    pathophysiology, 60
Facilitated diffusion, 5, 5f, 10
Falls, from heights, 45
Febrile seizures, 220, 314–315
Federal drug-related legislation, 20
Federal Food, Drug, and
        Cosmetic Act (1938), 20
Feet, rapid trauma assessment, 51
Fentanyl
    for pain management, 40t
    for rapid-sequence intubation, 106t
    for sickle cell disease, 261t
Fetus, FDA drug rating scale for, 22–23

Hyperosmolar hyperglycemic nonketotic syndrome,
205–206, 207t
Hypertension
definition of, 134, 178
pathophysiology, 134
during pregnancy, 289–290
Hypertensive emergencies
assessment/management, 135
obstetric, 289–291, 290t, 291t
pathophysiology, 134
signs/symptoms, 134
Hyperthyroidism, 209
Hypertonic fluid, 6, 10
Hyperventilation, 118–119, 279
Hyphema, 61, 62, 70
Hypocalcemia, 227
Hypocapnia, 118, 122
Hypoglycemia
assessment, 203
management, 203, 203t, 205t
pathophysiology, 202
pediatric, 315–316, 316t
signs/symptoms, 203
treatment, 37t
vs. hyperglycemia, 204t
Hypokalemia
definition of, 213, 229
pathophysiology, 226
signs/symptoms, 226–227
Hypomagnesemia, 227–228
Hyponatremic dehydration,
6, 10, 224–225
Hypoperistalsis, 234, 240
Hypopnea, 102t
Hypotension, 38t
Hypothalamus, 184f, 199
Hypothermia, 269–270
Hypothyroidism, 210
Hypotonic fluid, 6, 10
Hypoventilation, 119–120
Hypovolemia, 230, 312–313
Hypovolemic shock, 75, 78–79, 79t

I

Ibuprofen, for meningitis, 316t
ICP (intracranial pressure), 53–54, 188
Idioventricular rhythm, 165–166, 166t
IgA, 259
IgD, 259
IgE, 259
IgG, 259
IgM, 259
Immune response
nonspecific, 256–257
specific, 256, 257–260, 258f
Immune system
age-related changes, 325t
definition of, 256, 265
response, 256–260, 258f

Immunity
active vs. passive, 259
definition of, 256, 265
humoral, 257, 258–259, 258f, 265
Impacted fracture (impaction injury), 64, 65t
Impaled objects, 62, 68
Implied consent, 17, 19
Incomplete fracture, 64
Indications, in drug profile, 21
Infections
gastrointestinal, 230, 238–239
neurologic conditions and, 188
Infectious diarrhea, incidence/prevalence, 231t
Inferior dislocations, 67
Inflammation
definition of, 256, 265
gastrointestinal, 230
signs/symptoms of, 257
Informed consent, 17, 19
Ingestion, 241, 251
Inhalation, 241, 251
Inhalation injury, 90–91, 96
Inhalation poisoning, 89
Inherent firing rate, 129
Initial/primary assessment, 12–15
Injection, 241, 251
Injury patterns, from motor
vehicle collisions, 43–44
Inotropics, 31t
Insulin, 199, 200, 213
Integumentary system, age-related
changes, 325t
Interferon, 256, 257, 265
Internal bleeding, management, 73
Interstitial fluid, 5, 10
Interstitium, 110, 122
Intra-abdominal hemorrhage,
abdominal pain, 233t
Intracellular fluid, 5, 10
Intracranial pressure (ICP), 53–54, 188
Intraosseous infusion procedure,
pediatric, 319
Intrauterine fetal demise, 291
Intrinsic asthma, 114
Intrinsic control, of arterioles, 125
Intubation, 103–107
Ionization of drug, absorption and, 24
Ipratropium
for allergic reactions/anaphylaxis, 217t
for ARDS, 117t
for asthma, 115t
pharmacology, 121t
for respiratory distress, 38t
Irreversible shock, 74, 85
Irrigation of eye, 62, 63f
Irritable bowel syndrome,
incidence/prevalence, 231t
Ischemia, 135, 178
Isotonic dehydration, 6, 10, 224
Isotonic fluid, 6, 10
IV drip rate calculation, 35

J

Jacksonian seizure (simple partial seizures), 220
Junctional escape rhythms (escape rhythms)
    definition of, 178
    management, 156
    pathophysiology, 155–156
    signs/symptoms, 155t, 156, 156f
Junctional tachycardia
    definition of, 178
    pathophysiology, 156
    signs/symptoms, 156t, 157, 157f
    treatment, 157, 157t–158t

K

Kehr's sign, 58, 70, 233, 240
Kernig sign, 223, 229
Ketorolac
    for heat cramps, 37t
    for pain management, 40t
    for sickle cell disease, 261t
Kidnapping, 17, 19
Kidneys, in acid-base balance, 8
King LT-D airway, 109–110, 109f
Kinins, 257, 265
Kussmaul respirations, 8, 102t

L

Labetalol, for atrial fibrillation, 148t
Lactated Ringer's solution
    for dehydration, 225t
    for hypotension, 38t
    for metabolic acidosis, 209t
    for placenta previa, 294f
    for septic shock, 81t
Large intestines
    gastrointestinal bleeding, 232t
    injuries, 60
Laryngotracheobronchitis (croup), 306, 306t–307t, 322
Larynx, 98, 99f, 122
LeFort fractures, 60
Left-sided congestive heart failure, 132, 133t–134t
Legal issues, for EMS provider, 16–17
Legs, rapid trauma assessment, 51
Leukemias, 261–262
Leukocytes, 252, 266
Levalbuterol
    for allergic reactions/anaphylaxis, 217t
    for ARDS, 117t
    for asthma, 115t, 310t
    for bronchiolitis, 311t
    for COPD, 113t
    for emphysema, 114t
    for pediatric allergic reactions, 314t
    pharmacology, 120t
    for respiratory distress, 38t
LH (luteinizing hormone), 200t

Lidocaine
    dosing, 176
    pediatric administration, 320t
    for pediatric rapid-sequence
        intubation, 321t
    for premature ventricular complex, 160t
    for pulseless ventricular tachycardia, 39t
    for rapid-sequence intubation, 106t
    for tachycardia, 39t
    for ventricular fibrillation, 39t, 162t, 317t
    for ventricular tachycardia, 161t
Limb presentation, 287–288
Lipid solubility, drug absorption and, 24
Liver injuries, 59
Lorazepam
    pediatric administration, 320t
    for seizures, 38t, 221t
Lower airway pediatric emergencies,
        310–312, 311t
Lumbar plexus, 185
Lumbar spine, rapid trauma assessment, 50
Lund and Browder chart, 93, 93f, 96
Lungs
    anatomic differences between children
        and adults, 302
    injuries of, 55–57
    sounds, 100–101
Luteinizing hormone (LH), 200t
Lymphocytes, 253, 266
Lymphokines, 259
Lysosomes, 3, 3f

M

Macrophages, 259
Magnesium sulfate
    for asthma, 115t, 310t
    for bronchiolitis, 311t
    for COPD, 113t
    for croup, 307t
    dosing, 176
    for eclampsia, 291t
    for emphysema, 114t
    pediatric administration, 320t
    pharmacology, 121t
    for pulseless ventricular tachycardia, 39t
    for seizures, 38t
    for tachycardias, 40t
    for ventricular fibrillation, 39t, 317t
    for ventricular tachycardia, 161t
    for wide complex tachycardia, 40t
Magnesium sulfate, for respiratory
        distress, 38t
Mallory-Weiss syndrome, 235, 240
Mandibular fractures, 60
Mass-casualty incidents, 46–47, 46t
Massive hemothorax, 56
Maxillary fractures, 60
Mechanical energy, 43
Mechanisms of action, in drug profile, 21

Tricuspid valve, 124, 179
Tricyclic antidepressants overdose
   assessment, 248
   pathophysiology, 247
   signs/symptoms, 247–248
   treatment of, 39*t*, 242*t*, 248, 248*t*
Tripoding, 111, 123
TSH (thyroid-stimulating hormone), 200*t*
Tubular excretion, 25
Tumor, 108, 123
Turbinates, 98, 123
T wave
   interpretation, 130, 131, 168
   in normal sinus rhythm, 169*t*, 170
Type 1 diabetes, 201–202, 213
Type 2 diabetes, 202, 213

U

Ulcerative colitis, 231*t*, 233*t*, 235
Umbilical cord, prolapsed, 286–287, 300
Upper airway emergencies, pediatric,
   306–310, 306*t*–307*t*, 309*f*
Uterine rupture, 285–286
Uvula, 98, 123

V

Vacuoles, 3, 3*f*
Vagal stimulation
   for junctional tachycardia, 157*t*
   for supraventricular tachycardia, 144*t*
Vallecula, 98, 123
Vascular bed, 110, 123
Vascular causes, of neurologic
   conditions, 186, 187*f*
Vasodilators, 33*t*
Vasopressin
   for asystole, 165*t*
   for pulseless ventricular tachycardia, 39*t*
   for ventricular fibrillation, 39*t*, 162*t*
Vasopressors, 33*t*, 176, 179
Vecuronium, for rapid-sequence
   intubation, 106*t*
Veins, 126, 126*f*, 179
Ventricle, 124, 180
Ventricular antiarrhythmics, 33*t*
Ventricular arrhythmias, 138–139
   asystole, 164–165, 164*t*, 165*t*, 177
   fibrillation (*See* Ventricular fibrillation)
   idioventricular rhythm, 165–166, 166*t*
   premature ventricular complex,
      158–160, 158*t*, 159*f*, 160*t*, 179

   pulseless electrical activity, 163–164,
      163*t*, 179
   tachycardia (*See* Ventricular tachycardia)
Ventricular fibrillation
   assessment, 162
   definition of, 180
   pediatric, 317, 317*t*
   signs/symptoms, 162, 163*f*
   treatment, 162, 162*t*
Ventricular tachycardia
   definition of, 160, 180
   pathophysiology, 16, 160*t*
   with pulse, 160–161
   signs/symptoms, 160*f*, 161
   treatment, 161, 161*t*
Venules, 126
Vercuronium, for pediatric rapid-sequence
   intubation, 321*t*
Vesicants, burns from, 88*t*
Villi, 4
Viruses, 256, 266
Visceral pain, 234*t*
Visceral peritoneum, 234, 240
Visual acuity, 62
Vital signs, 304*t*
Vitamin B$_1$, 33*t*
Vitamin B$_{12}$ complex. *See* Thiamine
VITAMINS-CD, 331*t*
Volume on hand, 34
Vulnerable period of repolarization, 131

W

Wasp stings, 273–274
Water, retention, 6
WBCs (white blood cells), 253
Wenckebach block (type 1 second-degree AV block),
   149–151, 150*f*, 150*t*, 179
Wernicke encephalopathy, 250, 251
Wheezing, 101
White blood cells (WBCs), 253

Y

Yawning, 102*t*

Z

Zone of coagulation, 87
Zone of hyperemia, 87
Zone of stasis, 87
Zygomatic fractures, 60

Photo and Illustration Credits

Chapter 6

6-1A-B © Charles Stewart, MD.

Chapter 7

7-3 © Mediscan/Visuals Unlimited; 7-8 Courtesy of Covidien. Used with permission; 7-9 © Courtesy of King Systems.

Chapter 8

8-6, 8-7, 8-8, 8-9, 8-10, 8-12, 8-13, 8-14, 8-15, 8-16, 8-18, 8-19, 8-20, 8-21, 8-22, 8-25, 8-26, 8-31 From *Arrhythmia Recognition: The Art of Interpretation*, courtesy of Tomas B. Garcia, MD; 8-23, 8-24, 8-35, 8-36 From *12-Lead ECG: The Art of Interpretation*, courtesy of Tomas B. Garcia, MD; 8-34 From *Introduction to 12-Lead ECG: The Art of Interpretation*, courtesy of Tomas B. Garcia, MD; 8-39 Adapted from *12-Lead ECG: The Art of Interpretation*, courtesy of Tomas B. Garcia, MD.

Chapter 14

14-1 © Phototake/Alamy Images.

Chapter 17

17-3, 17-4 From *Arrhythmia Recognition: The Art of Interpretation*, courtesy of Tomas B. Garcia, MD.

Unless otherwise indicated, all photographs and illustrations are under copyright of Jones and Bartlett Publishers, LLC, courtesy of Maryland Institute for Emergency Medical Services Systems, provided by the American Academy of Orthopaedic Surgeons, or have been provided by the author(s).